PERSPECTIVES IN STEROID RECEPTOR RESEARCH

Perspectives in Steroid Receptor Research

Editor

Francesco Bresciani
Institute of General Pathology
First Faculty of Medicine and Surgery
University of Naples
Naples, Italy

Raven Press ■ New York

Raven Press, 1140 Avenue of the Americas, New York, New York 10036

Made in the United States of America

International Standard Book Number 0-89004-490-2
Library of Congress Catalog Card Number 79-5398

Dedicated to the memory of Tyra Korling Bresciani
(Chicago 1934—Naples 1979)

Preface

The discovery of steroid hormone receptors and the study of their role in the mechanism of hormone action have been a success story in recent biomedical research. This volume presents chapters by many of the scientists who have contributed to this success. Recent advances are assessed, and perspectives in steroid research are discussed.

The chapters in this volume pursue a global approach to steroid receptors. All major aspects of steroid receptor research are covered, from purification and structural and functional characterization of receptor to interaction of receptor with ligand and of the ligand–receptor complex with genomic structures; from changes that receptors undergo after such interactions ("activation" and "inactivation") to induced protein synthesis and other cell and tissue responses following steroid–receptor interaction; from methods of receptor assay to applications of receptor analysis to breast cancer prognosis and clinical investigation of postmenopausal endometrium. Biochemists, physiologists, pharmacologists, pathologists, and medical oncologists are among the contributors, and experts on different steroid receptors are freely intermixed. This global approach is pursued on the basis of the following facts and beliefs: although perculiarities do exist, steroid hormones share the same basic mechanism of action; specialists in the field can benefit from exchange of experience with different specific receptors; although for practical purposes on may distinguish between basic and applied research, there is in truth only one research, and progress is achieved as a whole.

The meeting on which this book is based marked the twentieth anniversary of the beginning of research that set a new course in the study of the mechanism of action of steroid hormones and prepared the ground for identification of steroid hormone receptors (1,2). The work by Jensen and Jacobson (2), with its elegant and clear-cut demonstration of ^{3}H-17 β-estradiol accumulation and retention in target organs, had the major impact on the thinking of fellow scientists and changed the course of research in the field. One may remember that before this work, the most advanced working hypothesis was that steroid hormones produce their effects on target tissues by interacting directly with enzymes.

The chapters in this volume clearly demonstrate how far we have progressed during the past 20 years and how steroid hormone receptors are no longer strictly a subject for research in endocrinology, but have become a focus of interest in biological and medical research in general. Unraveling the mechanism by which steroid hormones control protein synthesis may well furnish the key for a general understanding of control of gene expression in eukaryotic cells and, thereby, of the special case of control of gene expression which is control of cell replication. In turn, understanding of control of cell replication at a molecular level is a prerequisite for identifying the alteration(s) of this control mechanism which is responsible for neoplastic transformation. Thus, steroid receptors are at the center of the two major problems of biological and medical research today.

This volume will be of interest to endocrinologists, biochemists, cell biologists, and clinicians interested in the biological bases of endocrine disorders involving the steroid hormones.

Francesco Bresciani

REFERENCES

1. Glascock, R. F., and Hoekstra, W. G. (1959): Selective accumulation of steroid hormone tritium-labelled hexoestrol by the reproductive organs of immature female goats and sheep. *Biochem. J.*, 72:673–682.
2. Jensen, E. V., and Jacobson, H. I. (1960): Fate of steroid estrogens in target tissues. In: *Biological Activities of Steroids in Relation to Cancer*, edited by G. Pincus and E. P. Volmer, pp. 161–178. Academic Press, New York.

Acknowledgments

I would like to express my thanks to Dr. Vincenzo Sica for his collaboration in organization of the Sorrento meeting, on which this volume is based, as well as to Drs. Gianfredo Puca and Ernesto Nola and other colleagues at the Institute of General Patholgy, Università de Napoli, for their help with various aspects of the meeting. A special thanks goes to the secretaries, Mrs. Anna Maria Riccio and Adele Esposito, for their infinite patience and unfailing support. The Sorrento meeting was supported in part by the Consiglio Nazionale della Ricerche, Roma. Also, I thank Dr. Ermes Tornatore and acknowledge with gratitude a grant from SORIN BIOMEDICA, Saluggia. Finally, I express my appreciation to Raven Press for their collaboration and understanding in preparing this book.

Contents

xi

Contributors

Ferdinando Auricchio
Institute of General Pathology
First Faculty of Medicine and Surgery
University of Naples
80138 Naples, Italy

Carol A. Barnett
Department of Biology
San Diego State University
San Diego, California 92115, U.S.A.

L. V. M. Beex
Department of Medicine
Division of Endocrinology
University of Nijmegen
Nijmegen, The Netherlands

Th. J. Benraad
Department of Experimental
*   Endocrinology*
Division of Endocrinology
University of Nijmegen
Nijmegen, The Netherlands

Norman D. Bloom
Department of Surgery
Maimonides Medical Center
Brooklyn, New York 11219, U.S.A.

Rodolfo Bova
Institute of General Pathology
First Faculty of Medicine and Surgery
University of Naples
80138 Naples, Italy

Francesco Bresciani
Institute of General Pathology
First Faculty of Medicine and Surgery
University of Naples
80138 Naples, Italy

David J. Brigati
Department of Pathology
Memorial Sloan-Kettering Cancer
*   Center*
New York, New York 10021, U.S.A.

Franco Maria Buonaguro
Institute of General Pathology
First Faculty of Medicine and Surgery
University of Naples
80138 Naples, Italy

Anne C. Carter
Department of Medicine
Division of Endocrinology
State University of New York Downstate
*   Medical Center*
Brooklyn, New York 11203, U.S.A.

Chunshing Chen
Ben May Laboratory for Cancer
*   Research*
University of Chicago
Chicago, Illinois 60637, U.S.A.

James H. Clark
Department of Cell Biology
Baylor College of Medicine
Houston, Texas 77030, U.S.A.

L. E. Closs
Ben May Laboratory for Cancer
*   Research*
University of Chicago
Chicago, Illinois 60637, U.S.A.

John G. Compton
Department of Cell Biology
Baylor College of Medicine
Houston, Texas 77030, U.S.A.

George A. Degenshein
Department of Surgery
Maimonides Medical Center
Brooklyn, New York 11219, U.S.A.

J. Delettré
Laboratory of Mineralogy and
Crystallography
Pierre and Marie Curie University
75230 Paris, France

Eugene R. DeSombre
Ben May Laboratory for Cancer
Research
University of Chicago
Chicago, Illinois 60637, U.S.A.

Dennis M. DiSorbo
Department of Biochemistry
Temple University School of Medicine
Philadelphia, Pennsylvania 19140,
U.S.A.

Howard J. Eisen
National Institute of Child Health and
Human Development
National Institutes of Health
Bethesda, Maryland 20205, U.S.A.

Laszlo Endrenyi
Institute of General Pathology
First Faculty of Medicine and Surgery
University of Naples
80138 Naples, Italy

G. Fabris
Institute of Anatomy and Pathologic
Histology
University of Ferrara
44100 Ferrara, Italy

Eric Gaetjens
Department of Pathology
State University of New York Downstate
Medical Center
Brooklyn, New York 11203, U.S.A.

C. Gelly
C.N.R.S. Steroid Hormone Research
Unit
Foundation for Hormone Research
75014 Paris, France

G. L. Greene
Ben May Laboratory for Cancer
Research
University of Chicago
Chicago, Illinois 60637, U.S.A.

A. Gulino
C.N.R.S. Steroid Hormone Research
Unit
Foundation for Hormone Research
75014 Paris, France

S. Z. Haslam
Lady Davis Institute for Medical
Research
Sir Mortimer B. Davis Jewish General
Hospital
Montreal, Quebec H3T 1E2, Canada

Richard A. Hiipakka
Ben May Laboratory for Cancer
Research
University of Chicago
Chicago, Illinois 60637, U.S.A.

E. V. Jensen
Ben May Laboratory for Cancer
Research
University of Chicago
Chicago, Illinois 60637, U.S.A.

Alison D. Johnson
Department of Biochemistry
University of Leeds
Leeds LS2 9LS, England

Peter W. Jungblut
Max-Planck-Institute for Experimental
Endocrinology
3000 Hanover 61, West Germany

Dong S. Kim
Department of Pathology
State University of New York Downstate
Medical Center
Brooklyn, New York 11203, U.S.A.

R. J. B. King
Hormone Biochemistry Department
Imperial Cancer Research Fund
London WC2A 3PX, England

A. J. M. Koenders
Department of Experimental
Endocrinology
Division of Endocrinology
University of Nijmegen
Nijmegen, The Netherlands

Shutsung Liao
Ben May Laboratory for Cancer
Research
University of Chicago
Chicago, Illinois 60637, U.S.A.

Marc E. Lippman
Medical Breast Cancer Section
Medicine Branch
Division of Cancer Treatment
National Cancer Institute
National Institutes of Health
Bethesda, Maryland 20205, U.S.A.

Gerald Litwack
Fels Research Institute
and
Department of Biochemistry
Temple University School of Medicine
Philadelphia, Pennsylvania 19140,
U.S.A.

C. Richard Lyttle
Ben May Laboratory for Cancer
Research
University of Chicago
Chicago, Illinois 60637, U.S.A.

W. Ian P. Mainwaring
Department of Biochemistry
University of Leeds
Leeds LS2 9LS, England

E. Marchetti
Institute of Anatomy and Pathologic
Histology
University of Ferrara
44100 Ferrara, Italy

Barry M. Markaverich
Department of Cell Biology
Baylor College of Medicine
Houston, Texas 77030, U.S.A.

Radmila D. Marković
Department of Biochemistry and
Molecular Biology
University of Belgrade
Belgrade, Yugoslavia

A. Marzola
Institute of Anatomy and Pathologic
Histology
University of Ferrara
44100 Ferrara, Italy

William D. McGuire
Department of Medicine/Oncology
University of Texas Health Science
Center
San Antonio, Texas 78284, U.S.A.

Heinrich H. D. Meyer
Max-Planck-Institute for Experimental
Endocrinology
3000 Hanover 61, West Germany

Antimo Migliaccio
Institute of General Pathology
First Faculty of Medicine and Surgery
University of Naples
80138 Naples, Italy

Anna Maria Molinari
Institute of General Pathology
First Faculty of Medicine and Surgery
University of Naples
80138 Naples, Italy

J. P. Mornon
Laboratory of Mineralogy and
Crystallography
Pierre and Marie Curie University
75230 Paris, France

I. Nenci
Institute of Anatomy and Pathologic
Histology
University of Ferrara
44100 Ferrara, Italy

B. L. Nguyen
C.N.R.S. Steroid Hormone Research
Unit
Foundation for Hormone Research
75014 Paris, France

T. Ojasoo
Roussel-Uclaf Research Center
93230 Romainville, France

Bert W. O'Malley
Department of Cell Biology
Baylor College of Medicine
Houston, Texas 77030, U.S.A.

J. R. Pasqualini
C.N.R.S. Steroid Hormone Research
Unit
Foundation for Hormone Research
75014 Paris, France

Louis P. Pertschuk
Department of Pathology
State University of New York Downstate
Medical Center
Brooklyn, New York 11203, U.S.A.

David S. Phelps
Department of Anatomy
Temple University School of Medicine
Philadelphia, Pennsylvania 19140,
U.S.A

Giovanni Alfredo Puca
Institute of General Pathology
First Faculty of Medicine and Surgery
University of Naples
80138 Naples, Italy

J. P. Raynaud
Roussel-Uclaf Research Center
93230 Romainville, France

Gian Paolo Rossini
Ben May Laboratory for Cancer
Research
University of Chicago
Chicago, Illinois 60637, U.S.A.

Andrea Rotondi
Institute of General Pathology
First Faculty of Medicine and Surgery
University of Naples
80138 Naples, Italy

Patrizia Sampaolo
Institute of General Pathology
First Faculty of Medicine and Surgery
University of Naples
80138 Naples, Italy

Thomas J. Schmidt
Department of Biochemistry
Temple University School of Medicine
Philadelphia, Pennsylvania 19140,
U.S.A.

William T. Schrader
Department of Cell Biology
Baylor College of Medicine
Houston, Texas 77030, U.S.A.

G. Shyamala
Lady Davis Institute for Medical
Research
Sir Mortimer B. Davis Jewish General
Hospital
Montreal, Quebec H3T 1E2, Canada

Vincenzo Sica
Institute of General Pathology
First Faculty of Medicine and Surgery
University of Naples
80138 Naples, Italy

C. Sumida
C.N.R.S. Steroid Hormone Research
Unit
Foundation for Hormone Research
75014 Paris, France

Ellis H. Tobin
School of Medicine
State University of New York Downstate
* Medical Center*
Brooklyn, New York 11203, U.S.A.

Susan Upchurch
Department of Cell Biology
Baylor College of Medicine
Houston, Texas 77030, U.S.A.

Wayne V. Vedeckis
Department of Cell Biology
Baylor College of Medicine
Houston, Texas 77030, U.S.A.

Rüdiger K. Wagner
Max-Planck-Institute for Experimental
* Endocrinology*
3000 Hanover 61, West Germany

Alessandro Weizs
Institute of General Pathology
First Faculty of Medicine and Surgery
University of Naples
80138 Naples, Italy

M. I. Whitehead
Department of Obstetrics and
* Gynaecology*
King's College Hospital
London SE5 8RX, England

Perspectives in Steroid Receptor Research,
edited by F. Bresciani.
Raven Press, New York © 1980.

An Approach to the Mapping of the Steroid Hormone Receptor

J. Delettré, J. P. Mornon, *T. Ojasoo, and *J. P. Raynaud

*Laboratory of Mineralogy and Crystallography, Pierre and Marie Curie University, 75230 Paris, France; and *Roussel-Uclaf Research Center, 93230 Romainville, France*

The molecular aspects of the interaction between steroid hormones and cytoplasmic receptors are still unelucidated. An ever-increasing volume of information is available on the characteristics of steroids, but the receptor protein(s) remain(s) elusive. Little is known about its molecular weight (probably high (6,46)) and structure, let alone about the nature of the sites of interaction with the steroid. Are these sites at the surface of the protein (an unlikely hypothesis since steroids are highly hydrophobic molecules), in a pocket, or even between two domains ?

The recent progress made in the characterization and crystal structure determination of purified plasma proteins, to which some steroids also bind with high affinity (e.g. progesterone binding globulin (3,48) and uteroglobin (7,29)) and of enzymes such as Δ^5-3-keto-steroid isomerase (49) lends support to the conviction that a similar methodology may yet enlighten the study of the far more labile tissue receptor proteins. Attempts to isolate the estrogen (6) and progesterone (46) receptors have already led to their partial purification, but not to an extent permitting their detailed study. Until then, information on binding sites can only be deduced indirectly by correlating observations on well-known steroid structures and conformations with biochemical data on receptor binding, as illustrated in the present chapter.

GENERAL PROPERTIES OF THE BINDING SITE(S)

A large body of evidence suggests that the steroid binds to the receptor protein via at least two hydrogen

1

bonds (at O(3) at one extremity and at O(17) or O(20) and/or O(21) at the other) and via Van der Waals forces that stabilize this binding. The resultant interaction energy between steroid and protein (∿-12 kcal/mol) is more or less equally distributed between the hydrogen bonds (∿2 x -3 kcal) and the Van der Waals forces (∿-6 kcal). The latter energy corresponds approximately to the interaction of, for instance, two methyl groups with their immediate environment (24).

Since the binding of steroid and protein involves both bonds that engender strain (hydrogen bonds) and numerous, weaker, interchangeable interactions (Van der Waals forces), the binding site is characterized by both an element of rigidity and pliability. For a synthetic steroid to compete effectively with the natural hormone for binding to the receptor site, its polar groups probably have to occupy positions within the site similar to those of the natural hormone in order to meet the distance and direction requirements for hydrogen bonding. This is supported by the observation that superimposition of the skeletons of, for example, synthetic progestins and progesterone (obtained by X-ray crystallography or molecular geometry calculations (13)) reveals differences of the order of only 0.1-0.2 Å between homologous carbon atoms (15). It is furthermore substantiated by the experimental observation that, in the absence of direct interference with the polar groups, the effect of the introduction of various substituents into a steroid molecule on its relative binding affinity for a receptor is equivalent to the sum total of the effects of the introduction of each individual substituent (21,26,50). Such additivity is only compatible with a fairly well-defined positioning of the molecule within the binding site, always giving rise to the same substituent—protein interactions. Consequently, any deviations in the overall skeleton and/or polar groups of the natural hormone, which do not greatly reduce binding capacity compared to those that do (see below), constitute particularly valuable information for demarcating the boundaries of the binding site.

Both steroid and protein can undergo distortion and mutual adaptation. Steroid flexibility varies greatly with the degree of unsaturation and substitution of the steroid skeleton. It is always greatest in a direction perpendicular to the mean plane of the skeleton, being low for the more saturated steroids (e.g. progesterone and testosterone) but becoming marked for highly unsaturated derivatives such as the Δ4,9,11 trienes. The flexibility of these trienes may account for their ability to bind to the receptors of several steroid hormone classes (17,36,40,41). The flexibility of the protein is unknown and probably rather limited. Binding of the steroid to the protein very likely induces a transconformation of the protein, perhaps by the formation of a programmed sequence of interactions starting from a defined initial conformation. The influence of substitution at diverse points of the steroid skeleton on binding affinity suggests that the steroid is probably in relatively close contact with the protein at several points (Van der Waals interactions), as if it were in a hydrophobic pocket within the protein. The dual nature of steroids, part rigid, part flexible, suggests an interaction model situated somewhere between the lock-and-key and zipper models (8); binding could be initiated at one extremity of the steroid (e.g. the A ring (19,21,23)) via a hydrogen bond and then followed through by mutual moulding of steroid and protein.

INDIRECT MAPPING OF THE BINDING SITE(S)

In the absence of a purified receptor protein, some insight can be gained into the nature of the binding site(s) by correlating, for a wide selection of ligands, molecular conformation with binding data. It is assumed that, by identifying a sufficient number of *different* ligands interacting with the receptor, a mould of the volume occupied by the active conformations of these ligands would represent the binding site. Such an approach requires a knowledge of the contribution of each substituent of a steroid to binding and conformation by comparison of many pairs of steroids differing by that substituent only and a knowledge of the most probable conformations of these steroids. Furthermore, it necessitates the study of the thermodynamic properties of the binding of a large number of highly varied steroids to the five recognized classes of steroid hormone receptors. The interaction between steroid and protein being a dynamic process involving complex thermodynamic equilibria with different association and dissociation rates, only a dynamic estimate of binding can be ultimately correlated with conformational data. In the absence of the direct measurement of rate constants, this estimate can be given by a comparison of relative binding affinities (RBAs) measured under different incubation (time and temperature) conditions (4,35,37). We already possess a vast body of structural data (X-ray crystallography and molecular geometry calculations) and of biochemical data (RBAs). In the present chapter, we shall focus our attention on two points only, namely, the nature of the hydrogen bond at O(3) for estrogens and the preliminary mapping of the binding site for progestins.

Are steroid estrogens hydrogen bond donors at O(3) ?

Among the five steroid hormone classes (estrogen, progestin, androgen, mineralocorticoid and glucocorticoid), only the natural estrogens have a phenolic A ring and a hydroxy group at O(3), the other natural hormones (except for dihydrotestosterone) being characterized by a 3-keto-4-ene structure. Very little interference is encountered between binding to the estrogen receptor and the other steroid hormone receptors; phenolic steroids compete almost exclusively for binding to the estrogen receptor and 3-keto-4-ene steroids compete rarely for estrogen binding (31,32, 40,45,47). The 3-keto-4-ene steroids are acceptors, but not donors, of hydrogen bonds at O(3). Although phenolic steroids can theoretically be either donors and/or acceptors of such bonds, a simple explanation for the lack of cross-reactivity could be provided by the hypothesis that estrogens have to be donors of hydrogen bonds at O(3). The following results are in agreement with this hypothesis.

(a) Comparison of 19-nor-Δ4 steroids and of their 19-nor-Δ5(10) homologs.
When shifting the Δ4 double bond of nortestosterone or of norethindrone to a Δ5(10) position (prenortesterone and norethynodrel), the RBAs of these compounds for the progestin and androgen receptors are markedly and expectedly decreased (Table 1), but their RBAs for the estrogen receptor are hardly affected, in spite of a change in conformation (27,30,34,42) towards that of estradiol (9) as illustrated in Fig. 1 for prenortestosterone and as also observed for norethynodrel. Apart

TABLE 1. Relative binding affinities(RBAs)

	ES	PG	AND
Nortestosterone	⟨ 0.1	20 ± 3	154 ± 20
Prenortestosterone	⟨ 0.1	2.5	24
Norethindrone	⟨ 0.1	156 ± 18	43 ± 3
Norethynodrel	0.3 ± 0.1	9.1 ± 0.5	3.4 ± 0.7

ES, PG, AND : estrogen, progestin and androgen receptors in mouse uterus, rabbit uterus and rat prostate cytosol respectively. RBAs were measured after 2 hr incubation at 0°C as previously described (31). The RBAs of estradiol, progesterone and testosterone for their respective receptors were taken as equal to 100.

from the O(3) oxygen atom and the electronic properties of the A ring, little distinguishes estradiol from prenortestosterone or ethynyl estradiol from norethyno-drel.

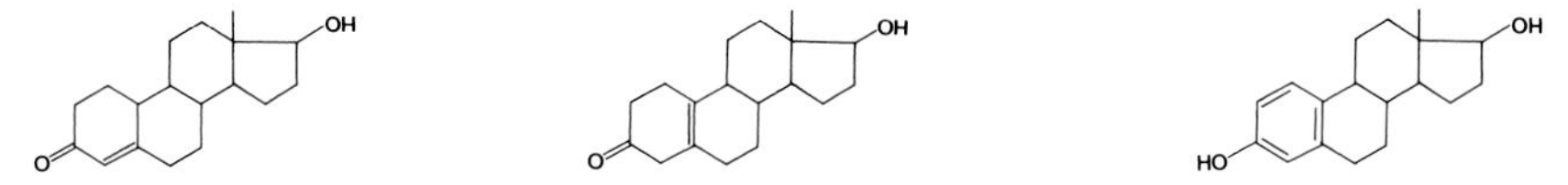

Nortestosterone   **Prenortestosterone**   **Estradiol**

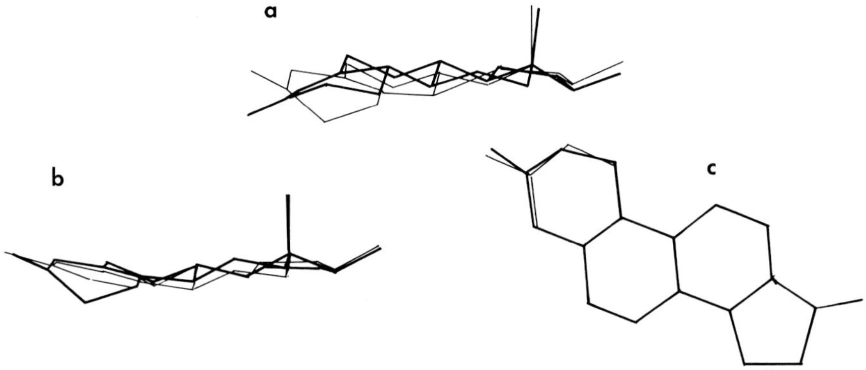

FIG. 1. Best-fit superpositions of crystalline conformations (a) Nortestosterone (dark lines) (34) and prenortestosterone (fine lines) (42); (b,c) Prenortestosterone (dark lines) and estradiol (fine lines) (9).

(b) Comparison of Δ4,9,11 steroids and of homologous or quasi-homologous estradiol derivatives.
    The lack of receptor specificity of Δ4,9,11 steroids, which is probably related to their high degree of flexibility, has been reported in some detail (17,41). However, even when these steroids bind effectively to the progestin, androgen, mineralocorticoid and gluco-corticoid receptors, they do no bind under standard incubation conditions to the estrogen receptor. Such lack of binding is difficult to explain if one compares their flat crystalline (or calculated minimum energy (15)) conformations with those of estradiol and ethynyl estradiol (24) (Fig. 2). The aromatic nature of the A ring has little influence on conformation and its electronic state is only little different since 4 of the 6 atoms of the A ring of 3-keto-Δ4,9,11-trienes are of the Sp^2 type (C(3), C(4), C(5), C(10)). Once again, only the O(3) atom is the distinguishing feature.

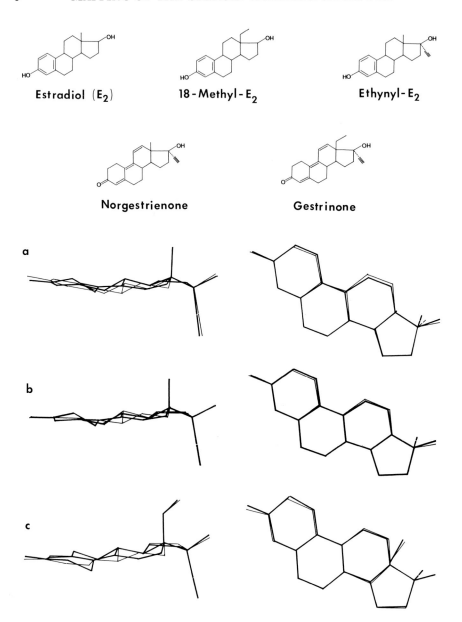

FIG. 2. <u>Best-fit superpositions of crystalline conformations</u>
(a) Norgestrienone (dark lines) (25) and ethynyl estradiol (fine
lines) (24); (b) Norgestrienone (dark lines) and estradiol (fine
lines) (18); (c) Gestrinone (dark lines) (16) and 18-methyl
estradiol (fine lines) (1).

(c) Affinity of ethynodiol, androstanediols and A-nor-
hydroxy derivatives.
Although the conformations of ethynodiol, of androst-
ane-3β,17β-diol and of several A-nor hydroxy derivatives
(12,33, unpublished data) are fairly different from that
of estradiol, these compounds can nevertheless bind to
the estrogen receptor. Ethynodiol has an RBA of 14
(compared to 100 for estradiol) for the estrogen receptor of mouse uterus cytosol after incubation for 2 hr
at 0°C, and the A-nor-hydroxy derivative, compound J
(see Appendix) (11), has an RBA of about 6 under the
same conditions. According to several reports (22,32),
androstane-3β,17β-diol also binds with weak affinity
to the cytosolic estrogen receptor. In the case of all
these compounds, the hydroxy groups at C(2 or 3) could
act as hydrogen bond donors and account for the estrogen binding in spite of the fairly unsuited geometry.

In conclusion, the hypothesis that estrogens are
hydrogen bond donors with regard to the estrogen receptor is supported by the following evidence :
Synthetic 3-keto-Δ4,9,11 steroids do not bind to the
estrogen receptor despite the high degree of similarity
between their conformations and those of homologous
estrogens and despite the overlap between the hydrogen
bond zones of the 3-keto and 3-hydroxy groups (see
Fig. 6); certain non-phenolic C(3) hydroxy derivatives
can bind to this receptor despite a different conformation. These results confirm, as previously suggested
(2), that the ability to form hydrogen bonds would
appear to be more crucial to binding than the chemical
nature of the A-ring.

Can information on unusual steroid progestins
help to demarcate the progestin binding site ?

Of the data available on the conformations of progestins (15,19,20,28), many are redundant insofar as they
yield the same, limited, information on the binding
site, presumably because they concern molecules differing only by the nature and orientation of substituents
partaking in Van der Waals interactions rather than
hydrogen bonds. Only data on unusual steroids can lead
to new information. In particular, the steroids in
Table 2 have enabled us to define the zones of the
progestin receptor which could interact with the oxygen
atoms at C(3) and C(20 or 17).

Table 2. Steroids used to map the progestin binding
site - Study of the hydrogen bond at O(3) -

	RBA for PG 2 hr	24 hr	Relevance of the chosen steroid
Progesterone	100	100	Reference compounds (10,30).
Norethindrone	156 ± 18	263 ± 10	
A-Nor-progesterone		1.4	Particular conformation of ring A(A-nor)(15).
RU 1479	117 ± 14	159	Particular conformations of rings A and B (A-nor and B-homo) (15,24).
RU 2992	229 ± 63	220 ± 60	Particular conformation of ring A (A-nor); flexibility due to 3 conjugated double bonds (15).
Isopregnanolone	0.7	1.5	Combination of 3β-OH and 5α-H (15).

Relative binding affinities (RBA) for the progestin receptor (PG)
in rabbit uterus cytosol were determined as described previously
after 2 hr or 24 hr incubation (31,40). Reference to conformations obtained by X-ray crystallography and/or molecular geometry
calculations is made in the right-hand column.

Table 2. (contd) - Study of the hydrogen bond at
O(20 or 17) -

	RBA for PG 2 hr	24 hr	Relevance of the chosen steroid
Compound B₁₉	220 ±45	403 ±12	Spirolactone ring at C-17 limiting interactions (43,44).
D-Nor-progesterone	3.3 ±1.3		Particular conformation of ring D (D-nor) (15).
RU 5098	6.7 ±0.5	7.2 ±1.0	
RU 5099	182 ±26	340 ±70	Influence of the OH and CH₃ groups on the orientation of the 17β side-chain (15,24,38).
RU 27988	14 ±1	11 ±4	
RU 27987	194 ±27	660 ±40	

All steroid conformations have, unless otherwise
indicated, been compared by using a program for the
best-fit superposition of the maximum number of homologous carbon atoms of the steroid skeletons. Simply
superposing the polar groups often gives mean displacements of as much as 0.3-0.5 Å for the synthetic steroid compared to the natural hormone. Such displacements
are considerably higher than the very slight variations
in steroid conformation known to influence binding (15).

Figure 3 illustrates the discrepancy between superposition of the O (3) and O (20) functions only and the
B, C, and D rings of the conformations of progesterone
(observed) and A-nor-progesterone (calculated).

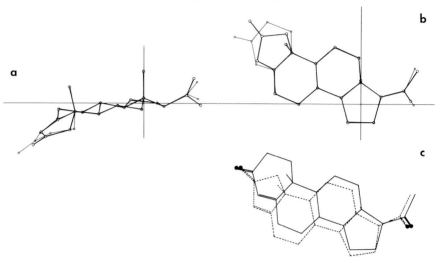

FIG. 3. Best-fit superpositions of the conformations of A-nor-
progesterone and progesterone
Best-fit superposition of the B,C, and D rings (a,b) and of the
O(3) and O(20) functions only (c) of the calculated conformation
of A-nor-progesterone (fine or dotted lines) and the observed
crystalline conformation of progesterone (dark lines).

(a) The O(3) zone
    A best-fit superposition of rings B, C and D of
A-nor-progesterone and of progesterone (Fig. 3) shows
that there is only a very slight difference between
homologous atoms but a marked difference in the orientation of the ketone groups. The weak RBA of A-nor-progesterone (Table 2) is thus probably due to the inability of its ketone group to form an adequate hydrogen
bond with the receptor and suggests that the receptor
interaction zone of the O(3) of A-nor-progesterone does
not include the receptor atom binding to progesterone,
when these two molecules are superposed.
    If the B ring of A-nor-progesterone is converted
into a B-homo ring and the ketone is shifted from C(2)
to C(3) (see RU 1479), the ketone group takes up a position closer to that observed for progesterone (Figs.
4 a,b) but the overall shape of the molecule (observed
experimentally or calculated) is less bent than that of
progesterone. The double-headed arrows in Figs. 4a,b
indicate the flexibility range of the calculated confor-

mations of RU 1479 (the upper lower energy positions
are the most probable). RU 1479 is furthermore characterized by an intramolecular O(5)...O(3) hydrogen bond
which stabilizes the conformation and prevents the
ketone from accepting intermolecular hydrogen bonds in
a region where the angle O(5)...O(3)...X (X being the
donor) is appreciably less than 90° (Fig. 4c). The
interaction zone of the ketone of RU 1479 is favorable
to binding to the progestin receptor since RU 1479 has
a high RBA (Table 2).

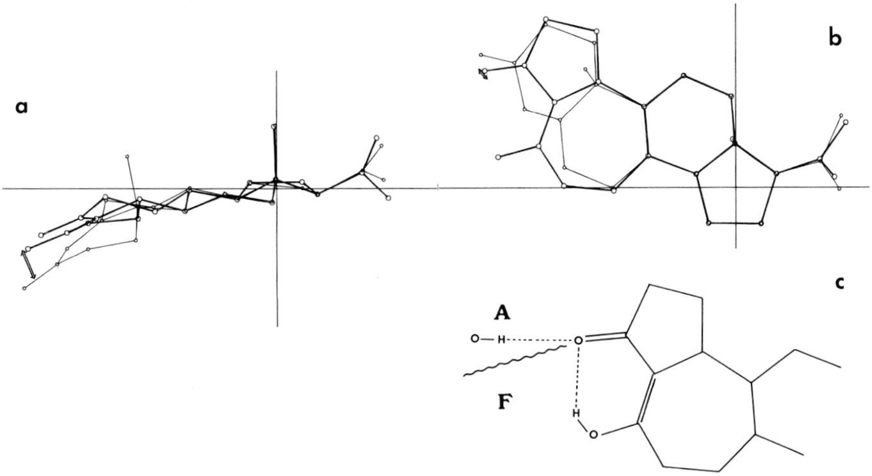

FIG. 4. Best-fit superpositions of the crystalline conformations
      of RU 1479 and progesterone
(a,b) Best-fit superpositions of the C(7) to C(18) atoms of
RU 1479 (dark lines) and progesterone (fine lines). (c) Schematic
representation of the allowed (A) and forbidden (F) areas of
intermolecular hydrogen bonding for RU 1479.

The introduction of Δ4,9,11 bonds into a molecule
confers a certain amount of flexibility (17,41) and
RU 2992, an A-nor-4,9,11-triene, although probably
rather less flexible than the corresponding 6-membered-
A-ring-Δ4,9,11 steroid, has the ability to adopt a
conformation allowing it to bind firmly to the progestin receptor (Table 2). Consequently, one would expect
this conformation to be different from that of A-nor-
progesterone which has little binding affinity. Molecular geometry calculations have in fact shown that
the preferential conformation of RU 2992 is markedly
less curved than that of progesterone or A-nor-progesterone (Fig. 5).

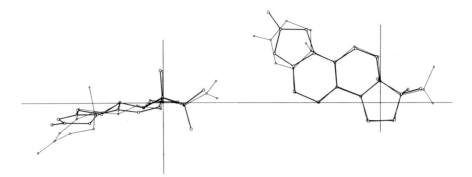

FIG. 5. <u>Best-fit superpositions of the conformations of RU 2992
and progesterone</u>
Superpositions of the calculated conformation of RU 2992 (dark
lines) and the observed crystalline conformation of progesterone
(fine lines).

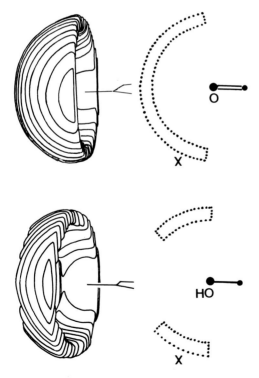

FIG. 6. <u>Observed hydrogen
bonding zones</u>

Possible locations for
H-bond donors (X) with
regard to the O(3) ketone
and H-bond acceptors or
donors (X) with regard to
the O(3) hydroxyl. The
X...O(3) distance for H-
bonding was taken to be
between 2.6 and 3.0 Å, since
greater distances considerably weaken the energy of
the H-bonds although bonds
of 3.3 Å have been observed.
In future studies, the
binding zones will be defined by probability gradients
taking variations in H-bond
length and in molecular
deformation into account.

By comparing the possible exchange zones for the hydrogen bonds involving the O(3) atoms of progesterone, A-nor-progesterone, RU 1479 and RU 2992 in relation to their different RBAs (Fig. 6 and Table 2), it is possible to define a small common volume, denoted Z, situated more towards the C(2) than the C(4) side of the ketone and above the β-face (Fig. 7). Although this zone has been defined with only 4 steroids, it has met all further requirements insofar as all subsequently studied progestins with affinity for the progestin receptor, unlike inactive steroids, have been shown to be able to form hydrogen bonds in this zone. For instance, the very low RBAs of 3β-OH,5α-H derivatives of progesterone (e.g. isopregnanolone) (Table 2) can be explained by the fact that their oxygen atom is far too close to this zone for the formation of a hydrogen bond.

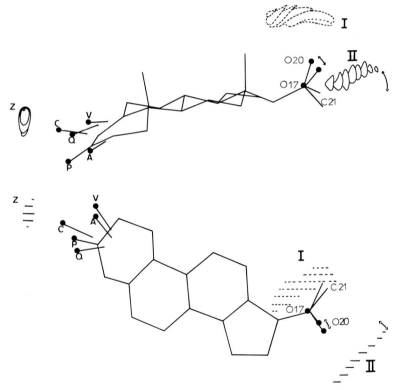

FIG. 7. Proposed hydrogen bonding zones
The proposed locations for hydrogen bond donors to the progestin receptor are indicated by "Z" for the O(3) steroid extremity and by "II" for the O(20 or 17) extremity. The O(3) positions of A-nor-progesterone, RU 1479, RU 2992, and isopregnanolone, after a best-fit superposition with progesterone (P), are denoted by A,Q,V and C, respectively.

(b) The O(20) or O(17) zone
   Steroids with a high RBA for the progestin receptor
have, as shown in Table 2, either a ketone, hydroxy
or lactone group at C(17). It is possible but unlikely
that these functions interact with different polar
groups of the progestin binding site (although some
such as the hydroxy group may also interact with polar
groups in the androgen (or other) binding sites); on
the contrary, the same active group of the progestin
receptor probably forms a hydrogen bond with the oxygen
atom of the lactone group of Compound B_{19}, the 17β-
hydroxy group of norethindrone, or the O(20) oxygen
of progesterone. The receptor thus acts as hydrogen
bond donor towards the O(20) or O(17) atom.

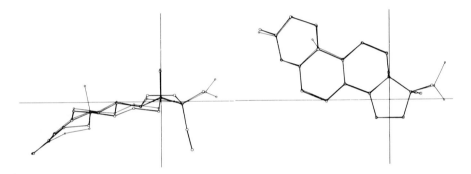

FIG. 8. Best-fit superpositions of the crystalline conformations
of norethindrone and progesterone
Norethindrone (dark lines) (30); progesterone (fine lines) (10).

   A best-fit superposition of the skeletons of progesterone and norethindrone (Fig. 8) reveals a difference
of about 1.2 Å between the O(20) atom of progesterone
and the O(17) atom of norethindrone, but this superposition does not take into account the possible rotation
of the 17β-acetyl side-chain. According to calculations
by quantum (CNDOII) and molecular (GEMO) mechanics, an
energy expenditure of less than 2 kcal would allow
variations of about -10° to -50° in the dihedral C(16)-
C(17)-C(20)-O(20) angle. Figure 7 indicates the receptor zone (denoted II) which could form hydrogen bonds
with both progesterone and norethindrone. The double-
headed arrows illustrate the mobility of this zone as
a function of the possible orientations of the 17β-ace-
tyl side-chain of progesterone. Zone I (shown in dotted
lines) could also form hydrogen bonds with both progesterone and norethindrone but is drastically influenced
by steric hindrance from the C(18) methyl.
   According to published crystallographic data (43,44),
the position and orientation of the 17 β-oxygen atom of a

spiro-oxathiolane function are very close to those of
the hydroxy group of norethindrone. However, owing to
the presence of the other atoms in the spiro-oxathiolane ring, this oxygen atom is less capable of forming
hydrogen bonds. This reduced hydrogen bond capacity is
illustrated in Fig. 9 and confirms the importance of
zone II.

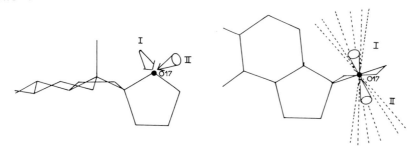

FIG. 9. Possible hydrogen-bond interactions of the O(17) atom of
steroids with a C(17) spiro-oxathiolane function

Finally, a great number of both structural and biochemical data further support the importance of zone
II. Thus, D-nor progesterone has little binding affinity
(Table 2) because its 17β-side-chain cannot form hydrogen bonds in this zone (Fig. 10). Of the two isomers,
RU 5098 & RU 5099 (15,24,38) and RU 27987 & RU 27988
(38), in each case only one binds appreciably to the
progestin receptor (Table 2) because only its 17β-side-
chain is able to adopt a position (on the β-face above
ring D towards C(16)) compatible with hydrogen bonding
within this zone.

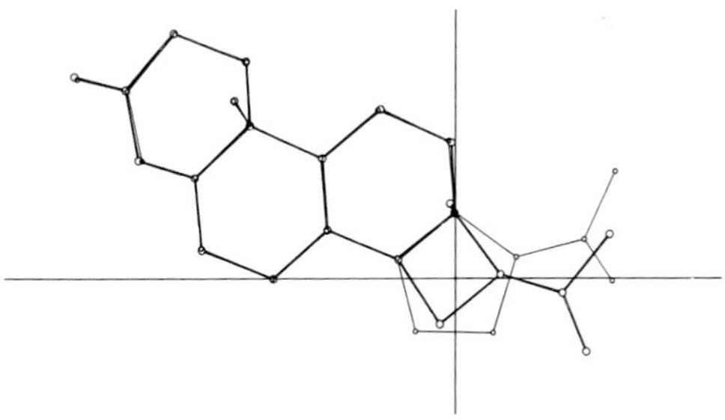

FIG. 10. Best-fit superposition of the conformations of D-nor-
progesterone and progesterone
Superposition of the calculated conformation of D-nor-progeste-
rone (dark lines) and the observed crystalline conformation of
progesterone (fine lines).

Can steroid conformation be related to binding kinetics?

As shown in Table 2, the steroids used to map the progestin binding site either bind strongly to the receptor, forming complexes which dissociate more slowly than the natural hormone complex (their RBAs increase with incubation time) (35,37), or bind very weakly forming complexes the RBAs of which are low and vary little. The first set of compounds can form hydrogen bonds within zones Z and II, whereas the remaining compounds are probably unable to do so and only bind to the receptor via weak Van der Waals forces differently affected by incubation conditions. Since, in many instances, it would appear that the kinetics of the binding between ligand and receptor determine the life-span of the complex and consequently the biological response (5,35), it was thought of interest to confront results obtained on conformation and binding kinetics. Figure 11 shows that the replacement of a C(13)methyl by an ethyl has no effect on overall molecular conformation, whereas Fig. 12 shows that this change can affect the dissociation rate of the steroid-receptor complex. Whereas in the case of norgestrienone and gestrinone, the RBAs recorded after 2 hr and 24 hr are about the same for both compounds, in the case of norethindrone and RU 2420 the replacement of the C(13) methyl by an ethyl leads to compounds (norgestrel and RU 4841 respectively) with much higher RBAs after 24 hr than 2 hr, i.e. compounds which dissociate much slower from the receptor.

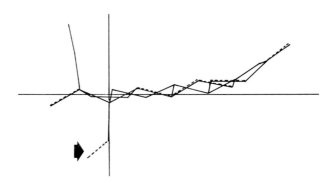

FIG. 11. Best-fit superpositions of the crystalline conformations of norethindrone and norgestrel
Norethindrone (dark lines); norgestrel (14) (dotted lines). The position of the C(18) methyl group (see arrow) is the same for both steroids.

Best-fit superpositions of progesterone with norethindrone (or norgestrel) and of progesterone with
$\Delta4,9$ or $\Delta4,9,11$ steroids (e.g. the trienes norgestrienone or gestrinone) have revealed that, as a result
of the twist of the skeleton of the dienes and trienes,
the orientation of the 17α-ethynyl substituent may be
quite different in the case of norgestrienone and gestrinone compared to norethindrone and norgestrel and
may differ by as much as 1 Å (15). Thus, this twist in
the skeleton could interfere with the interaction possibilities of the 13-ethyl group, even though the position of this group relative to the C-D ring junction
remains the same, and modify the kinetics of the interaction. This may thus constitute an attractive explanation for the change in kinetics of the ethynylated
trienes compared to the non-ethynyl trienes and ethynyl mono-enes. That the effects of the ethynyl substi-

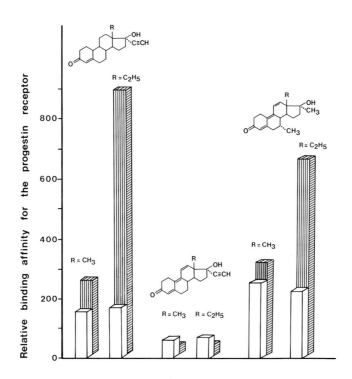

FIG. 12. RBA of progestins for the progestin receptor
The relative binding affinities of (from left to right) norethindrone, norgestrel, norgestrienone, gestrinone, RU 2420 and
RU 4841 for the progestin receptor were measured after 2 hr □
or 24 hr ▨ incubation with rabbit uterus cytosol as previously
described (31).

tuent and of unsaturation ($\Delta 4,9,11$) are not independent was first evident in studies (15,26) which showed that this is one of the rare cases where additivity of RBA increments does not strictly apply.

The examples in Fig. 12 illustrate the complexity of steroid-receptor interactions and emphasize the importance of considering kinetic factors in the mapping of a binding site, since several successive and probably non-independent interactions lead to the formation of the final stable complex. This may be totally different however, in the case of plasma proteins for which very much faster dissociation rates have been recorded than for steroid receptor complexes (48). Furthermore, in these examples, we have considered the kinetics of the binding of these compounds to the progestin receptor only; some of these compounds in particular the 17-hydroxy derivatives, can bind to the receptors of other hormone classes (e.g. the androgen receptor) (31,39,40) though generally to form somewhat less stable complexes (39). Comparative binding and conformational data suggest that the receptor binding sites of at least all 3-keto-$\Delta 4$ steroids are very closely related (17). A profitable future approach to binding site mapping is thus probably one that analyses the reasons why, for a particular steroid, one class of binding is more stable than others.

APPENDIX : CHEMICAL NAMES OF TEST-SUBSTANCES

A-Nor-progesterone	: A-Nor-pregn-3-ene-2,20-dione
D-Nor-progesterone	: D-Nor-pregn-4-ene-3,20-dione
Compound B 19	: (17R)4',5'-Dihydro-spiro[estr-4-ene-17,2' (3'H)-furan]3-one
Compound J	: 2α-Ethynyl-A-nor-androstane-2β,17β-diol
Estradiol	: Estra-1,3,5(10)-triene-3,17β-diol
Ethynodiol	: 19-Nor-17α-pregn-4-en-20-yne-3β,17β-diol
Ethynyl estradiol	: 19-Nor-17α-pregna-1,3,5(10)-trien-20-yne-3, 17β-diol
Gestrinone	: 13β-Ethyl-17β-hydroxy-18,19-dinor-pregna-4, 9,11-trien-20-yn-3-one
Isopregnanolone	: 3β-Hydroxy-5α-pregn-20-one
18-Methylestradiol	: 13β-Ethyl-gona-1,3,5(10)-triene-3,17β-diol
Norethindrone	: 17β-Hydroxy-19-nor-17α-pregn-4-en-20-yn-3-one
Norethynodrel	: 17β-Hydroxy-19-nor-17α-pregn-5(10)-en-20-yn-3-one
Norgestrel	: 13β-Ethyl-17β-hydroxy-18,19-dinor-17α-pregn-4-en-20-yn-3-one
Norgestrienone	: 17β-Hydroxy-19-nor-17α-pregna-4,9,11-trien-20-yn-3-one

Nortestosterone : 17β-Hydroxy-estr-4-en-3-one
Prenortestosterone : 17β-Hydroxy-estr-5(10)-en-3-one
Progesterone : Pregn-4-ene-3,20-dione
RU 1479 : A-Nor-B-homo-19-nor-pregna-3,6,20-trione
(enolized form).
RU 2420 : 7α,17α-Dimethyl-17-hydroxy-estra-4,9,11-trien
-3-one
RU 27987 : 17β-[(2S)2-hydroxy-1-oxo-propyl]-17α-methyl-
estra-4,9-dien-3-one.
RU 27988 : 17β-[(2R)2-hydroxy-1-oxo-propyl]-17α-methyl-
estra-4,9-dien-3-one
RU 2992 : 17β-Hydroxy-17α-methyl-A-nor-estra-3(5),9,11-
trien-2-one
RU 4841 : 7α,17α-Dimethyl-13β-ethyl-17-hydroxy-gona-4,
9,11-trien-3-one
RU 5098 : (20RS)20-Hydroxy-17α-methyl-19-nor-pregna-4,
9-dien-3-one
RU 5099 : (20SR)20-Hydroxy-17α-methyl-19-nor-pregna-4,
9-dien-3-one

REFERENCES

1. Barrans, Y., Courseille, C., Busetta, B., and Précigoux, G. (1976): Acta Cryst., B32: 1296-1298.
2. Bergink, E.W., Jansen, A.E.M., and de Winter, M.S.(1976): Endocrinology, Suppl.102, 282.
3. Blanford, A.T., Wittman, W., Stroupe, S.D., and Westphal, U. (1978): J. Ster.Biochem., 9: 187-201.
4. Bouton, M.M. and Raynaud, J.P.(1978): J. Ster.Biochem., 9,9-15
5. Bouton, M.M. and Raynaud, J.P.(1979): Endocrinology, 105, 509-515.
6. Bresciani, F., Sica, V., and Weisz, A.(1979): In: Biochemical Actions of Hormones, Vol.VI, edited by G.Litwack, pp.461-480, Academic Press, New York.
7. Buehner, M. and Beato, M.(1978): J.Mol.Biol., 120: 337-341.
8. Burgen, A.S.V., Roberts, G.C.K., and Feeney, J.(1975): Nature, 253: 753-755.
9. Busetta, B. and Hospital, M.(1972): Acta Cryst., B28: 560-567.
10. Campsteyn, H., Dupont, L. and Dideberg, O.(1972): Acta Cryst., B28, 3032-3042.
11. Canceill, J., Azadian-Boulanger, G., Philibert, D., Raynaud, J.P., and Jacques, J.(1977): C.R.Acad.Sci.(Paris), C285, 37-40.
12. Canceill, J.Gasc, J.C., Nédélec, L., Baert, F., Foulon, M., and Jacques, J.(1979): Bull.Soc.Chimique, part2, 157-164.
13. Cohen, N.C.(1971): Tetrahedron, 27: 789-797.
14. DeAngelis, N.J., Doyne, T.H., and Grob, R.L.(1975): Acta Cryst. B31, 2040-2043.

15. Delettré, J.(1978): In: Interaction "Hormone Steroïde-Protéine Cytoplasmique" au travers d'une Approche Structurale des Steroïdes Oestrogènes, Progestogènes, Androgènes. Le Steroïde à l'Etat Isolé, Correlations Paramètres Structuraux-Réponse Biologique, Ph.D. Thesis, Université Paris VI.
16. Delettré, J., Mornon, J.P., Lepicard, G.(1975): Acta Cryst., B31, 450-453.
17. Delettré, J., Mornon, J.P., Lepicard, G., Ojasoo, T., and Raynaud, J.P. J.Ster.Biochem.(in press).
18. Duax, W.L.(1972): Acta Cryst., B28, 1864-18 71
19. Duax, W.L., Cody, V., Griffin, J.F., Rohrer, D.C., and Weeks, C.M.(1978): J. Toxicol.Env.Health, 4, 205-277.
20. Duax, W.L. and Norton, D.A.(1975) Atlas of Steroid Structure, Vol.I, Plenum Press, New York.
21. Fanchenko, N.D., Sturchak, S.V., Shchedrina, R.N., Pivnitsky, K.K., Novikov, E.A., and Ischkov, V.L.(1979): Acta Endocr. (Kbh), 90: 167-175.
22. Garcia, M. and Rochefort, H.(1979): Endocrinology, 104: 1797-1804.
23. Hähnel, R., Twaddle, E., and Ratajczak, T.(1973): J.Ster. Biochem., 4, 21-31.
24. Lepicard, G.(1978): In: Interaction "Hormone Steroide-Protéine Cytoplasmique" au travers d'une Approche Structurale des Steroïdes Oestrogènes, Progestogènes, Androgènes. Le Steroïde à l'Etat Cristallin, Ph.D. Thesis, Université Paris VI.
25. Lepicard, G., Delettré, J., and Mornon, J.P.(1974): Acta Cryst. B30, 2751-2753.
26. Lepicard, G., Mornon, J.P., Delettré, J., Ojasoo, T., and Raynaud, J.P. (1978): J.Ster.Biochem., 9, 830.
27. McPhail, A.T., Luhan, P.A., Tschang, P.S.W., and Onan, K.D. (1977): J.Chem.Soc. Perkin Trans.II, 1977, 379-383.
28. Mornon, J.P., Delettré, J., Lepicard, G., Bally, R., Surcouf, E., and Bondot, P.(1977): J.Ster.Biochem., 8, 51-62.
29. Mornon, J.P., Fridlansky, F., Bally, R., and Milgrom, E.: J.Mol.Biol.(in press).
30. Mornon, J.P., Lepicard, G., and Delettré, J.(1976): C.R. Acad. Sci.(Paris), C282, 387-390.
31. Ojasoo, T. and Raynaud, J.P.(1978): Cancer Res., 38, 4186-4198.
32. Poortman, J., Vroegindewey-Jie, D., Thijssen, J.H.H., and Schwarz, F.(1977): Mol.Cell.Endocr., 8, 27-34.
33. Précigoux, G. and Fornies-Marquina, J.(1973): Cryst.Struct. Comm., 2: 287-290.
34. Précigoux, G., Busetta, B., Courseille, C., and Hospital, M. (1975): Acta Cryst., B31, 1527-1532.
35. Raynaud, J.P.(1978): In: Advances in Pharmacology and Therapeutics, Vol.I, Receptors, edited by J. Jacob, pp.259-278, Pergamon Press, Oxford.
36. Raynaud, J.P., Bouton, M.M., Moguilewsky, M.M., Ojasoo, T., Philibert, D., Beck, G., Labrie, F. and Mornon J.P.(1979): J.Ster.Biochem.(in press).

37. Raynaud, J.P., Bouton, M.M., and Ojasoo, T.(1979): Biochem. Soc.Trans., 7, 547-551.
38. Raynaud, J.P., Brown, N., Coussedière, D., Pottier, J., Delettré, J.. and Mornon, J.P.: In: Steroid-induced Uterine Proteins, edited by M. Beato, Elsevier, Amsterdam (in press).
39. Raynaud, J.P., Fortin, M., and Tournemine, C.(1980): In: Actualités de Chimie Thérapeutique (in press).
40. Raynaud, J.P., Ojasoo, T., Bouton, M.M., and Philibert, D. (1979): In: Drug Design, Vol.VII, edited by E.J. Ariëns, pp.169-214, Academic Press, New York.
41. Raynaud, J.P., Ojasoo, T., Mornon, J.P., Delettré, J. and Lepicard, G.(1980): In: Pharmacological Modulation of Steroid Action, edited by Genazzani et al., pp.171-180, 1980.
42. Sobti, R.R., Levine, S.G., and Bordner, J.(1972): Acta Cryst., B28, 2292-2297.
43. Surcouf, E.(1979): Acta Cryst., B35, 1922-1925.
44. Surcouf, E.(1979): Acta Cryst., B35, 1925-1928.
45. Terenius, L.(1974), Steroids, 23, 909-918.
46. Vedekis, W.V., Schrader, W.T., and O'Malley, B.W.(1978): In: Biochemical Actions of Hormones, Vol.V., edited by G.Litwack, pp.321-372, Academic Press, New York.
47. Watson, G., Korach, K.S., and Muldoon, T.G.(1977): Endocrinology 101, 1733-1743.
48. Westphal, U., Stroupe, S.D., Kute, T., and Cheng, S.L.(1977): J.Ster.Biochem., 8, 367-374.
49. Westbrook, E.M., Piro, O.E., Yonath, A., and Sigler, P.B.(1979): In: Abstracts, 1979 Winter Meeting of American Crystallographic Association, Honolulu.
50. Wolff, M.E., Baxter, J.D., Kollman, P.A., Lee, D.L., Kuntz, I.D., Bloom, E., Matulich, D.T, and Morris, J.(1978): Biochemistry, 17, 3201-3208.

Perspectives in Steroid Receptor Research,
edited by F. Bresciani.
Raven Press, New York © 1980.

Immunochemical Probes for Receptor Structure and Function

E. V. Jensen, G. L. Greene, L. E. Closs, and E. R. DeSombre

*Ben May Laboratory for Cancer Research, University of Chicago,
Chicago, Illinois 60637, U.S.A.*

INTRODUCTION

Ever since the first demonstration of specific binding substances for hexestrol (4) and for estradiol (13) in female reproductive tissues, the detection, measurement and characterization of steroid hormone receptors has depended on the use of a radioactively labeled hormone as a marker for the receptor protein to which it binds. During the past two decades, this experimental approach has provided a wealth of information concerning steroid hormone receptors, including an elucidation of the general nature of the intracellular interaction pathway by which the hormonal action is mediated. In the case of the estrogens (5,11), the hormone, without chemical change, binds to an extranuclear receptor protein (estrophilin), inducing its conversion to an active form. The activated steroid-receptor complex is translocated to the nucleus where it associates with chromatin and in some way alleviates restrictions on the synthesis of various types of RNA that are characteristic of hormone-dependent tissues.

Despite our knowledge of the overall pattern of hormone-receptor interaction, detailed understanding of the processes of receptor synthesis, activation, translocation and nuclear binding is still far from complete. To provide fresh insight concerning these phenomena, there has been need for methods to recognize the receptor protein that do not depend on its binding to labeled steroid. One such approach is the use of specific antibodies to the receptor itself. To this end, we have generated antibodies to estrophilin in the rabbit, the goat and the rat by immunizing them with purified estrogen-receptor complex of calf uterus, and we have prepared monoclonal antiestrophilin antibodies by culturing hybridoma cell lines obtained by the fusion of splenic lymphocytes from an immunized rat with cells of various mouse myeloma lines. The availability of these antibodies permits the application of immunochemical and immunocytochemical techniques for the detection and study of estrogen receptors in target cells.

ANTIBODIES TO ESTROPHILIN

Preparation of Antiestrophilin

After attempts to immunize rabbits with purified preparations of the calcium-stabilized (16) estradiol-receptor complex (E*R) of calf uterine cytosol proved unsuccessful, immunization was accomplished as described elsewhere (6-8) using the E*R complex extracted from calf uterine nuclei, after incubation with calf uterine cytosol containing tritiated estradiol (E*), and purified to 20 to 30% of the theoretical specific radioactivity by a sequence of salt precipitation, gel filtration and polyacrylamide gel electrophoresis. During the course of purification the receptor loses its tendency to aggregate in low salt medium, and its sedimentation rate changes from 5.2 S in sucrose gradients containing 400 mM KCl to 4.8 S in either high or low salt gradients. With the exception of the Lewis rat, who received three intraperitoneal injections of immunogen followed by one intradermal injection, immunizations were carried out by the intradermal procedure of Vaitukaitis et al. (20), using 20 to 60 μg of immunogen for each injection in the rats and rabbits and 80 to 150 μg for the goat. Antiestrophilin titer usually was observed in the serum 2 to 4 months after the primary injection, followed by booster injections at 3 to 4 week intervals. From the serum of the immunized animals a crude immunoglobulin fraction (i-Ig) was prepared by precipitation with ammonium sulfate, 40% of saturation; similar immunoglobulin preparations from non-immunized animals (n-Ig) served as controls.

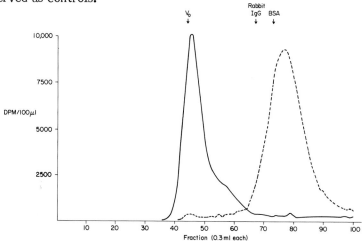

FIG. 1. Elution pattern from Sephadex G-200 of calcium-stabilized (16) E*R of calf uterine cytosol treated with rabbit i-Ig (——) or n-Ig (- - -). Gel filtration was carried out in 400 mM KCl in 10 mM Tris, pH 7.4. Vo = the void volume of the column as determined with blue dextran; bovine serum albumin (BSA) and rabbit immunoglobulin (IgG) were chromatographed separately in the same column to serve as markers. Reproduced from Jensen et al. (12).

Although the interaction of estrophilin with these antibodies does not require the presence of estrogen, the antibody does not prevent the binding of hormone to receptor, so the radioactive steroid can serve as a convenient marker for the association of receptor with antibody. Because the antiestrophilin antibodies thus far obtained all form non-precipitating immune complexes, the usual immunodiffusion methods are not applicable, although double antibody precipitation techniques, as well as the binding of E*R to Sepharose-linked i-Ig or to immobilized Staphylococcus aureus protein-A in the presence of i-Ig, can be used to detect the presence of antiestrophilin in immune serum or immuno-globulin preparations (8).   A convenient criterion for demonstrating antiestrophilin antibodies is their ability to increase the size of the soluble estradiol-receptor complex, as evident either by an acceleration of its elution on gel filtration (Fig. 1) or an increase in its rate of sedimentation on ultracentrifugation in a sucrose gradient (Fig. 2).

The sucrose gradient sedimentation technique has proved especially informative in detecting these antibodies and in recognizing different patterns of interaction with receptors.   In the sedimentation profiles illustrated, ^{14}C-labeled ovalbumin (3.6 S), rabbit immunoglobulin (6.6 S) and amylase (9.2 S) were used as internal markers, while non-radioactive

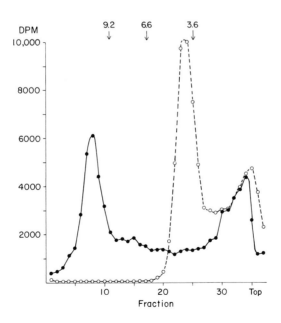

FIG. 2. Sedimentation pattern of purified E*R complex from calf uterine nuclei in 10 to 30% sucrose gradients containing 10 mM KCl in the presence of rabbit i-Ig (●) or n-Ig (O). Reproduced from Greene et al. (6).

bovine plasma albumin (4.6 S), bovine immunoglobulin (7.0 S) and ribosomal RNA from E. coli (16 S) served as external markers. Antibody generated in the rabbit reacts with the purified nuclear E*R from calf uterus to increase its sedimentation rate from 4.8 S to 10-11 S (Fig. 2), and with the 4 S complex of either calf or rat uterine cytosol to form a product sedimenting at about 7.5 S (Fig. 3). The 5.2 S estradiol-receptor complex present in crude extracts of either calf or rat uterine nuclei reacts with rabbit i-Ig to form an 11 S immune complex, always accompanied by a second entity sedimenting at about 8 S. Formation of this double peak with rabbit i-Ig is characteristic of all activated estradiol-receptor complexes studied, whether extracted from the nucleus after exposure to hormone in vitro or in vivo, or produced in the cytosol by warming with hormone or treatment with salt (as illustrated in Fig. 4 for hen oviduct cytosol). Whether the 8 S peak represents cytosol receptor that is incompletely transformed to the activated state or that is bound within the nuclear pellet is not entirely clear, although sucrose gradients run in the absence of antibody show no evidence of contamination of the 5 S complex with untransformed receptor.

Reactivity of Antiestrophilins

As is evident from the foregoing examples, rabbit antibody to nuclear calf uterine estrophilin reacts not only with the receptor used as

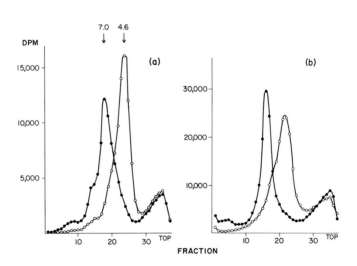

FIG. 3. Sedimentation pattern in 10 to 30% sucrose gradients containing 400 mM KCl of: (a) calf uterine cytosol and (b) rat uterine cytosol, each made 20 nM in E* with subsequent removal of unbound steroid by dextran-coated charcoal, in the presence of rabbit i-Ig (●) or n-Ig (○). Reproduced from Greene et al. (8).

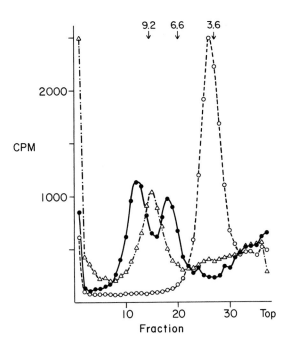

FIG. 4. Sedimentation pattern in 10 to 30% sucrose gradients containing 400 mM KCl of activated E*R of hen oviduct cytosol, in the presence of rabbit i-Ig (●), goat i-Ig (△) or rabbit n-Ig (O). Reproduced from Greene et al. (7).

immunogen but also with extranuclear as well as nuclear E*R complexes from every source tested (Table 1), including human breast cancers (Fig. 5b) and the non-mammalian species, hen (Fig. 4). Similar cross reactivity with hen oviduct has been reported with antibodies obtained by immunizing a rabbit with trypsin-treated estrogen receptor of calf uterine cytosol (17). Despite this lack of tissue and species specificity, there is no reaction between rabbit i-Ig and either androgen or progesterone receptors from a variety of sources. Thus, the rabbit antibody appears to recognize a common determinant that is conserved in estrophilin across a wide range of animal species, but which is not present in receptors for other steroid hormones.

Antiestrophilin antibodies generated in the goat react with either the cytosol or nuclear (Fig. 6) forms of calf uterine receptor to cause a greater increase in sedimentation rate (14 S) than that observed with the rabbit antibody. This effect appears to be specific for calf estrophilin, inasmuch as nuclear E*R from other species, such as rat uterus or hen oviduct (Fig. 4), form immune complexes sedimenting at 8-9 S. The

TABLE 1. Cross reactivity of rabbit i-Ig with estrophilin of various species

Receptor	Tissue	Species
Nuclear	Uterus	Calf, rat, rabbit, sheep
	Breast cancer	Human, MCF-7 cell line
	Endometrial tumor	Rat
	Pituitary tumor	Rat
Cytosol	Uterus	Calf, rat, rabbit, sheep, mouse, guinea pig, monkey
	Oviduct	Monkey, hen
	Breast cancer	Rat, human, MCF-7 cell
	Endometrial tumor	Rat
	Pituitary tumor	Rat

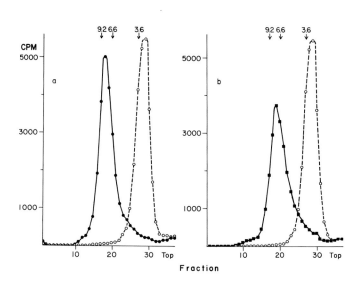

FIG. 5. Sedimentation pattern in 10 to 30% sucrose gradients containing 400 mM KCl of human breast cancer cytosol, made 2.5 nM in E* with removal of unbound steroid by dextran-coated charcoal, in the presence of: (a) ACI rat i-Ig (●) or n-Ig (O) and (b) rabbit i-Ig (■) or n-Ig (O). Reproduced from Greene et al. (7).

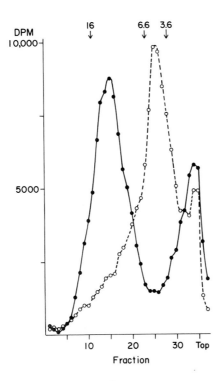

FIG. 6. Sedimentation pattern in 10 to 50% sucrose gradients containing 400 mM KCl of E*R from calf uterine nuclei in the presence of goat i-Ig (●) or n-Ig (O). Reproduced from Greene et al. (6).

reactivity of goat i-Ig has been examined with most of the E*R complexes listed in Table 1, and in every case tested, cross reactivity was observed. Thus, goat i-Ig appears to recognize an antigenic determinant common to estrophilin of most if not all species, as well as an additional determinant that is specific for calf receptor.

Antiestrophilin antibodies generated in the ACI rat have been found to cross react with E*R from those species tested, and their reaction with the cytosol receptor of human breast cancer resembles that of the rabbit antibody, forming an immune complex that sediments at about 8 S (Fig. 5a). In contrast, i-Ig from the Lewis rat, while reacting readily with both nuclear and extranuclear E*R of calf uterus (Fig. 7), did not recognize estrophilin derived from other species. Whether the fact that this animal, unlike the rabbit, goat and ACI rat, received the first three injections of immunogen by the intraperitoneal route played any role in the species-specificity of the antibody produced is not known.

On the basis of the foregoing results, there appears to be an antigenic determinant common to estrophilin from a variety of sources that is recognized by antibodies to calf estrophilin generated in the rabbit, the goat and the ACI rat. Whether it is the same determinant that is recognized by all three antibody preparations is not yet certain, nor is it clear whether i-Ig from the goat and the Lewis rat recognize the same specific determinant in calf estrophilin.   Though interaction of the receptor with antibody does not prevent its ability to bind estradiol, the common determinant recognized by the rabbit antibody is located in the same region of the receptor molecule as is the estradiol binding site (Fig. 8), inasmuch as collaborative experiments with Merry Sherman have established that the mero receptor (18) of human breast cancer cytosol retains the ability to react with rabbit i-Ig.

MONOCLONAL ANTIBODIES TO ESTROPHILIN

Hybridization and Cloning Experiments

The hormone specificity and cross reactivity of the foregoing antibody preparations make them attractive as probes for receptor structure and function and as reagents for their immunochemical purification, assay and intracellular localization. For many of these purposes, however, the usefulness of the antibody preparations is limited by their heterogeneity.   To obtain antiestrophilin uncontaminated by other immunoglobulins, we have employed the techniques of Köhler and Milstein (14), as modified by McKearn et al. (15), to obtain monoclonal cell lines secreting specific antibodies to estrophilin (9).

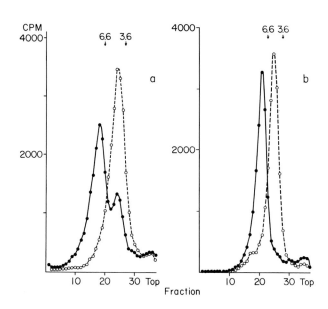

FIG. 7. Sedimentation pattern in sucrose gradients containing 400 mM KCl of: (a) E*R in calf uterine cytosol (10-30% sucrose) and (b) E*R from calf uterine nuclei (10-50% sucrose), in the presence of Lewis rat i-Ig (●) or n-Ig (O). Reproduced from Greene et al. (9).

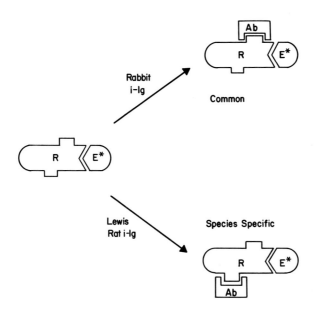

FIG. 8. Schematic representation of the reaction of rabbit i-Ig with common determinant of calf uterine estrophilin and of Lewis rat i-Ig with species-specific determinant.

As summarized in Table 2, the polyethylene glycol-mediated fusion of splenic lymphocytes from the immunized Lewis rat was carried out with cells of three different mouse myeloma lines (3,14,19) to yield proliferating hybridomas in over 50% of the original microtiter wells (485/912). Nearly 10% of the derived hybridoma lines (44/485) secreted anti-estrophilin antibody as determined by double antibody precipitation, using goat anti-Lewis rat immunoglobulin with crude nuclear E*R from calf uterus as the labeled antigen. Hybrid lines were successfully derived from all three mouse myeloma cell lines, although the P3 and NSI myelomas produced more viable hybrids then did the Sp2/0 myeloma. However, hybridomas from the Sp2/0 myeloma have the advantage that this line does not synthesize any mouse myeloma immunoglobulin (19), so the antibody secreted by Sp2/0 hybridomas is entirely that derived from the rat lymphocytes.

Several of the hybrids, including lines derived from all three myeloma mutants, were cloned by limiting dilution. About 15% of the total wells (79/510) produced viable clusters of hybridomas, and approximately 70% of these proliferating clones (56/79) secreted antiestrophilin. Several of the clones were expanded in spinner cultures to volumes of 350 ml or greater, producing milligram amounts of rat immunoglobulin. Viable antibody-secreting hybridomas have been recovered after storage in liquid nitrogen for at least six months.

TABLE 2. Monoclonal hybridoma lines obtained by fusion of spleen cells
of immunized Lewis rat with cells of three different mouse
myeloma lines.

Mouse myeloma used		Hybridomas		
Cell line	Ig Chains[a]	Positive Wells	Positive Clones	Ig Class[b]
P3-X63-Ag8	Heavy + light	14/187	16/23	1 IgM
P3-NSI/1-AG4-1	Light	20/188	19/23	2 IgM
Sp2/0-Ag14	None	10/110	21/33	4 IgM
				3 IgG2a

[a]Immunoglobulin produced by myeloma cells themselves.
[b]So far the type of immunoglobulin produced has been characterized
for 10 of the 56 hybridoma clones found to make antiestrophilin.

Properties of Monoclonal Antiestrophilin

As summarized in Table 2, three of the expanded antiestrophilin-
secreting clones, all derived from the Sp2/0 myeloma, were found to
secrete rat IgG of the γ_{2a} subclass (1), which was purified by a sequence
of two precipitations from ammonium sulfate (40% of saturation)
followed by chromatography on DEAE-cellulose.   Seven additional
expanded clones, derived from all three myeloma lines, were found to
secrete IgM, which was purified by similar salt precipitation followed by
filtration through Bio-Gel A-1.5 M agarose.   As shown in Fig. 9,
monoclonal i-IgG, like the original Lewis rat i-Ig, reacts with either the
4 S cytosol or 5 S nuclear E*R of calf uterus to produce 8 S immune
complexes, whereas i-IgM formed complexes sedimenting at 12-13 S with
both cytosol and nuclear E*R.   The latter observation is unusual, since
rat IgM is reported to sediment at 18-19 S (2).   However, the IgM
produced by the hybridoma clones, though giving an immunological test
for µ chains (1), was found to sediment itself in the 12 S region.
Monoclonal antiestrophilin of the IgG class shows comparable affinity for
both the cytosol and nuclear forms of calf uterine estrophilin, whereas
the IgM antiestrophilin reacts preferentially with the nuclear receptor,
so higher antibody concentrations must be employed to demonstrate
reaction with cytosol E*R (Fig. 9a).   These monoclonal antibodies do not
interfere with the binding of E* to the Ig-receptor complex, as demonstrated by postlabeling (with E*) fractions from sucrose gradients
containing unoccupied receptor and either IgG or IgM.
By inclusion of [^{35}S] methionine in the culture medium of an IgG-
secreting hybridoma clone, we have obtained radiolabeled antiestrophilin, recognized by sedimentation of the isotope at about 7 S (Fig.
10a).   When treated with an excess of calf nuclear E*R, the sediment-

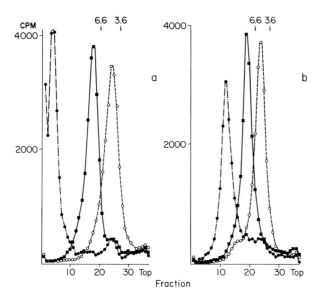

FIG. 9. Sedimation pattern in sucrose gradients containing 400 mM KCl of E*R (0.6 pmol) from: (a) calf uterine cytosol (10-30% sucrose) and (b) calf uterine nuclei (10-50% sucrose), in the presence of Lewis rat n-Ig (O), 20 μg clonal i-IgG (■) or clonal i-IgM (●), 200 μg in (a) and 20 μmg in (b). Reproduced from Greene et al. (9).

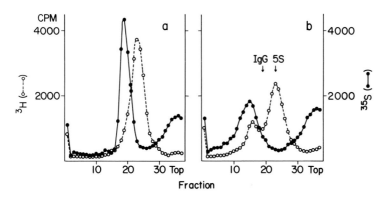

FIG. 10. Interaction between ^{35}S-labeled monoclonal antiestrophilin and excess calf nuclear E*R. Sedimentation pattern in 10 to 30% sucrose gradients containing 400 mM KCl of nuclear calf uterine E*R (O) and a limiting amount of monoclonal [35S] IgG (●): (a) in separate tubes and (b) after incubation together for 1 hr at 4°C. The arrows in (b) indicate the sedimentation positions of E*R (5 S) and labeled IgG (7 S) corresponding to the peaks in (a). Reproduced from Greene et al. (9).

ation peak of the [^{35}S] IgG is completely shifted to the 8-9 S region, along with that portion of the excess E*R that reacted (Fig. 10b). This observation, as well as the fact that on repeated cloning antiestrophilin antibody is produced by 100% of the recloned cultures, indicates that the hybridoma cell lines obtained are actually monoclonal.

Like the total i-Ig from the serum of the parent Lewis rat, the monoclonal antiestrophilin antibodies secreted by the hybridoma cells, react specifically with estrogen receptors from calf tissues but not with receptors from other species. Thus, the monoclonal antibodies provide useful reagents for the purification of calf uterine estrophilin by immunoadsorption and for the immunocytochemical localization of receptor in calf uterus, but they cannot be used for the study of receptors in target tissues of other species, in particular for the assay of estrophilin in human breast cancers as a guide to selection of therapy (10). Because i-Ig from the ACI rat, immunized with calf uterine estrophilin, does cross react with estrogen receptors from human breast cancers as well as from MCF-7 human breast cancer cells, it seems likely that fusion of myeloma cells with splenic lymphocytes of the ACI rat may provide hybridoma lines secreting cross reacting monoclonal antiestrophilin, useful in the immunoradiometric assay of receptors in human breast cancers. Alternatively, if the receptor protein of MCF-7 cancer cells can be purified and concentrated to the point that it is immunogenic in a host animal whose cells can hybridize with those of mouse myeloma, the monoclonal antibodies thus produced should react directly with both occupied and unoccupied estrogen receptors of human breast cancers, eliminating the need for species cross reactivity. Such investigations are now under way in our laboratory, in the hope of expanding the applications of immunochemical techniques in investigations of the measurement and function of estrogen receptors in target tissues.

SUMMARY

Antibodies to the estrogen receptor protein have been generated in the rabbit, the goat and the rat by immunization with purified preparations of nuclear estradiol-receptor complex of calf uterus. Because these antibodies form non-precipitating immune complexes, their interaction with estrogen receptors can be demonstrated and characterized by their effect on the sedimentation properties of tritiated estradiol-receptor complexes in sucrose gradients. Antiestrophilin antibodies raised in the rabbit, goat and ACI rat cross react with estrophilin from hormone-responsive tissues and tumors of a wide variety of animal species, whereas antibodies raised in the Lewis rat were found to react specifically with calf estrophilin. Fusion of splenic lymphocytes from the immunized Lewis rat with cells of three different mouse myeloma lines, followed by cloning by limited dilution, yielded several hybridoma cell lines secreting monoclonal antibody to estrophilin. These monoclonal antibodies, of either the IgM or IgG2a types, resemble the antiserum of the parent Lewis rat in reacting specifically with calf estrophilin. Radiolabeled monoclonal antibody can be prepared biosynthetically by inclusion of [^{35}S] methionine in the hybridoma culture medium. These cross reacting and species-specific antiestrophilin antibodies provide useful reagents for the detection, purification, assay and study of estrogen receptors in target cells, independent of the binding of labeled hormone by the receptor.

ACKNOWLEDGEMENTS

These investigations were supported by research grants from the American Cancer Society (BC-86) and Abbott Laboratories, by a research grant (CA-02897) and contract (CB-43969) from the National Cancer Institute, and by the Women's Board of the University of Chicago Cancer Research Foundation. During part of this investigation, L.E. Closs was a Helena Rubinstein Scholar. We are grateful for the excellent technical assistance of Peter Engler, Sophia Mirviss, Therese Francoeur and Solomon Wiseman, as well as the cooperation of Professor Frank Fitch and the help of Nancy Sobel.

REFERENCES

1. Bazin, H., Beckers, A., and Querinjean, P. (1974): Europ. J. Immunol., 4:44-48.
2. Bloch, K.J., Morse, H.C., and Austin, F. (1968): J. Immunol. 101:650-657.
3. Cowan, N.J., Secher, D.S., and Milstein, C. (1974): J. Mol. Biol., 90:691-701.
4. Glascock, R.F., and Hoekstra, W.G. (1959): Biochem. J., 72:673-682.
5. Gorski, J., and Gannon, F. (1976): Ann. Rev. Physiol., 38:425-450.
6. Greene, G.L., Closs, L.E., DeSombre, E.R., and Jensen, E.V. (1979): J. Steroid Biochem., 11:333-341.
7. Greene, G.L., Closs, L.E., DeSombre, E.R., and Jensen, E.V. (1980): J. Steroid Biochem., 12:159-167.
8. Greene, G.L., Closs, L.E., Fleming, H., DeSombre, E.R., and Jensen, E.V. (1977): Proc. Nat. Acad. Sci. USA, 74:3681-3685.
9. Greene, G.L., Fitch, F.W., and Jensen, E.V. (1980): Proc. Nat. Acad. Sci. USA, 77:157-161.
10. Jensen, E.V., Block, G.E., Smith, S., Kyser, K., and DeSombre, E.R. (1971): Nat. Cancer Inst. Monogr., 34:55-70.
11. Jensen, E.V., and DeSombre, E.R. (1973): Science, 182:126-134.
12. Jensen, E.V., Greene, G.L., Closs, L.E., and DeSombre, E.R. (1979): In: Steroid Hormone Receptor Systems, edited by W.W. Leavitt and J.H. Clark, pp. 1-16. Plenum Publishing Corp., New York.
13. Jensen, E.V., and Jacobson, H.I. (1960): In: Biological Activities of Steroids in Relation to Cancer, edited by G. Pincus and E.P. Vollmer, pp. 161-178. Academic Press, New York.
14. Köhler, G., and Milstein, C. (1975): Nature (London), 256:495-497.
15. McKearn, T.J., Fitch, F.W., Smilek, D.E., Sarmiento, M., and Stuart, F.P. (1979): Immunol. Rev., 47:91-115.
16. Puca, G.A., Nola, E., Sica, V., and Bresciani, F. (1972): Biochemistry, 11:4157-4165.

17. Radanyi, C., Redeuilh, G., Eigenmann, E., Lebeau, M.C., Massol, N., Secco, C., Baulieu, E.E., and Richard-Foy, H. (1979): C.R. Acad. Sci. [D] (Paris), 288:255–258.
18. Sherman, M.R., Pickering, L.A., Rollwagen, F.M., and Miller, L.K. (1978): Fed. Proc., 37:167–173.
19. Shulman, M., Wilde, C.D., and Köhler, G. (1978): Nature (London), 276:269–270.
20. Vaitukaitis, J., Robbins, J.B., Nieschlag, E., and Ross, G.T. (1971): J. Clin. Endocrinol. Metab., 33:988–991.

Perspectives in Steroid Receptor Research,
edited by F. Bresciani.
Raven Press, New York· © 1980.

The Interrelationship of Estrogen Receptors Extracted from Various Subcellular Compartments

Peter W. Jungblut, Heinrich H. D. Meyer, and Rüdiger K. Wagner

Max-Planck-Institute for Experimental Endocrinology, 3000 Hanover 61, West Germany

Abstract

"Acidic" cytosol and nuclear estradiol receptors can be degraded to a product indistinguishable from "basic" microsomal receptor by hyaluronidases from testes (hydrolase) and streptomyces hyaurolyticus (eliminase). The estradiol-binding site and the sites partaking in receptor dimerization reside in the "basic" receptor core, which is different from the tryptic receptor fragment. The entity removed from "acidic" receptors is responsible for the tendency to aggregate, the disaggregating effects exerted by salt and acidic polysaccharides, the Mg^{++}-promoted adsorption to heparin-sepharose, the precipitability by protamine and facilitates receptor-retention on hydroxyapatite. Its involvement in receptor translocation into the nucleus is discussed and evidence for a similar hyaluronidase-sensitivity of other steroid receptors is presented.

Introduction

Uterine estrogen receptors have been found in the soluble phase of the cytoplasm (25), in the nucleus (6,7) and in the microsomal fraction of homogenates (13). An unique feature of the microsomal receptor is its somewhat lower net charge. It migrates in agargel electorphoresis at pH 8.2 towards the cathode and can thus be easily distinguished from the cytosol- and nuclear receptors, which both move to an anodic position adjacent to the origin. Another remarkable

Dedicated to Ulrich Westphal at the occasion of his 70th birthday.

difference between the "basic" microsomal and the
"acidic" cytosol/nuclear receptors is, that the former
lacks the tendency to aggregate, even in low-salt
media. Properties shared by all three receptors are
their identical affinities to estrogens and the estra-
diol-facilitated dimerization of their respective
monomers. The temperature-dependent dimerization of
the 3.5S microsomal receptor proceeds in low ionic
strength buffers (14), that of the salt-dispersed 4S
cytosol receptor (2,15,17,26) requires the continued
presence of salt. However, the same ionic bonds seem
to be involved in the process, since the two dimers
can be reversibly dissociated by lowering the pH from
7.0 to 6.5, a phenomenon also seen with the salt-ex-
tracted nuclear 5S receptor dimer (14,15).

This suggests, that the steroid-binding site and
the sites partaking in the dimerization process are
compounded in a common receptor substructure. Considering the origin, the smaller size and the lower
net charge of the microsomal receptor, it could represent such a receptor core, onto which another moiety
is attached before release, as known for the posttranslational glycosilation of proteins in cytoplasmic
membranes. Our first attempt to prove this hypothesis
by reverting "acidic" to "basic" receptor with the aid
of neuraminidase failed (14). A variety of other exo-
and endoglycosidases tried were also unsuccessful.
These did not include hyaluronidase, since hyaluronic
acid was unknown to us as a constituent of intracellular glycoproteins. The initial experiment of this
study, therefore, was aimed at a different purpose.
We wanted to investigate, whether the admixture of
extracellular hyaluronate could give rise to the formation of receptor aggregates, which are frequently
found in cytosols. The result came as a surprise. We
report here on the conversion of "acidic" to "basic"
receptor by two different hyaluronidases and on properties of the "acidic" receptor, which reside in the
enzymatically removeable portion of the molecule.

Materials and Methods

Radioactive substances.
$17\beta(6,7-^3H)$ estradiol, spec.act. 43 Ci/mmol,
purity > 97 % and dexamethasone, spec.act. 28 Ci/mmol,
purity > 98 %, were purchased from NEN. $(15,16-^3H)$ D-
norgestrel, spec.act. 39 Ci/mmol, purity > 95 %, was
a gift of Schering AG.
Enzymes.
Hyaluronoglucosidase (Strept. hyalurolyticus),

homogeneous and proteinase-free, was obtained from
Seikagaku Fine Biochemicals, Tokyo; testes hyaluronidase (bovine type VI, ovine type II) from Sigma and
trypsin from Boehringer, Mannheim.
All other chemicals were commercial products of analytical grade.

Extraction and analyses of receptors.
Cytosol receptor: Uteri from calves, pigs or rats
were extracted with 1-6 volumes of either 0.01 M phosphate, 0.005 M NaN$_3$ pH 7.5 or 0.01 M glycylglycine,
0.005 M NaN$_3$, pH 7.5 buffers, containing dithiothreitol (DTT), where indicated in the figure legends. Suspensions of fresh tissue in buffer were homogenized
with the Utraturrax (Janke & Kunkel), frozen tissue
in a Microdismembrator (Braun, Melsungen) after pre-
cooling in liquid nitrogen. Particles were removed by
centrifugation for 1 h at 140,000 x g$_{av}$.
Extractions of microsomal and nuclear receptors
were performed as previously described (11,13).

Saturating concentrations of labelled steroids
were used as detailed in the results section. Excess
free steroid was adsorbed to sieved charcoal (40μm
nylon netting) prior to receptor analysis by agargel
electrophoresis (24) and density gradient centrifugation. Gradients were sampled in constant-volume fractions by upward displacement (8). Protein was assayed
according to Bradford (1). Measurement of radioactivity: 15 ml of fluor (80 g naphthalene, 5 g PPO, 50 mg
POPOP/1000 ml xylene-dioxane 1 : 2) were added to
0.05 - 0.3 ml aqueous samples in polyethylene vials
and counted in Tri-Carb Spectrometers models 3310-3330
with ³H-efficiencies between 30 and 40 %.

Interaction of receptors with heparin-sepharose.
Heparin-sepharose was prepared by the method of
Molinari et al. (16). All operations were carried out
at 0 - 2°C. The adsorbent was equilibrated with a pH
7.5 buffer "A" (0.01 M glycylglycine, 0.005 M NaN$_3$,
0.005 M MgCl$_2$, 0.001 M DTT). Receptor-containing extracts were preincubated with saturating concentrations of labelled estradiol and MgCl$_2$ was added to
give a final concentration of 0.005 M prior to exposure to the adsorbent. Proportions of 1 ml of packed
adsorbent to 9 ml of extract were used in batch operation. Consecutive adsorptions were carried out after
intermittent washings with 1) 0.1 M KCl in buffer A
and 2) buffer A. For receptor purification, the adsorbent was washed in columns with buffer "B" (buffer A
without MgCl$_2$) containing 0.18 M KCl until no protein
could be detected in the effluent. This was followed
by a wash with 0.4 M KCl in buffer B. The bulk of receptor was then eluted with 0.1 % heparin in buffer B.

The comparative binding of cytosol and microsomal receptors and the sensitivity of adsorbed receptor to
hyaluronidase was studied in stirred suspension.

Precipitation of estradiol-receptor complex by
protamine (12).
0.05 ml aliquots of solutions containing labelled
"basic" or "acidic" receptor were diluted with 0.15 ml
0.01 M glycylglycine, 0.01 M KH_2PO_4/K_2HPO_4, 0.005 M
NaN_3 pH 7.2 to which 0.25 ml of a 0.1 % solution of
protamine chloride in the same buffer was added drop-
wise. The suspension was shaken for 10 minutes and
then spun for 5 min at 9,500 x g_{av}. The sediment was
washed twice with buffer containing 0.1 % protamine
chloride and 1 % TWEEN 80, transferred to counting
vials and extracted for 5 days at 40°C with scintillation fluor.

Binding of estradiol-receptor complex to
hydroxyapatite (4).
Batch operation: Hydroxyapatite (Biogel HTP,
Bio-Rad) was equilibrated and then suspended in pH 7.2
and pH 7.7 buffers (0.01 M glycylglycine, 0.01 M
KH_2PO_4/K_2HPO_4, 0.005 M NaN_3). To 0.1 ml aliquots of
the suspensions 0.1 ml of samples (dialyzed against
buffer) were added, shaken for 30 minutes and the
hydroxyapatite collected by centrifugation. The
pellets were washed twice with the respective buffers
containing 1 % TWEEN 80 before counting.
Column operation: 100 mg quantities of hydroxyapatite were equilibrated with pH 7.2, pH 7.7 and pH
8.2 buffers and filled into Pasteur-pipet columns.
2 ml of dialyzed samples were applied (flow rate
0.7 ml/h), followed by a buffer wash of 2 ml. The
samples were analyzed for receptor content by agargel
electrophoresis before and after column-passage.

Treatments of receptor preparations with enzymes.
Cytosols and microsomal extracts were incubated
for 20 - 48 h at 2°C with varying concentrations of
testes- or streptomyces hyaluronidase. The effect of
hyaluronidase on nuclear receptor was studied by
addition of the enzyme to the extraction buffer. The
incubations of purified receptor with either streptomyces hyaluronidase or trypsin were carried out at
30°C for varying times.

Results

1. Dissolution of receptor aggregates and conversion of "acidic" to "basic" receptor by
hyaluronidase treatment of cytosols.
The tendency of estradiol receptors to form large
aggregates varies from extract to extract, even when

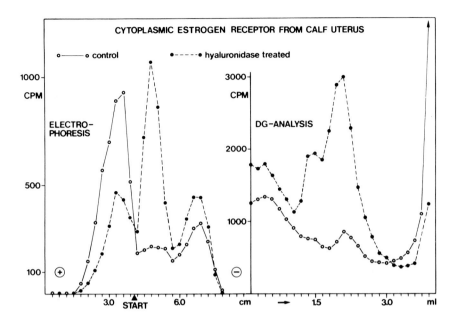

FIG. 1. Cytosol from frozen tissue; 1 part + 4 volumes 0.01 M
phosphate pH 7.5; incubated 20 h at 0-2°C with 4 x 10⁻⁸ M ³H-
estradiol in the presence or the absence of 3,000 NFU/ml bovine
testes hyaluronidase VI Sigma; charcoal-treated before analysis.
Agargel electrophoresis: 0.05 ml applied; 3 h; 3°C; 140 mA.
Density gradient centrifugation: 0.2 ml layered on 5-20 % sucrose
in 0.05 M Na-barbital/acetate pH 8.2, 0.3 M KCl; 14 h; 2°C;
56,000 rpm; SW 56; L2-65B.

analyzed immediately after preparation. Prolonged
storage of extracts generally increases this tendency
and cytosols prepared from frozen tissue are prone to
contain a sizeable fraction of aggregated receptors.
These aggregates can be remarkably resistant to salt
as shown in the right-hand panel of figure 1. In agargel electrophoresis, they are responsible for the
asymmetry of the anodic receptor peak (left-hand panel
of figure 1). Treatment of the same extract prepared
from frozen calf uteri with hyaluronidase resulted in
strikingly different patterns, both on density gradient and electrophoretic analyses (figure 1).
   Most of the macromolecular-bound estradiol now
sedimented in two clearly discernible peaks in the
3-5 S region and in electrophoresis, a major peak of
radioactivity migrated to the position of the "basic"
microsomal receptor (13), while the remaining acidic
peak attained a more symmetrical shape. The enzyme
-promoted changes can be interpreted as a dissolution

of aggregates by removing an acidic receptor constituent. The smaller 3.5S peak corresponds to the position of monomer "basic" microsomal receptor, the larger 4.5-5S peak is likely to contain a mixture of
"basic" microsomal receptor dimer and "acidic" cytosol
monomer.
    2. Disintegration of cytosol 9S receptor by hyalu-
ronidase.
    In fresh uterine extracts, prepared with low salt
media, receptor-bound estradiol sediments preferably
in the 9S region (23) and gives rise to an anodic peak
in agargel electrophoresis (24). Similar to its effect
on larger aggregates, hyaluronidase disintegrates the
9S receptor into smaller entities and changes its
electrophoretic mobility (figure 2). Although in this
experiment with rat uterus cytosol the digestion was
not carried out to completion, the result emphasizes
the importance of the acidic constituent for the formation of 9S receptor. It again raises the question,
whether this receptor species is an in-vivo reality or
rather an in-vitro artefact.

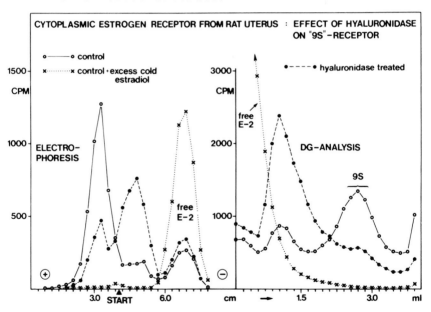

FIG. 2. Cytosol from fresh tissue; 1 part + 6 volumes 0.01 M
phosphate pH 7.5 + 0.05 M DTT; incubated 24 h at 0-2°C with
4 x 10⁻⁸ M ³H-estradiol in the presence or the absence of 205
NFU/ml ovine testes hyaluronidase Sigma; charcoal-treated before
analysis. Agargel electrophoresis: see legend figure 1. Density
gradient centrifugation: 0.2 ml on 5-20 % sucrose in 0.01 M
phosphate pH 7.5; 10 h; 2°C; 56,000 rpm; SW 56, L2-65B.

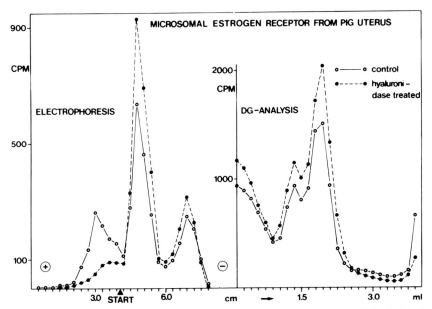

FIG. 3. Lyophylized microsomal sediment extracted with 0.01 M phosphate pH 7.5; incubated 20 h at 0-2°C with 4 x 10⁻⁸ M ³H-estradiol in the presence or the absence of 3,000 NFU/ml bovine testes hyaluronidase VI Sigma; charcoal-treated before analysis. Agargel electrophoresis: see legend figure 1. Density gradient centrifugation: 14 h; other conditions as in legend to figure 1.

3. Sensitivity of "acidic" receptor present in microsomal extracts to hyaluronidase treatment.

We have previously described the presence of "basic" and "acidic" receptors in extracts of uterus microsomes (13). The proportion of the latter was always lower and continued to decrease with further improvements in the extraction procedure. An unequivocal decision as to their biosynthetic sequence could not be reached. It appears now, that the fraction of "acidic" receptor present in microsomal extracts is not different from the cytosol (and the nuclear) receptor. After incubation of an extract prepared from lyophylized pig uterus microsomes with hyaluronidase (figure 3), the "acidic" receptor peak decreased to the same extent as that of the cathodically migrating, bound estradiol increased. The density gradient analyses before and after enzyme treatment furthermore showed, that the increase of both the 3.5S (monomer) and 4.5S (dimer) peaks could be accounted for by processed ("acidic") receptor aggregates.

Unless the "acidic" receptor entity in the

extract was an impurity of the microsome pellet, it can be considered as a still membrane-bound follow-up product of its "basic" precursor.

   4.Degradation of nuclear receptor by hyaluronidase.
   The assignment of a nuclear origin to receptors relies on the purity of the nuclear fraction isolated from homogenates (11). An essential requirement is the removal of the outer layer of the nuclear envelope, which is part of the rough ergastoplasm and contains "basic" receptor. Extraction of purified, stripped uterine nuclei with buffered salt solutions in the presence of estradiol at elevated temperature yields an "acidic" hormone-receptor-complex, which sediments at 5S. This dimer complex can be reversibly disso- ciated into 4S monomers by proton addition and with- drawal (10,15). When hyaluronidase is present during the extraction, subsequent analysis reveals a degra- dation of the "acidic" to the "basic" receptor variety and a small but discernible decrease in sedimentation velocity, provided the density gradient centrifugations

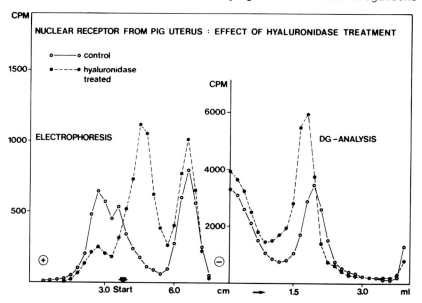

FIG. 4. Purified, stripped pig uterus nuclei extracted for 23 h at 0°C followed by 40 min at 30°C with 0.01 M phosphate pH 7.5, 0.3 M KCl, 0.03 M DTT, 6 x 10⁻⁷M ³H-estradiol in the presence or absence of 410 NFU/ml ovine testes hyaluronidase II Sigma; charcoal-treated before analysis. Agargel electrophoresis: 0.05 ml applied; 1-3°C; 1 h at 40 mA; 1 h at 60 mA; 3 h at 100 mA. Density gradient centrifugation: 0.2 ml on 5-20 % sucrose in 0.01 M phosphate pH 7.5; 0.3 M KCl; 14 h; 2°C; 56,000 rpm; SW 56; L2-65B.

were performed simultaneously in the same centrifuge (figure 4). The 5S peak represents the typical dimer of acidic nuclear receptor, the 4.5S peak the dimer of its "basic" degradation product. It is also noticeable from figure 4, that more receptor was extracted in the presence of the enzyme. Up to fourfold higher yields could be obtained (table 1).

TABLE 1. Improvement of receptor yields from pig uterus nuclei by hyaluronidase

Ablative Treatment	Number of Binding Sites/Nucleus Extracted by	
	Salt only	Salt + Hyaluronidase
Ovariectomy	2,690	12,630
"	3,010	8,420
"	2,910	9,220
"	2,170	11,100
"	2,230	8,500
Ovariectomy and Adrenalectomy	2,230	4,760

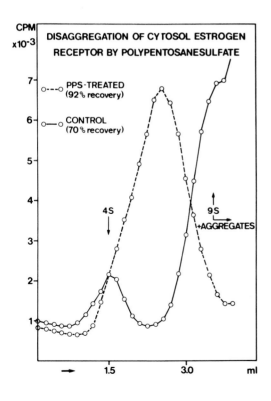

FIG. 5. Calf uterus cytosol; 1:1 homogenate with 0.05 M phosphate pH 7.5, 0.005 M NaN$_3$; incubated for 30 min at 25°C with 6 x 10^{-8} M ^{3}H-estradiol with or without the addition of 0.25 mg/ml Thrombocid^R (polypentosanesulfate MW$_{av}$ 4,000; 1.7 SO$_3^-$ / monosaccharide),chilled and charcoal-treated before density gradient centrifugation: 0.2 ml layered on 5-20 % sucrose in buffer(s.a.) 12 h; 1°C; 56,000 rpm; SW 56; L2-65B (July-16-1973).

5. Properties attributable to the hyaluronidase -sensitive portion of the "acidic" receptor.

Several years ago, we observed that semisynthetic polypentosanesulfates and heparin exert a disaggregating effect on "acidic" receptor aggregates when added to cytosols (figure 5). This observation and the description of heparin-sepharose as a suitable adsorbent for "native" receptor (16) aroused the suspicion that the tendency to aggregate and the potency to interact with sulfonated carbohydrate polymers might reside in the very portion of the "acidic" receptor which is split-off by hyaluronidase. "Basic" receptor, in contrast to its "acidic" counterpart, should then lack the capacity to adsorb to heparin-sepharose. This is indeed the case (table 2). Only a minor fraction of "basic" receptor was removed from a microsomal extract (devoid of "acidic" receptor) during batch incubation with the adsorbent and this was readily eluted by 0.1 M KCl, pointing to an ion-exchange phenomenon. ("Basic" receptor is eluted from CM-cellulose by pH 7.5 buffers, ionic strength μ = 0.015). The Mg^{++}-promoted complexing of "acidic" receptor with heparin -sepharose, obviously, proceeds by a different mechanism.

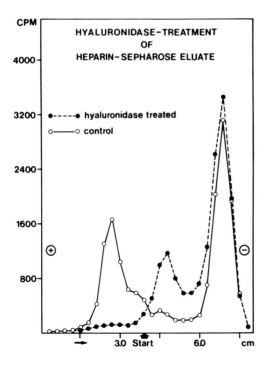

FIG. 6. Purified "acidic" cytosol receptor from pig uterus (eluted with 0.1 % heparin from heparin -sepharose, 0.09 mg/ml protein, 6×10^{-9} M binding sites), saturated with ^{3}H-estradiol (1.2×10^{-8} M), incubated for 3 h at 30°C without or with 18 TRU/ml streptomyces hyaluronidase. Agargel electrophoresis: see legend figure 1.

TABLE 2. Binding of "acidic" and "basic" estrogen receptor to heparin-sepharose.

	"Acidic" Receptor $\times 10^{-12}$ moles	%	"Basic" Receptor $\times 10^{-12}$ moles	%
Content in 2 x 9 ml extract	88.7	100	26.5	100
Adsorbed after 2 x 90 min to 1 ml heparin-sepharose	70.3	79	7.5	29
Elution 2 x 15 min, 2 x 4.5 ml 0.01 M glycylglycine pH 7.5, 0.005 M NaN_3, 0.001 M DTT, 0.005 M $MgCl_2$, 0.1 M KCl	7.9	9	7.3	27
Elution 3 x 60 min, 4 x 6 ml 0.01 M glycylglycine pH 7.5, 0.005 M NaN_3, 0.001 M DTT, 0.18 M KCl	16.8	19	0	0
Elution 1 x 6 h, 1 x 12 h, 1 x 24 h, 3 x 4.5 ml 0.01 M glycylglycine pH 7.5, 0.005 M NaN_3, 0.001 M DTT, 0.1 % heparin	29.7	33.5	0	0
Elution 1 x 24 h, 9 ml 0.01 M glycylglycine pH 9.0, 0.005 M NaN_3, 0.001 M DTT, 0.02 M EDTA, 1 M KCl	11.8	13	0	0

"Acidic" receptor eluted from heparin-sepharose (after washing with 0.4 M KCl), by 0.1 % heparin is at least 200-fold enriched over the original extract. Incubation of the eluate with hyaluronidase has the same effect on the electrophoretic mobility of the receptor as seen in enzyme-treated tissue extracts (figure 6). It should be noted, that the experiment shown in figure 6 was performed with an eluate which had been stored for 8 days at 2-4°C. In fresh eluates, the small basic peak visible in the untreated control is missing. It can be interpreted as the product of a slow degradation of "acidic" receptor by coeluted endogeneous enzyme.

The same stored eluate was used for studying the kinetics of hyaluronidase action by incubation with the enzyme at 30°C. Aliquots were taken out at various times after enzyme addition, chilled, and immediately thereafter analyzed. The transition of "acidic" to "basic" receptor apparently follows 0-order kinetics (figure 7). This can hardly be explained by a substrate saturation of the enzyme.

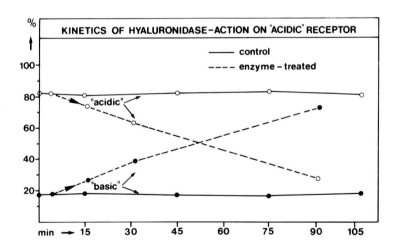

FIG. 7. Time course of hyaluronidase action on "acidic" receptor. Same preparation and conditions as in figure 6. 0.05 ml aliquots chilled at times indicated and analyzed by agargel electrophoresis. Results expressed in % of total receptor content.

Another strong hint for the kind of interaction taking place between heparin-sepharose/Mg^{++}/"acidic" receptor is provided by the effect of hyaluronidase on the complex. After batch adsorption of "acidic" receptor from a cytosol, the adsorbent was exhaustively washed and then exposed to hyaluronidase, without changing the pH or the ionic strength of the medium. The result was a liberation of "basic" receptor (figure 8). Part of the enzyme could not be removed from the adsorbent by the intermittent washings, since the "basic" receptor form prevailed in the subsequent elution with 0.1 % heparin. (Heparin is neither a substrate for streptomyces hyaluronidase nor a competitive inhibitor of the enzyme.)

We also investigated, whether the adsorption of estradiol-receptor complex to hydroxyapatite (4) and the precipitation by protamine (12) are due to interactions with the basic receptor core or must be attributed to the hyaluronidase-sensitive portion of the acidic receptor (table 3). Using a batch procedure, no unequivocal answer could be obtained with respect to hydroxyapatite adsorption. At pH 7.2, similar proportions of "acidic" and "basic" receptor were bound,

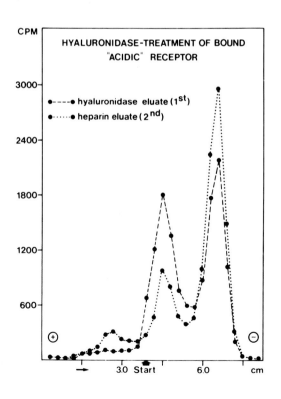

FIG. 8. To 1 ml of packed heparin-sepharose complexed with "acidic" receptor, washed with 0.18 M KCl in buffer B, 100 TRU streptomyces hyaluronidase in 0.5 ml 0.05 M KCl in buffer B were added and the suspension stirred for 4 days at 2°C. 1st eluate: soluble phase + 3 ml wash with buffer B; 2nd eluate: 3 ml 0.1 % heparin in buffer B for 1 day. Eluates reincubated with 1.2×10^{-8} M ^{3}H-estradiol overnight at 2°C; analyzed by agargel electrophoresis.

TABLE 3. Comparative binding of the estradiol complexes of "acidic" and "basic" receptor to hydroxyapatite and protamine.

	"Acidic" Receptor DPM/0.05 ml	"Basic" Receptor DPM/0.05 ml
Specifically bound in electrophoresis	40,312 = 100 %	41,026 = 100 %
Adsorbed to hydroxyapatite pH 7.2	18,018 = 45 %	19,701 = 48 %
Adsorbed to hydroxyapatite pH 7.7	19,338 = 48 %	13,047 = 32 %
Precipitated by protamine chloride	22,788 = 57 %	4,624 = 11 %

"Acidic" receptor: eluted from heparin-sepharose with 0.1 % heparin, 0.08 mg protein/ml, binding site concentration 1.04×10^{-8} M.

"Basic" receptor: liberated from heparin-sepharose by streptomyces hyaluronidase, 0.15 mg protein/ml, binding site concentration 1.07×10^{-8} M.

which however amounted to less than 50 % of the receptor concentrations measured by agargel electrophoresis. At pH 7.7, the adsorbed fraction of "acidic"
receptor remained unchanged, while that of the "basic"
receptor was reduced by one third. Passage over
hydroxyapatite columns at low flow rates raised the
adsorption of both receptors to the 80 % level at pH
7.2; 57 % of the "acidic" and 36 % of the "basic" receptor were retained in pH 7.7 operation and at pH 8.2
the retained proportions were 46 % for the "acidic"
and 10 % for the "basic" receptor, respectively. Again,
an ion-exchange phenomenon could be responsible for
the adsorption of the "basic" receptor, but the same
mechanism might also prevail in the binding of the
"acidic" receptor to hydroxyapatite.

A more pronounced difference between the two receptors is seen on protamine precipitation. From virtually equimolar solutions, only 11 % of "basic" receptor were precipitated, while in the parallel experiment 57 % of "acidic" receptor coprecipitated
with protamine chloride. Notwithstanding the reservation that the precipitation of "acidic" receptor by
protamine remained incomplete, as had been previously
observed (9), the resemblance to the interaction of
the basic protein with linear polyanions appears
striking.

6. Differentiation between the "basic" receptor
core and the tryptic receptor fragment.

Preparations of testes hyaluronidase can be contaminated with acrosin (5,25,27), a seryl-endopepti-
dase of similar specificity to trypsin. Although the
hyaluronidase-promoted transition of "acidic" to
"basic" receptor could not be inhibited by 0.2 mM diiso-
propylfluorophosphate, we proceeded to compare the
effects exerted by hyaluronidase and by trypsin on the
receptor. Aliquots of a solution of "acidic" receptor,
eluted from heparin-sepharose, were subjected to
either hyaluronidase- or trypsin treatment or sequentially treated with the two enzymes. The results
(figure 9) showed, that the tryptic fission product
is different from that following hyaluronidase action.
Furthermore, the tryptic receptor fragments derived
from either the "acidic" or the "basic" receptor are
indistinguishable. This allows for the conclusion,
that the same lysyl- or arginyl peptide bond is
attacked by trypsin in the two receptors and that
the hyaluronidase-sensitive portion of the "acidic"
receptor is a compounded "satellite" of the "basic"
receptor core.

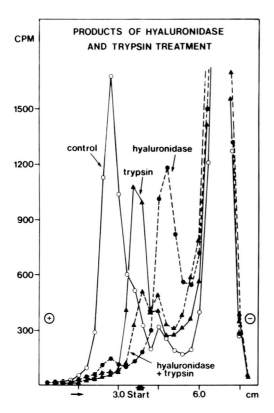

FIG. 9. "Acidic" receptor preparation as in figure 6, incubated with 1.2×10^{-8} M ^{3}H-estradiol at 30°C in the absence or presence of 1) 27 TRU/ml streptomyces hyaluronidase for 1 h; 2) 10 µg/ml trypsin for 15 min; 3) hyaluronidase and trypsin (as before) consecutively.

Discussion

Proteo(-hyalurono) glycans are rarely found intracellularly and no evidence has as yet been published on a glycoprotein nature of the estrogen- or other steroid hormone receptors. We have therefore hesitated to immediately describe the initial observation made two years ago and instead continued to accumulate supporting evidence. At this stage, we feel that the claim is sufficiently substantiated, although final proof, such as the carbohydrate analysis of pure receptor remains to be provided.

In discussing the objections, two major points could be raised: 1. the possible presence of endopeptidases in the enzyme preparations and 2. the apparent absence of sugars in another member of the steroid receptor family, the progesterone receptor from chicken oviduct.

A contamination of particle-free tissue extracts ("cytosols") with intra- and extracellular endopeptidases is very likely to occur. It is however less likely, that these contaminating enzymes are highly receptor-specific. They should rather attack all proteins present and thus liberate a measurable number of carboxyl anions and protons, which is not the case. The existence of specific receptor "clipases" has been concluded from the retarding effect of high concentrations of basic, low molecular endopeptidase inhibitors on the degradation of "native" progesterone receptor to smaller entities in tissue extracts (21). Assuming, that the progesterone receptor - like the estrogen receptor - is hyaluronidase-sensitive, an alternative explanation for the inhibitory effect of leupeptin and aprotinin could be their complexing with the carboxyls of hyaluronic acid. This would protect the "acidic" receptor against extra- and intracellular hyaluronidases, which are present, at least in uterine extracts. The evidence for a true hyaluronidase action on "acidic" receptor appears to be more convincing than that for the "clipase" hypothesis: the conversion of "acidic" to "basic" receptor is accomplished by hyaluronate-4-glycanohydrolase from testes and by the eliminase from streptomyces hyalurolyticus, both of which would have to be contaminated with the same specific receptor "clipase", if the hyaluronidases are ineffective themselves.

The absence of sugars in the isolated progesterone receptor from chick oviduct was concluded from a negative periodic acid/Schiff reaction (19). This reaction requires vicinal hydroxyls. Although these are present in hyaluronate, the intense negative electrostatic field of the acid polysaccharide excludes the negatively charged periodate ions from the reactive domain (20). The investigators most probably were aware of this, but understandably could not expect the receptor to be an intracellular proteoglycan as indicated by the sensitivity of D-norgestrel/receptor complex from pig uterus to hyaluronidase (figure 10). In contrast to the binding of estradiol by freshly prepared extracts, D-norgestrel (also progesterone and R 5020) gives rise to an "acidic" and a "basic" peak of radioactivity in agargel electrophoresis, but only to a single ~ 4.5S peak in density gradient centrifugation. After exposure of the extract to hyaluronidase, both electrophoretic peaks decline in size while concomitantly the peak of radioactivity in the position of "free" steroid increases. This peak cannot be accounted for by free steroid left after charcoal treatment, as revealed by the appearance of a smaller ~ 3.5S peak in the density gradient analysis. The core protein of the progestin receptor apparently is of higher basicity than that of the estrogen receptor and the "native" progestin receptor from pig uterus - like the one from chick oviduct (18) - seems

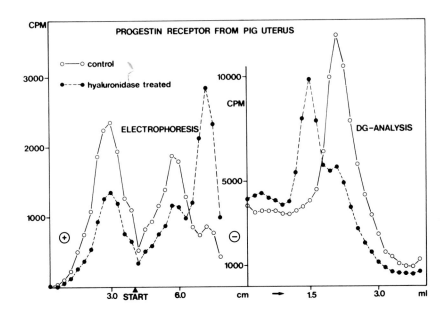

FIG. 10. Cytosol from fresh tissue; 1 part + 4 volumes 0.01 M phosphate pH 7.5; incubated 20 h at 0-2°C with 4×10^{-8} M ^{3}H-D-norgestrel in the presence or absence of 1,500 NFU/ml bovine testes hyaluronidase VI Sigma; charcoal-treated before analyses. Agargel electrophoresis: see legend figure 1. Density gradient centrifugation: 0.2 ml layered on 5-20 % sucrose in 0.01 M phosphate pH 7.5, 0.3 M KCl; 14 h; 2°C; 56,000 rpm; SW 56; L2-65B.

to exist in two forms.

We have also preliminary data on a hyaluronidase-sensitivity of the androgen- and the glucocorticoid receptor. An example for the latter is given in figure 11. Hyaluronidase-treatment of mouse lymphoma receptor results in a decrease of the major acidic peak at 3.3 cm and the appearance of both a faster migrating and a cathodic peak (4.5 - 6 cm) of specifically bound steroid, different from that seen after tryptic digestion. (Free steroid peaks at 6.9 cm).

In favor of a proteo-(hyalurono)glycan nature of the estrogen receptor speaks, that it offers reasonable explanations for some poorly understood features of the "acidic" receptor: the tendency to aggregate, the aggregate-dispersing effects of salt and polyanionic polysaccharides, the adsorption to heparin-sepharose, the precipitation by protamine. The parallel alignment of linear acid polysaccharides by complexing with divalent cations is a well-known phenomenon (3) and the spatial requirement of the Mg^{++}

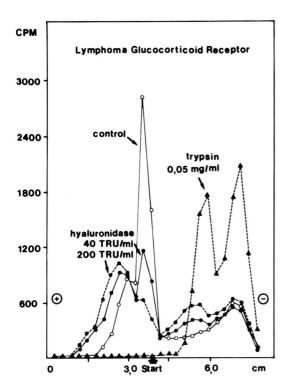

FIG. 11. Effects of streptomyces hyaluronidase and trypsin on glucocorticoid receptor. 2.5 x 10⁹ mouse lymphoma cells (S 491 TB 4) homogenized in 4 ml buffer (0.02 M Tricine, 0.05 M KCl, 0.01 M DTT, 10 % glycerol, pH 7.4). Cytosol incubated in the absence or presence of hyaluronidase with 6 x 10⁻⁸ M ³H-dexamethasone for 16 h at 0°C. Trypsin digestion for 30 min at 20°C after incubation with 6 x 10⁻⁸ M ³H-dexamethasone for 15.5 h at 0°C. Charcoal-treatment and electrophoresis see legend to figure 1. (In cooperation with U. Gehring and M. Spindler.)

-cation allows for a "mixed" interaction with carboxyl and sulfate anions, the probable mechanism of receptor adsorption to heparin-sepharose. This adsorption, the relative homogeneity of polypentosanesulfate-complexed "acidic" receptor (figure 5) and the common tryptic product of "acidic" and "basic" receptor, furthermore, lend proof to a discrete insertion point of the hyaluronate on the "basic" receptor core. As to the kind of their interaction, both a covalent bond and a lectin-type attachment are theoretically possible. However, if the basic receptor core would be a lectin for hyaluronate, in-vitro complexing with hyaluronate should be possible, which we could not accomplish. It is also difficult to envisage, that a preparation of purified nuclei devoid of the outer layer of the nuclear envelope should still contain sufficient quantities of extraneous hyaluronate to give rise to solely "acidic" receptor in salt extracts.

The absence of "basic" receptor in uterine nuclei and the residence of the estradiol-binding site as well as of the ionic residues involved in dimerization in the "basic" receptor core allow for the speculation that the carbohydrate tail attached to the core before its release into the cytosol is instrumental in nuclear entry and not necessarily in nuclear action. This seems to be the case, since estrone - which in contrast to estradiol does not facilitate receptor dimerization - is equally efficient in receptor-translocation from the cytosol into the nucleus (12). That the receptor translocated by estrone - again in contrast to estradiol - is not retained by the nucleus, almost precludes a pivotal role of the carbohydrate moiety in the specific enhancement of transcription. In which way the carbohydrate executes its "nucleotropic" action is unknown. An unfolding of the polysaccharide as a consequence of estrogen-binding to the receptor core could be the first step, if the different affinities of steroid-free and estrogen-saturated receptor to heparin-sepharose are any guide (16). A conceivable second step would then be the interaction of the "sticky" tail with a structure of the nuclear envelope.

We are aware, that all evidence presented is circumstantial rather than conclusive. It by no means identifies the estrogen-, lest the other steroid hormone receptors as "classical" proteo(-hyalurono)glycans. There might be only short stretches of hyaluronidase-sensitive structures present in an otherwise different "nucleotropic tail". It can also not entirely be excluded, that the two enzymes - in spite of their different modes of action - attack similar atypic sites. (The unimpaired effect of the streptomyces enzyme in the presence of heparin, however, speaks not in favour of a nuclease-like action.)

Attempts to label the presumable carbohydrate moiety of the estrogen receptor with the goal of identifying the specific products of the eliminase (saccharides with Δ 4,5 - unsaturated glucuronic acid residues at the non-reducing ends) are in progress. They might provide a quicker answer, than can be hoped for by conventional analysis of a large quantity of pure "acidic" receptor. Another realistic possibility is the search for cell lines which have lost the capacity of receptor glycosylation.

Despite these deficiencies, our results invite for a critical reevaluation of some in-vitro experiments.

Our view of the complex structure of the estrogen

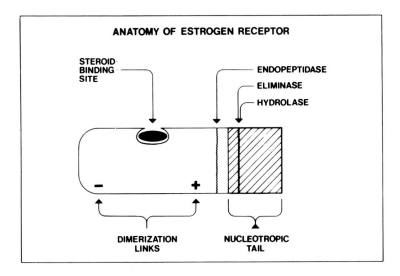

FIG. 12.

receptor is illustrated in figure 12. It is based on
the following conclusions:
    1. Purified hyaluronidase preparations from
testes (hydrolase) and from streptomyces hyalurolyticus (eliminase) convert nuclear and cytosol estrogen
receptors to products indistinguishable from the
microsomal estrogen receptor, which already contains
the steroid-binding site and the sites partaking in
receptor dimerization.
    2. Judging from the absence of "microsomal-type"
receptor in purified nuclei, the hyaluronidase-sensitive portion of the "holo" (cytosol, nuclear)-receptor
appears to be linked to nuclear entry.
    3. "Holo"-receptors for progestins, glucocorti-
coids and androgens contain similar, hyaluronidase
-sensitive structures.
    4. A contamination of the two differently acting
enzymes from entirely different sources with receptor
-specific endopeptidases is unlikely.
    5. The apparent proteoglycan-nature of "holo"-
steroid receptors with the implications of a membrane
-associated, posttranslational finishing and a final
intracellular destination are in contrast to current
views.
    The last statement invites for reenacting a
custom, which used to be Elwood Jensen's trademark.

Rather than summarizing experimental results and their
interpretation in own lyrics - as he did with his
pointed limericks - I resort to the last lines of a
famous poem by Christian Morgenstern:
"......Und er kommt zu dem Ergebnis
         Nur ein Traum war das Erlebnis
         Weil - so schließt er messerscharf -
         Nicht sein kann, was nicht sein darf!"
Translated and adapted in a way:
      .....After thorough contemplation
           Of the upsetting observation,
           He arrives at the conclusion,
           All this must have been illusion!
           "Facts" that our vision fool
           Are non-existing...as a rule!

Acknowledgment

We thank Linda Görlich and Jutta Heider for excellent technical assistance.

References

1. Bradford, M.M. (1976): Anal.Biochem. 72: 248-254.
2. Brecher, P.I., Numata, M., DeSombre, E.R., Jensen,
   E.V. (1970): Fed. Proc. 29: 249.
3. Dunstone, J.R. (1972): Biochem.J. 85: 336-351.
4. Erdos, T., Bessada, R. (1979): J.Steroid Biochem.
   10: 267-275.
5. Fritz, H., Förg-Brey, B., Fink, E., Schiessler,H.,
   Jaumann, E., Arnhold, M. (1972): Hoppe-Seyler's Z.
   Physiol.Chem. 353: 1007-1009.
6. Jungblut, P.W., Jensen, E.V. (1966): Endocrinology
   78: 30 abstr.
7. Jungblut, P.W., Hätzel, J., DeSombre, E.R.,Jensen,
   E.V. (1967): Berlin-Heidelberg-New York: Springer,
   Wirkungsmechanismen der Hormone, 55-86.
8. Jungblut, P.W., McCann, S., Görlich, L., Rosenfeld, G.C., Wagner, R.K. (1972): Research on
   Steroids IV: 213-231.
9. Jungblut, P.W., Hughes, Sh., Hughes, A., Wagner,
   R.K. (1972): Acta Endocrinologica 70: 185-195.
10. Jungblut, P.W., Gaues, J., Hughes, A., Kallweit,
    E., Sierralta, W., Szendro, P., Wagner, R.K.
    (1976): J.Steroid Biochem. 7: 1109-1116.
11. Jungblut, P.W., Kallweit, E., Sierralta, W.,
    Truitt, A., Wagner, R.K. (1978): Hoppe-Seyler's Z.
    Physiol.Chem. 359: 1259-1268.

12. Jungblut, P.W., Hughes, A., Gaues, J., Kallweit, E., Maschler, I., Parl, F., Sierralta, W., Szendro, P., Wagner, R.K. (1979): J.Steroid Biochem. 11: 273-278.
13. Little, M., Rosenfeld, G.C., Jungblut, P.W. (1972) Hoppe-Seyler's Z.Physiol.Chem. 353, 231-242.
14. Little, M., Szendro, P.I., Jungblut, P.W. (1973): ibid 354, 1599-1610.
15. Little, M., Szendro, P.I., Teran, C., Hughes, A., Jungblut, P.W. (1975): J.Steroid Biochem. 6: 493-500.
16. Molinari, A.M., Medici, N., Moncharmont, B., Puca, G.A. (1977): Proc.Nat.Acad.Sci. USA 74: 4886-4890.
17. Notides, A.C., Nielsen, S. (1974): J.Biol.Chem. 249: 1866-1873.
18. Schrader, W.T., O'Malley, B.W. (1972): J.Biol.Chem. 247: 51.
19. Schrader, W.T. (1978): personal communication.
20. Scott, J.E., Harbinson, R.J. (1968): Histochemie 14: 215-220.
21. Sherman, M.R., Pickering, L.A., Rollwagen, F.M., Miller, L.K. (1978): Fed.Proc. 37: 167-173.
22. Steggles, A.W., Vertes, M., King, R.J.B. (1969): Biochem.J. 115: 48.
23. Toft, D., Gorski, J. (1966): Proc.nat.Acad.Sci. Wash. 55: 1574-1581.
24. Wagner, R.K. (1972): Hoppe-Seyler's Z. Physiol. Chem. 353: 1235-1245.
25. Waldschmidt, M., Karg, H. (1964): Ber.V.Int.Congr. on Anim.Reproduct. and Art. Insem.Trento VII: 316. Waldschmidt, M., Karg, H., Hoffmann, B. (1964): Naturwiss. 51:18.
26. Yamamoto, K.R., Alberts, B.M. (1972): Proc.Nat. Acad.Sci.USA 69: 2105-2109.
27. Zanefeld, L.J.D., Dragoje, B.M., Schumacher, G.F.B. (1972): Science 177: 702-703.

Perspectives in Steroid Receptor Research,
edited by F. Bresciani.
Raven Press, New York © 1980.

Cytochemical Evidence for Steroid Binding Sites in the Plasma Membrane of Target Cells

I. Nenci, G. Fabris, E. Marchetti, and A. Marzola

Institute of Anatomy and Pathologic Histology, University of Ferrara, 44100 Ferrara, Italy

Modern molecular cytochemistry has developed several probes sensitive enough to detect steroid–cell interactions and may provide insight into so far undefined events of the steroid action mechanism. Though the visual localization may be expected to materialize the biochemical findings (4,5) it may challenge them as well so that revising of some previously accepted concepts may be called for. It is generally assumed that steroids enter target cells by simple diffusion, even if the mode of transition of steroids through the plasma membrane is not known and specific surface binding and interaction sites have been repeatedly invoked (see 6 for the most recent literature).

The plasma membrane structure and dynamics have been investigated extensively by means of visual tracer technique (7), also as far as the hormone–membrane interplay is concerned (8).

In this paper we have summarized our recent findings on the presence and kinetic characteristics of estradiol binding sites in the plasma membrane of target cells.

MATERIALS AND METHODS

Cells.

Isolated human breast cancer cells were obtained by spontaneous spillage after mechanical disruption of surgical specimens.

ZR-75-1 breast cancer cell line was obtained by Dr. G. Bussolati (Istituto di Anatomia Patologica, Università di Torino, Italy) and maintained in Eagle's minimum essential medium supplemented with 5% fetal calf serum.

Mouse fibroblast, BHK and HEp-2 cell lines were maintained in standard cell culture conditions.

17β–Fluorescent Estradiol (FE).

The 1 –(N)– fluoresceinyl estrone thiosemicarbazone was a gift of Dr. W.B. Dandliker (Department of Biochemistry, Scripps Clinic and Research Foundation, La Jolla, Cal., USA) and its interaction with specific estradiol receptor has been fully characterized (1).

Cells harvested in phosphate buffered saline (PBS) were centrifuged and resuspended in 4×10^{-8} M fluorescent estradiol for 45'-60' at 4°C. After prolonged washing in several changes of cold PBS, part of the cell suspension was collected, dropped on slides and immediately inspected.

The remaining washed cells were resuspended in PBS and kept at 37°C for variable gaps of time. At times the incubation was performed at room temperature or at 37°C from the beginning.

Control tests:
- pre and coincubation of breast cancer cells with estradiol and anti-estrogens (diethylstilbestrol and tamoxifen) in excess (10^{-5} M).
- incubation of estradiol non-target cells (mouse fibroblast, BHK and HEp-2 cell lines) with FE as above.

Estradiol-6-CMO-BSA-FITC (E-BSA-F).

The 17β-Estradiol-6-carboxymethyloxime-bovine serum albumin-fluorescein isothiocyanate conjugate was synthesized by Dr. S.H. Lee (3) (Department of Pathology, Hospital of St. Raphael, New Haven, Conn., USA).

Cells suspended in PBS were centrifuged and incubated with E-BSA-F for 45'-60' at 4°C. Cells were then washed thoroughly in cold PBS; part of the cells were then dropped on slides and immediately inspected, the remaining cells were resuspended in PBS at 37°C, collected and inspected after a varying length of time.

Control tests:
- incubation with E-BSA-F reacted with specific estradiol antibody in excess.
- pre and coincubation with estradiol, polyestradiol phosphate in excess.
- incubation of estradiol non-target cells with the fluorescent probe as above specified.

Immunocomplexed polyestradiol phosphate (IcPEP).

Polyestradiol phosphate has been reacted with rabbit estradiol-6-CMO-BSA antibody according to the primoflocculation technique (10) to obtain soluble immunocomplexes. The persistence of estradiol reactive groups in the soluble immunocomplexed polyestradiol has been tested by double immunodiffusion technique (Fig. 1).

Cells harvested in PBS were centrifuged and resuspended in IcPEP for 30'-45' at 4°C and 37°C. After several washes in cold PBS, cell suspensions were divided in two groups for immunofluorescence and immunoperoxidase processing, respectively.

Immunofluorescence. Cell suspensions were centrifuged and incubated for 30' at 4°C with fluorescein-labeled swine antiserum against rabbit immunoglobulins G. Cells were then thoroughly washed in cold PBS, dropped on slides and immediately inspected under U.V. microscope.

Immunoperoxidase. Cells suspended in PBS were smeared on slides and allowed to dry at 4°C. Slides were then incubated for 30' at room

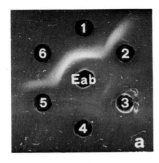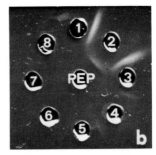

FIG. 1. Double immunodiffusion technique shows that the IcPEP with a slight antigen excess maintains estradiol groups reactive to estradiol antibody, with identity lines with native polyestradiol. PEP: polyestradiol phosphate; Eab: anti-estradiol-6-CMO-BSA; IcPEP: immunocomplexed polyestradiol (μg PEP/ml Eab).

Fig. 1a. 1: PEP; 2: Eab/2; 3: IcPEP (2.5); 4: IcPEP (25) + anti-Ig; 5: Eab/2; 6: IcPEP (25).

Fig. 1b. 1: IcPEP (25); 2: Eab; 3: IcPEP (25); 4: IcPEP (2.5); 7: IcPEP (2.5); 8: non-immune serum.

temperature with horseradish peroxidase-labeled swine antibody against rabbit immunoglobulins G. After several washes in PBS, cell preparations were reacted for 15' with 3-3' diaminobenzidine tetrahydrochloride in 0.05 M Tris-HCl buffer, pH 7.6, containing 0.01% H_2O_2. After being thoroughly washed in distilled water some slides were reacted with 1% OsO_4 in PBS for 1'.

For light microscopy cell preparations were dehydrated, cleared and mounted in Eukitt.

For transmission electron microscopy cell preparations were dehydrated and flat embedded in Araldite. Ultrathin sections were obtained by an Ultratome III LKB; some grides were counterstained with uranyl acetate or lead citrate. All grides were inspected with an Hitachi HS8 electron microscope.

For scanning electron microscopy cell preparations were dehydrated through graded alcohols and critical-point dried with liquid CO_2, gold-coated and examined with a Siemens Autoscan electron microscope. Electron probe X-ray microanalysis was performed on osmicated specimens by a Wavelength dispersive X-ray Spectrometer Siemens Autospec to obtain a modulated X-ray scan image and a "y" modulated X-ray line-scan.

Control tests:

Cells harvested in PBS were centrifuged and preincubated with
- N-ethylmaleimide 10^{-3} M for 30' at room temperature, or
- neuraminidase (500 U/ml) for 45' at 37°C, or

- estradiol $17\beta 10^{-5}$ M, or testosterone 10^{-5} M, or diethylstilbestrol 10^{-5} M, or tamoxifen 10^{-5} M for 60' at room temperature, or
- polyestradiol phosphate 50 µg/ml,

then washed and resuspended in IcPEP (as above).

- Cells harvested in PBS were centrifuged and resuspended for 60' at 4°C in heat–aggregated rabbit estradiol antibody (2). After washing, cells were reacted with fluorescein–labeled swine antiserum against rabbit immunoglobulins G.
- Cells harvested in PBS were centrifuged and incubated for 60' at 4°C with heat–aggregated fluorescein–labeled swine antiserum against rabbit immunoglobulins G.
- Estradiol non–target cells (mouse fibroblast, BHK and HEp–2 continuous cell lines) were incubated with IcPEP in the same way as target cells.

RESULTS AND DISCUSSION

17β– Fluorescent Estradiol (FE).
Incubation of isolated target cells with FE has permitted the visualization of estradiol uptake, transport and distribution.

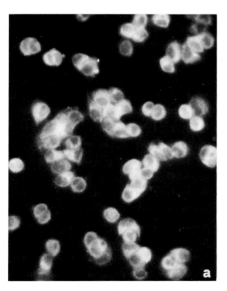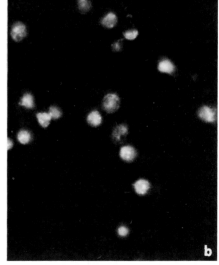

FIG. 2. Fluorescent estradiol is taken up, bound to cytoplasmic receptors at 4°C (a) and translocated into the nucleus at 37°C (b). ZR–75–1 breast cancer cell line.

Infact, while at 4°C only a cytoplasmic positivity was displayed, the raising of the temperature of incubation has allowed the translocation process and the redistribution of the hormone in the nuclear compartment to take place (Fig. 2). Pre and coincubation of cells with estradiol and anti-estrogens in excess has prevented any positivity, thus giving evidence of the specific interaction between FE and cytosol estradiol receptors.

Non-target cells did not take up this estradiol analogue, also when exposed to high concentrations of the labeled hormone (Fig. 3).

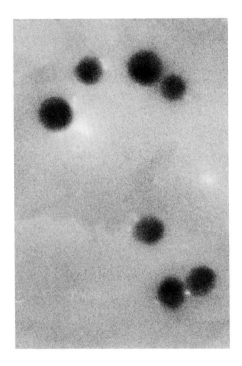

FIG. 3. Mouse fibroblasts do not take up the fluorescent e-stradiol and look like "black holes" in the fluorescent back-ground.

Only when the plasma membrane of non-target cells had been damaged, the fluorescent estradiol was allowed to get into non-target cells and to react aspecifically with cell structures.

This selective cell penetration is in contrast with the expected absence of permeability barrier according to the simple diffusion mechanism of entry of steroid hormones into cells and needs a specific recognition site for the hormone on the plasma membrane of target cells.

Estradiol-6-CMO-BSA-FITC (E-BSA-F).

In order to visualize specific "docking" sites for steroid hormones over the target cell surface, E-BSA-F, a protein carrier double-labe-led with both estradiol and fluorescein, which is hindered by its size from getting through the plasma membrane, has been exploited.

Moreover, at scanning electron microscopy, this macromolecular hormonal probe was bound homogeneously over the surface of the cells incubated at 4°C. Also electron probe X-ray microanalysis revealed a
random distribution of the bound macromolecule on the cell surface
(Fig. 6a, b).

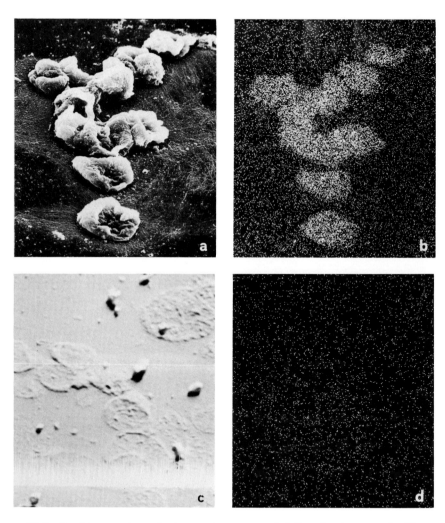

FIG. 6. At scanning electron microscopy (a) the electron probe X-ray
microanalysis displays a homogeneous distribution of IcPEP on breast
cancer cells reacted at 4°C (b). Control cells (c) do not display significant positivity over the emission background (d).

No surface positivity has been ever observed in cells incubated with heat–aggregated immunoglobulins, by either the direct or the indirect immunocytochemical technique. Only lymphocytes and macrophages present in the cell suspension displayed some peripheral positivity through the surface receptor for the Fc fragment of immunoglobulins.

When cells incubated at 4°C in IcPEP were then warmed, the surface bound macromolecular probe formed microclusters, first scattered over the cell surface, then coalesced in large aggregates which migrated towards one pole of the cell (Fig. 7a), thus forming crescent or polar–like caps (Fig. 7b).

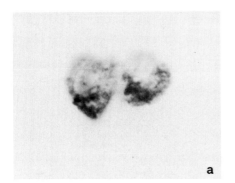 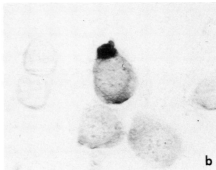

FIG. 7. When breast cancer cells are incubated at 37°C, the surface positivity traced by horseradish peroxidase–labeled anti–Ig G looks at light microscopy like polarized clusters (a) or a dense cap (b), according to the incubation time.

This redistribution of the bound ligand was evident in immunofluorescence– and immunoperoxidase–processed cells at light and scanning electron microscopy, and further testified also by X–ray microanalysis performed at scanning electron microscopy (Fig. 8).

The temperature–dependent phenomenon of capping is known to occur when multivalent ligands bind to some constituents of the plasma membrane of freely suspended cells. Since capping results from crosslinking between multivalent ligands – as these macromolecular probes – with membrane constituents, obviously this process does not occur in the physiological interplay between univalent steroids and the plasma membrane of target cells.

As the two–dimensional translational diffusion is a well known property of membrane intrinsic constituents according to the Singer's fluid mosaic membrane model (9), the observed surface binding sites for estra–

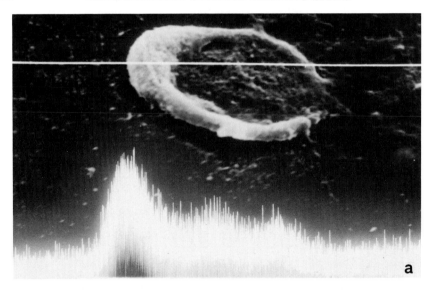

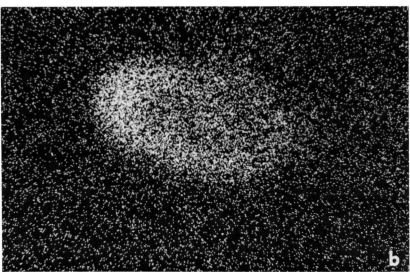

FIG. 8. When breast cancer cells are incubated at 37°C the polar redistribution of the bound IcPEP is very apparent at scanning electron microscopy (a) coupled with electron probe X-ray microanalysis (b).

diol could be considered intrinsic membrane components, either because they are themselves integral membrane proteins or because they are steadily linked to such proteins. So that, this estradiol binding site on the surface of target cells appears to conform to the dynamic properties of a potential receptor mechanism.

CONCLUDING COMMENTS

The meaning of these membrane docking sites with respect to the mechanism of steroid hormone action, is not immediately obvious. The binding capacity of these surface sites was abolished by pretreating the cells with estradiol in excess and chiefly polyestradiol (Table 1.).

TABLE 1. Inhibitory effect on surface binding of labeled estradiol

Polyestradiol	+++
Estradiol	++
Tamoxifen	−+
Diethylstilbestrol	−
N−Ethylmaleimide	−
Neuraminidase	−
Testosterone	−

The location of cytoplasmic receptors at the surface level has been already hypothesized, nevertheless these membrane binding sites, unlike estradiol cytoplasmic receptors, were neither saturated by diethylstilbestrol and tamoxifen, nor inactivated by N−ethylmaleimide and neuraminidase.

Since testosterone did not prevent in our conditions estradiol binding, also the sex−steroid binding globulin does not seem to be involved in this interaction.

The possibility has to be taken into consideration that these surface sites be involved in the internalization of the hormone and, namely, act as a channel for estradiol toward its cytoplasmic receptor within target cells.

Lastly, an alternative hypothesis is that these surface binding sites, by analogy with other systems, are involved in a direct interplay between the hormone and some specific membrane functions like, for instance, the permeability to ions.

ACKNOWLEDGEMENTS

   The authors thank Prof. G.B. Lanza, Director of the Institute, for the
institutional support; Dr. G. Battaglia and Dr. A. Aleotti of the Electron
Microscopy Department, for excellent technical assistance for the scanning electron microscopy; Dr. E. Cassai of the Institute of Microbiology,
for the management of the cell lines. This study was in part supported by
"Progetto Finalizzato del C.N.R.: Controllo della Crescita Neoplastica.
Sottoprogetto: Controllo Endocrinologico". Dr. Elisabetta Marchetti is
recipient of a fellowship from "Fondazione Anna Villa Rusconi", Varese,
Italy.

REFERENCES

1. Dandliker, W.B., Brawn, R.J., Hsu, M.-L., Brawn, P.N., Levin,
   J., Meyers, C.Y., and Kolb, V.M. (1978): Cancer Res., 38: 4212-
   -4224.
2. Dickler, H.B., and Kunkel, H.G. (1972): J. Exp. Med., 136:191-
   -196.
3. Lee, S.H. (1978): Am. J. Clin. Pathol., 70:197-203.
4. Nenci, I. (1978): Cancer Res., 38:4204-4211.
5. Nenci, I., Beccati, M.D., Piffanelli, A., and Lanza, G. (1976): J.
   Steroid Biochem., 7:505-510.
6. Pietras, R.J., and Szego, C.M. (1979): J. Cell Biol., 81:649-663.
7. Poste, G., and Nicholson, G.L., editors (1977): Dynamic Aspects
   of Cell Surface Organization. North-Holland, Amsterdam.
8. Schlessinger, J., Shechter, Y., Willingham, M.C., and Pastan, I.
   (1978): Proc. Natl. Acad. Sci. USA, 75:2659-2663.
9. Singer, S.J. (1974): Ann. Rev. Biochem., 43:805-833.
10. Sternberger, L.A., Hardy, P.H., Cuculis, J.J., and Meyer, H.G.
    (1970): J. Histochem. Cytochem., 18:315-333.

Perspectives in Steroid Receptor Research,
edited by F. Bresciani.
Raven Press, New York © 1980.

Progesterone Receptor Proteins: Studies of the Relationship Between the A and B Forms

William T. Schrader, John G. Compton, Wayne V. Vedeckis, and Bert W. O'Malley

Department of Cell Biology, Baylor College of Medicine, Houston, Texas 77030, U.S.A.

SUMMARY

Progesterone receptor B protein (110,000 g/mole) of chick oviduct was tested as a potential precursor to receptor A (79,000 g/mole) which is present in the same tissue in equivalent amounts. Neither exposure to warming, dialysis, storage, increased salt concentration, precipitation nor other treatments were successful in converting receptor B to receptor A as assayed by DEAE-cellulose and DNA-cellulose chromatography. The failure to detect conversion of receptor B to receptor A in vitro suggests that receptor B is not a precursor to A and that the receptor A protein is not an artifact of isolation.

INTRODUCTION

We have been studying the progesterone receptor of chicken oviduct (for review see ref. 17). Two distinct progesterone-binding proteins have been described and isolated to apparent homogeneity from this tissue (4,11,14). Structural (1,13) and functional (3,9) studies have led us to postulate that these two proteins are subunits of a larger complex. Due to the similarity of their proteolytic digestion products (18,20), it has remained a possibility that the larger B protein (M_r = 110,000) is the natural precursor of the smaller A protein (M_r = 79,000). Since receptor B is a single polypeptide chain, its conversion to the smaller protein would involve a proteolytic step. Furthermore, receptor A has been shown to bind to DNA at physiological ionic strength. Hence, conversion of receptor B to receptor A might account for the phenomenon of receptor "activation" in which the receptor becomes able to interact with genomic components.

73

Alternatively, it is possible to view receptor A as a degradative form derived from receptor B. Partly for these reasons, the receptor A-B subunit model has not been widely accepted.[1]

To shed further light on the question of the relationship between receptors B and A, we have conducted a series of studies aimed at detecting conversion of B to A. In this communication we report our inability to find any evidence for the formation of receptor A from receptor B in either crude or purified preparations.

METHODS

Receptor Preparations

Methods for labeling and isolating chick oviduct progesterone receptors have been reported in detail elsewhere (10). Oviduct cytosol from estrogenized immature chicks was prepared in TESH Buffer (0.01 M Tris-HCl, 0.001 M Na_2EDTA, 0.012 M 1-thioglycerol, pH 7.4 (25°)) at ratios of buffer to tissue (ml/g) of 4:1. Receptors were labeled at 0° with $2x10^{-8}$ M [1,2-^{3}H]progesterone (50 Ci/mmole) for at least 60 min, or with nonradioactive progesterone at the same molarity. Ammonium sulfate precipitation (0% to 35% saturation) and resolution of receptors A and B by DEAE-cellulose column chromatography have been described elsewhere (10).

Hormone-Receptor Binding

Binding of [^{3}H]R5020 to chick oviduct cytosol was carried out as described for [^{3}H]progesterone (10). After 1 hour, aliquots (100 μl) were diluted by addition of 1.0 ml TESH buffer, and applied to Whatman DE-81 filters. The filters were washed with 3 ml of TESH, dried and counted for tritium.

Chromatographic Assays of Receptor Forms

DEAE-cellulose chromatography

Salt gradient elution of DEAE-cellulose columns using linear KCl gradients (11) has shown that receptor A elutes at 0.15 M KCl and receptor B at 0.2 M KCl. Free [^{3}H]progesterone and receptor mero-protein, a proteolytic degradation product of both A and B containing the hormone-binding domain ($M_r \sim 23,000$) (18,20) both pass through the resin unretarded. DEAE-cellulose columns were loaded and washed at 0.03 M KCl and then eluted

[1]In this regard, we have recently obtained data with other receptors suggesting that such a structure may be of general applicability to all steroid receptors (15).

stepwise with 0.15 M KCl to yield receptor A and with 0.5 M KCl to elute receptor B in the analytical experiments below. In some experiments, a 0.03 to 0.4 M KCl gradient was substituted for stepwise elution.

DNA-cellulose chromatography

Receptors A and B differ markedly in their adsorption to this resin. The column was prepared and run as described elsewhere (4). Receptor B binds weakly to DNA cellulose, eluting at 0.03 M KCl; whereas receptor A elutes at 0.18 M KCl-TESH (20). In the analytical experiments below, receptor samples were applied at 0.1 M KCl at which only receptor A is adsorbed. Free progesterone, mero-receptor and receptor B all flow through the column unretarded under these conditions. The receptor A fraction was then eluted stepwise by applying 0.5 M KCl-TESH.

Gel Filtration

A gel filtration column (2.6 cm x 90 cm) containing A-1.5 M agarose beads (Bio-gel) was calibrated with Blue Dextran 2000 (V_0), KCl (V_T) and [^{3}H]progesterone-receptor complexes prepared by labeling oviduct cytosol in TESH containing 0.3 M KCl. Samples of cytosol (3 ml) in the absence or presence of labeled progesterone were chromatographed at 15 ml/h and collected in 1 ml fractions. Each fraction from elutions not containing hormone was post-labeled by addition of 100,000 cpm/tube of [^{3}H]progesterone and labeled receptor-hormone complexes were adsorbed to hydroxylapatite slurries. The slurries were collected and washed on glass fiber filters (2.4 cm; Reeve-Angle 934AH) and counted for tritium.

Treatment of Receptor with Protease

Chick tissues contain a calcium-activated neutral protease (7,19) which hydrolyzes both receptors B and A into discrete fragments (20). The potential participation of this enzyme in converting B to A was tested with the following protocol. Labeled receptor B from DEAE-cellulose was added to unlabeled oviduct cytosol (as a source of the protease) and the mixture was brought to 1 mM in CaCl$_2$ and maintained at 4° for 30 min. This time is sufficient to cause the conversion of some receptor B to mero-protein (in the presence of calcium). The preparations were then assayed for the presence of labeled receptor A by DEAE-cellulose and DNA-cellulose chromatography. Endogenous proteolytic activity was also tested for by warming non-radioactively labeled cytosol containing labeled receptor B. The mixtures were warmed to 25° for 60 min and then cooled to 4° before assaying on DEAE and DNA-cellulose columns.

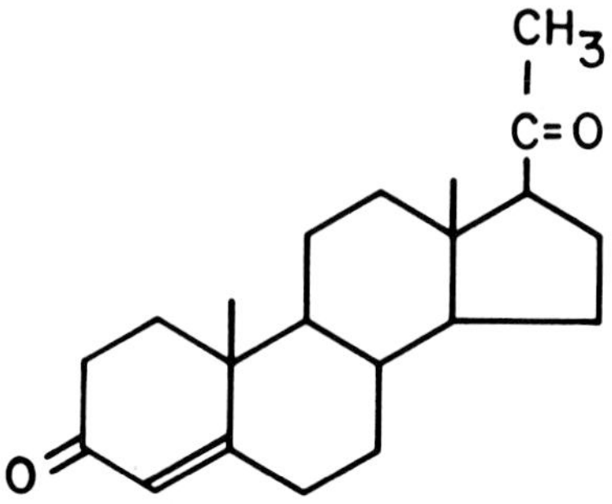

Progesterone

A_{max} = 249 nm

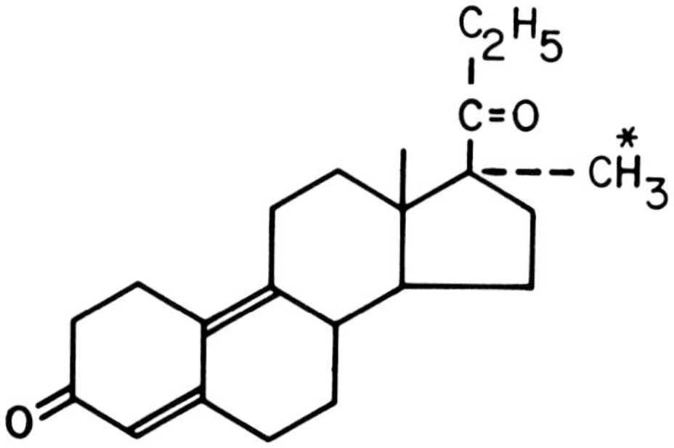

R5020

A_{max} = 320 nm

FIG. 1. Choice of radioactive ligand for progesterone receptor photoaffinity labeling. Top structure, progesterone showing measured absorption maximum wavelength. Lower structure, R5020 (17α, 21-dimethyl-19-nor-pregn-4,9-diene-3,20-dione) and its observed adsorption maximum.

Finally, a partially-purified sample (2000-fold) of chick calcium-activated neutral protease (19) was incubated with labeled receptor B protein in the absence of cytosol. Incubation was for 30 min at 4° in the presence of 1 mM $CaCl_2$, the optimum concentration for the purified enzyme. After incubation, the samples were assayed by DEAE and DNA-cellulose chromatography for their labeled receptor A content.

Photoaffinity Receptor Labeling

Receptors in cytosol were complexed with the synthetic progestin R5020 (Roussel-Uclaf) labeled with ^3H at 80 Ci/mmole. This compound can covalently attach to the progesterone receptor (5) when photoactivated by ultraviolet light at 320 nm. The cytosol was labeled with R5020 for one hour at 0° and the receptors were precipitated by addition of ammonium sulfate to 40% saturation. The precipitates were redissolved in TESH buffer, placed in an ice bath and irradiated by use of an 85 watt low-pressure mercury vapor lamp for 1 hour. The sample vials were covered by a borosilicate glass plate to absorb the strong UV emission of the lamp at 254 nm. The protein solutions were lyophilyzed, redissolved in TESH, dialyzed against 1% sodium dodecyl sulfate and analyzed by polyacrylamide gel electrophoresis according to the method of Laemmli (8). Tube gels (6mm x 10cm) contained 7.5% total acrylamide (0.2% N, N'-methylene-bis-acrylamide). After fractionating each gel into slices 2mm thick, the fractions were minced and counted for tritium.

RESULTS

Photoaffinity Labeling

We have recently demonstrated that the progesterone receptor of chick oviduct can be resolved into two distinct polypeptide chains after photoaffinity labeling with the synthetic steroid R5020, in vitro. Our choice of R5020 for the photoaffinity experiments was based on a comparison of the structure of R5020 with that of progesterone (Figure 1). The critical additional conjugated double bond in the B ring of R5020 shifts the ultraviolet absorption maximum wavelength of this derivative closer to the visible when compared to that of progesterone. Since ultraviolet radiation at these wavelengths are not strongly absorbed by proteins in solution, the potential damage to the receptors themselves is greatly reduced. The compound R5020 is not strictly a progestin, possessing affinity for androgen receptors as well. However, the concentration of progesterone receptors is so much higher than that of other steroid receptors in oviduct cytosol that potential reaction of the ligand with these other receptor proteins could be ignored in the present experiments.

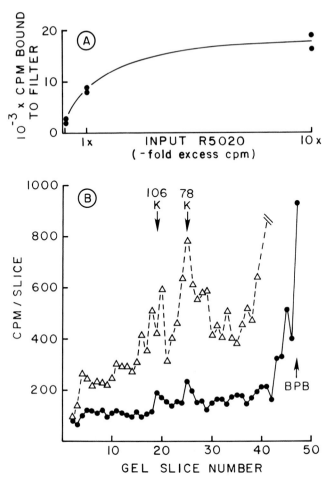

FIG. 2. Interaction of [³]R5020 (80 Ci/mmole) with chick progesterone receptor. Panel A, DEAE-cellulose filter assay of [³H]
R5020 binding to cytosol receptors before photoactivation. Receptor-hormone complexes were detected as described in text using
Whatman DE-81 filters. Input concentrations of ligand are given
in Methods; results of duplicate samples as shown (●). Panel B,
SDS-polyacrylamide gel electrophoresis of photoaffinity-labeled
receptor preparations. Incubation, precipitation and photoactivation steps were as described in text. Gel slices were counted
for ³H and migration was compared to companion gels containing
stained protein of known molecular weight (data not shown).
Results of two companion gels are presented: △——△ , sample from
10x incubation of Panel A; ●——●, sample from 1x incubation of
Panel A. BPB, from bromphenol blue tracking dye locus after
electrophoresis.

As shown in the top panel of Figure 2, [³H]R5020 binds saturably to the progesterone receptor. On the abcissa, 1x refers to a concentration of 2x10⁻⁸ M, an amount equal to that normally used for progesterone binding studies (as described in Methods). Identical samples (1.0 ml) containing either 0.1x, 1x or 10x [³H]R5020 bound were irradiated and analyzed on polyacrylamide gels as described in Methods. Slices of the gels were counted for tritium and the results are shown in the bottom panel of Figure 2 for the 1x and 10x experiments (analysis of the 0.1x experiment was not possible since insufficient radioactivity was present). In the experiment at 1x steroid concentration, two bands of radioactivity are found at positions on the gel corresponding to molecular weights of 106K and 78K, as reported in an earlier communication where these two peaks were shown to be receptors B and A, respectively (5). The 10x gel showed a considerable broadening of the peaks, consistent with significant labeling of additional proteins when saturation of the receptor sites was exceeded. In both profiles, there is equivalent labeling of the 106K and 78K bands. Thus, the two receptor bands B and A can be resolved by this photoaffinity technique, just as they were in purification (14) and ion-exchange studies published earlier (11).

Gel Filtration

The demonstration that two forms of the progesterone receptor exist in photoaffinity labeled solutions leaves open the possibility that the presence of steroid bound to the protein causes the resulting receptor heterogeneity. This question could be answered by analyzing the elution profile of unlabeled receptors during gel filtration on A 1.5 M at 0.3 M KCl. As shown in Figure 3, two peaks of equal size are resolved from a control sample of cytosol incubated for 2 hr with [³H]progesterone. These two peaks have previously been identified as the receptor B and receptor A forms isolated by DEAE-cellulose ion-exchange chromatography (11); their elution positions are indicated in Figure 3. Brief labeling (2 min) with progesterone yielded a pattern similar to that of longer incubation; a peak representing a mixture of equal amounts of receptor B and receptor A forms. Furthermore, the presence of two receptor forms is not dependent on the formation of a hormone-receptor complex, as seen from the pattern obtained when unlabeled cytosol was chromatographed on the same column at 0.3M KCl. Post-labeling of the apo-receptor in each column fraction revealed a pattern similar to those obtained with prelabeled cytosol and consisting of equal amounts of B and A receptor forms. Thus, detection and/or production of both B and A receptor forms was independent of the presence of the ligand. Companion experiments, not presented here, showed that a variety of protease inhibitors added during cytosol preparation did not alter the gel filtration

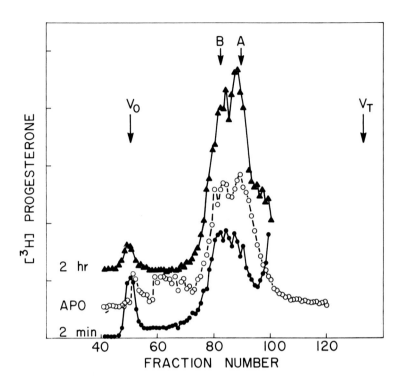

FIG. 3.   Receptor component analysis by gel filtration in Agarose
A-1.5m.   The column was run in TESH-0.3M KCl and calibrated as
outlined in the text. ▲——▲ , analysis of labeled cytoplasmic
receptors B and A obtained by treatment of cytosol with 0.5M KCl
during 2-hour labeling period. o——o, companion analysis of
unlabeled cytosol sample also incubated 2 hours in 0.5M KCl before the chromatogram. Radioactive progesterone added to each
fraction after collection, stored at 0° for 3 hours and then
bound [³H]progesterone-receptor complexes determined by hydroxylapatite adsorption assay as described in the text. ●——●,
companion cytosol sample labeled for 2 min with [³H]progesterone
before start of chromatography; V_O, void volume; V_T, total
volume, both determined as outlined in Methods. Radioactivity
scales of the three runs have been adjusted graphically to permit
plotting of all three runs on a single pair of coordinates for
 mparison.

profiles.

Conversion Studies

The tests above established that receptors B and A could be detected as we had earlier described under different conditions. However, there remained the possibility that receptor A, the smaller protein, was a product of receptor B digestion or degradation during tissue disruption or preparation of cytosol. Table I summarizes several experiments which directly tested for conversion of receptor B into receptor A. Two methods were used to distinguish between receptor B and receptor A: DEAE-cellulose chromatography in which receptor A elutes at 0.1 to 0.15 M KCl while receptor B elutes at 0.2M KCl; and DNA-cellulose chromatography in which receptor B elutes at 0.03M KCl and receptor A at 0.18 M KCl (10,20).

Since the property of tight binding to DNA-cellulose resides solely in the receptor A form, this property can be used as a rigorous test for identifying the presence of this protein. In contrast, elution of receptor A from DEAE-cellulose between 0.1 and 0.15 M KCl is not unique; a smaller proteolytic fragment called form IV (20), produced from receptor B or receptor A by limited digestion with an enzyme endogenous to the chick oviduct, also binds weakly to this resin. Extensive digestion leads to the appearance of the mero-hormone receptor fragment which does not adsorb to either DEAE- or DNA-cellulose.

[3H]progesterone-labeled receptor B protein prepared as described in Methods, was precipitated by 50% saturation of ammonium sulfate and redissolved in TESH buffer at a final concentration of 2×10^{-8}M. This preparation of [3H]receptor B was analyzed for receptor A content by rechromatography on DEAE-cellulose and DNA-cellulose using stepwise elution from 1.0 ml columns of these resins. Table I shows results of this control experiment; only 3% of the tritium eluted as A by DEAE and only 9% of radioactivity eluted as A by DNA assay.

A rigorous test for the in vitro conversion was performed as follows: the [3H]receptor B solution in TESH was used as the homogenization buffer to prepare cytosol from fresh oviducts. Non-radioactive progesterone (2×10^{-8}M) was added during homogenization to prevent apo-receptors in the tissue extract from binding any [3H]progesterone released from the exogenous [3H]receptor B. After preparation of cytosol by high-speed ultracentrifugation, the resulting solution was assayed for its receptor forms (Table I). Fifteen percent of the radioactivity migrated on DEAE as receptor A but only 6% in the DNA cellulose assay. Thus, this protocol showed negligible conversion of [3H]receptor B to receptor A.

TABLE I

TESTS OF [3H]RECEPTOR B PROTEIN AS PRECURSOR TO RECEPTOR A

| EXPERIMENT[a] | INCUBATION CONDITIONS | ASSAY OF [3H]RECEPTOR FORMS PRODUCED[b] | | | | |
| | | DEAE-CELLULOSE ASSAY | | | DNA ASSAY | |
		.03M KCl (mero)	.15M KCl (form IV+A)	.5M KCl (B)	.1M KCl (mero+B)	.5M KCl (A)
Control	Rechromatograph	3%	3%	94%	91%	9%
Expose B to whole tissue	Use B as buffer to make cytosol	25	15	60	94	6
Expose B to cytosol	B + cytosol 25° 60 min	45	18	37	94	6
Endogenous protease activation	B + cytosol 4° 30 min + 1 mM CaCl2	62	20	18	93	7
Expose B to purified protease	B + protease 4° 30 min + 1 mM CaCl2	6	5	89	88	12

a [3H]Receptor B protein prepared by DEAE-cellulose chromatography was precipitated at 50% sat. (NH4)2SO4 and redissolved in TESH.
b Receptor form present in each fraction shown in parentheses

As shown on the next line of Table I, continued incubation of this cytosol containing [3H]receptor B at 25° for up to 60 min failed to alter the amount of radioactivity in the receptor A fraction by either test. Radioactivity did increase to 45% in the DEAE 0.03 M KCl wash, probably due to production of mero-receptor fragments during this incubation (18). Thus, the proportion of A protein in the extract did not increase, a result contrary to that expected if an enzymatic conversion mechanism was operative in vitro.

Activation of the endogenous calcium-activated neutral protease at 0° was attempted next. As shown in Table I, this method produced 62% conversion of [3H]receptor B to mero-protein, but again there was no increase in the amount of receptor A. In this experiment, it was possible that the endogenous protease was too active under these conditions, and degraded newly-created receptor A to mero-protein very quickly. Therefore, a partially-purified sample of the protease was added directly to an additional sample of fresh [3H]receptor B protein alone. As shown by the bottom line of Table I, again only negligible conversion to receptor A was seen. From these experiments we conclude receptor B is not a precursor for production of receptor A, at least by endogenous proteases as tested here under in vitro conditions.

Since our protocols for characterization and purification of receptors B and A invariably have included ammonium sulfate precipitation of the receptor complexes from cytosol, it was of interest to test whether this treatment might cause conversion of B to A. For this study [3H]receptor B was again employed and the results are shown in Table II. When a [3H]receptor B preparation was precipitated alone by 35% saturation of ammonium sulfate, redissolved and chromatographed again on DEAE-cellulose, as a control experiment, only 4% of the tritium eluted in the receptor A fraction. DNA-cellulose characterization was not undertaken. Labeled receptor B was added to fresh cytosol (containing 2×10^{-8}M non-radioactive progesterone) at two different ratios of [3H]B to endogenous receptors, 1:1 and 10:1. Then the mixtures were subjected to 35% saturation with ammonium sulfate precipitation and analyzed by both DEAE- and DNA-cellulose chromatography. Each column was eluted with a KCl gradient and yields of receptor forms were obtained by pooling fractions over the ranges of KCl molarity indicated in Table II. Negligible amounts of radioactivity eluted as receptor A from DEAE-cellulose in either the 1:1 or 10:1 experiments, while the values are only 4% and 2% receptor A by the more discriminating DNA-cellulose assay. Thus, this protocol also fails to detect formation of the DNA-binding receptor A protein from receptor B.

TABLE II

EFFECT OF AMMONIUM SULFATE PRECIPITATION UPON [3H]RECEPTOR B INTEGRITY

EXPERIMENT[a]	RATIO[c] [3H]B : [1H]B	ASSAY OF [3H]RECEPTOR FORMS PRODUCED[d]				
		DEAE-CELLULOSE ASSAY			DNA ASSAY	
		DROPTHRU (mero)	<.15M (form IV+A)	.15-.4M (B)	<.15M (B)	.15-.4M (A)
Re-chromatograph [3H]B	---	4%	<1%	96%	---	---
[3H]B + [1H]cytosol[b]	1:1	9	<1	81	96%	4%
[3H]B + [1H]cytosol[b]	10:1	10	<1	90	98%	2

a [3H]B prepared by DEAE-cellulose was mixed with cytosol or buffer alone and precipitated at 35% sat. ammonium sulfate.

b Receptors in cytosol were first complexed with non-radioactive progesterone (2 X 10^{-8}M) before addition of [3H]B.

c Input molar ratio of [3H]B to [1H]B monomer present in cytosol sample.

d Receptor form present in each pool shown in parentheses.

DISCUSSION

The experiments described above were designed to test for the in vitro conversion of receptor B protein to receptor A. All previous experiments we have done, including extensive re-chromatography, purification, and analysis by gel electrophoresis under denaturing conditions have failed to detect such conversion. Thus, we have hypothesized that B and A are closely-related, but non-identical proteins which do not share a precursor-product relationship. The early experiments had not, however, directly tested for such a conversion in both crude and purified systems.

We felt that the most direct and crucial test of this idea would be to have labeled receptor B present during homogenization of fresh oviduct tissue. In this way, the protein would be exposed to both intra- and extra-cellular enzymes or other factors. This would be at least as deleterious an environment as that experienced by the tissue's own intracellular receptors under normal disruption conditions. Two independent assays of receptor forms, one a charge method (DEAE-cellulose) and the other a selective binding assay (DNA-cellulose) would be used simultaneously to detect B to A conversion.

Table I shows clearly that such conversion did not occur. Furthermore, continued incubations in cytosol at several temperatures, times and with activated endogenous proteases also failed to elicit conversion. Table II shows that the ammonium sulfate protocol itself is not a converting stimulus. Figures 2 and 3 were included to show the results obtained with other detection methods on the relative abundancy of receptors B and A. In both of these experiments, one utilizing a novel photoaffinity labeling technique, the same result is always obtained: there is no evidence for conversion of receptor B to receptor A.

It is important to note that these results do not eliminate the possibility that the receptor A protein is derived in vivo from the same polypeptide chain as receptor B by proteolytic cleavage. However, we have demonstrated that if an enzyme or enzymes exist with this activity, they do not utilize exogenous receptor B as a substrate. Perhaps the larger forms of the receptor, sedimenting at 6-8S as isolated from cytosol, are the proper substrate. Since relatively mild treatments such as dilution, dialysis, 0.3 M KCl, precipitation with ammonium sulfate, etc., result in the appearance of receptors B and A in equal amounts, the putative enzymes would have to be "activated" very easily, and yet their activity be precise and self-limiting. We consider that this model is less likely than our hypothesis that receptors B and A pre-exist in chick oviduct cells in vivo.

The concept of receptors B and A being subunits of a larger, functional complex (9) has always seemed the most plausible explanation for their nearly-equal concentrations we observe in both cytoplasm and nuclei. The fact that receptor B does not bind to DNA at physiological salt concentrations has led others to speculate that the "activated" receptor might be protein A, produced from receptor B by proteolysis. In this regard, it is of interest to note that the conditions of time and temperature used in Table I (25° 60 min) are sufficient to optimally "activate" receptor-hormone complexes of cytosol for binding to nuclei (2). Yet, no conversion to A protein was seen. This finding is also consistent with our observation that the ratio of B to A in cytosol does not vary during the time course of warming to elicit nuclei binding.

Rather, we feel that the best explanation for the data on chick oviduct progesterone receptor is that both B and A are pre-formed in the cell and await encounter with progesterone to act in a concerted fashion. Studies with bifunctional cross-linking agents (1), sedimentation studies (13), and recent reconstitution studies (6) all support the concept of hetero-complexes of A and B.

We are, as yet, unable to directly determine whether receptor A derives from its own gene, or is instead produced in vivo from the same gene product as receptor B. Nevertheless, the relationship between the two proteins should be investigated by amino acid sequencing procedures, especially in view of the similarities of the two proteins in their susceptibility to digestion by specific proteases. However, the studies presented above make it extremely doubtful that receptor A might arise, for example, merely as an experimental artifact. The structural studies necessary to further extend these arguments are now under way in our laboratory.

ACKNOWLEDGEMENTS

This research was supported by NIH grants HD-07857 and HD-07495 to the Baylor Center for Population Research and Studies in Reproductive Biology. W.V.V. was recipient of an NIH post-doctoral fellowship. J.G.C. is supported by a post-doctoral grant from the American Cancer Society.

REFERENCES

1. Birnbaumer, M. E., Schrader, W. T., and O'Malley, B. W. (1979): Biochem. J., 181:201-213.
2. Buller, R. E., Toft, D. O., Schrader, W. T., and O'Malley, B. W. (1975): J. Biol. Chem., 250:801-808.
3. Buller, R. E., Schwartz, R. J., Schrader, W. T., and O'Malley, B. W. (1976): J. Biol. Chem., 251:5178-5186.
4. Coty, W. A., Schrader, W. T., and O'Malley, B. W. (1979): J. Steroid Biochem., 10:1-12.
5. Dure, L. S. IV, Schrader, W. T., and O'Malley, B. W. (1980): Nature, (in press).
6. Grody, W. W., Schrader, W. T., and O'Malley, B. W. (in preparation).
7. Ishiura, S., Murofushi, H., Suzuki, K., and Imahori, K. (1978): J. Biochem., 84:225-230.
8. Laemmli, U. (1970): Nature, 227:680-685.
9. O'Malley, B. W., Spelsberg, T. C., Schrader, W. T., Chytil, F., and Steggles, A. W. (1972): Nature, 235:141-144.
10. Schrader, W. T. (1975): Methods in Enzymol., 36:187-211.
11. Schrader, W. T. and O'Malley, B. W. (1972): J. Biol. Chem., 247:51-59.
12. Schrader, W. T., Toft, D. O., and O'Malley, B. W. (1972): J. Biol. Chem., 247:2401-2407.
13. Schrader, W. T., Heuer, S. S., and O'Malley, B. W. (1975): Biology of Reproduction, 12:134-142.
14. Schrader, W. T., Coty, W. A., Smith R. G., and O'Malley, B. W. (1977): Ann. N.Y. Acad. Sci., 286:64-80.
15. Schrader, W. T., Seleznev. Y., Vedeckis, W. V., and O'Malley, B. W. (1980): In: Gene Regulation by Steroid Hormones, edited by A. K. Roy and J. H. Clark, (in press). Springer-Verlag, New York.
16. Sherman, M. R., Corvol, P. L., and O'Malley, B. W. (1970): J. Biol. Chem., 245:6085-6096.
17. Vedeckis, W. V., Schrader, W. T., and O'Malley, B. W. (1978): In: Biochemical Actions of Hormones, Vol. V, edited by G. Litwack, pp. 321-372. Academic Press, New York.
18. Vedeckis, W. V., Schrader, W. T., and O'Malley, B. W. (1979): In: Steroid Hormone Receptor Systems, edited by W. W. Leavitt and J. H. Clark, pp. 309-327. Plenum Press, New York.
19. Vedeckis, W. V., Freeman, M. R., Schrader, W. T. and O'Malley, B. W. (1980): Biochemistry (in press).
20. Vedeckis, W. V., Schrader, W. T., and O'Malley, B. W. (1980): Biochemistry, (in press).

Perspectives in Steroid Receptor Research,
edited by F. Bresciani.
Raven Press, New York © 1980.

Use of the Affinity Label
17β-Bromoacetoxytestosterone in the Purification
of Androgen Receptor Proteins

W. Ian P. Mainwaring and Alison D. Johnson

Department of Biochemistry, University of Leeds, Leeds LS2 9LS, England

As widespread interest has grown in elucidating the mechanism
of action of steroid hormones at the molecular level, the need
for the extensive purification of the steroid "receptor"
proteins is now universally acknowledged. Purified receptor-
steroid complexes are absolutely essential if we are to probe
their regulatory roles, particularly in genetic transcription,
with accuracy and authenticity.

Receptor purification has proved to be an extremely difficult
undertaking, for apart from the inherent instability of the
receptor proteins, conventional methods of protein fractionation
have been found wanting in terms of resolution and specificity.
Despite these technical problems, conspicuous success has been
achieved in the purification of the receptors for oestradiol-17β
(3, 18, 21) and progesterone (5, 6). In these cases, investigators have exploited the particular advantages of affinity
chromatography either on immobilized steroid ligands or other
matrices with a marked selectivity for steroid-receptor complexes
(e.g. immobilized heparin). The purification of androgen
receptor complexes is particularly difficult, because they seem
to be perhaps the most unstable of all steroid hormone receptors
(8). Indeed, there has been little, if any, real progress in
androgen receptor purification since the publication of the work
of Mainwaring and Irving (9, 10) some five years ago. In common
with the experience of others, the present investigators found
that androgen receptors could not be purified by affinity
chromatography on matrices containing immobilized androgens,
because these receptors degrade so rapidly in the absence of
their favoured ligands; affinity chromatography by this method
essentially requires the receptor to be presented to the matrix
in steroid-free conditions. Androgen receptors simply do not
survive this manipulation. Clearly, other approaches were
indicated.

Affinity labelling has proved to be an invaluable technique for probing the structure of enzymes engaged in steroid metabolism (1, 17, 20). In this procedure, structural analogues of the substrate are bound covalently to the active site, thus facilitating structural and sequence analysis. More recently, le Gaillard and Dautrevaux (7) successfully applied affinity labelling for identifying unequivocally the single steroid-binding site in human transcortin. Encouraged by this important paper (7), we have recently shown that 17β-bromoacetoxytestosterone can be used to label the single binding site in human SBG (sex steroid-binding β globulin), both covalently and specifically (11). Here, we report the use of this affinity label in the purification of the androgen receptors from rat prostate and mouse kidney. Much of our purification procedure is based on the excellent work of Molinari et al. (14), developed originally for the oestrogen receptor of calf uterus.

MATERIALS AND METHODS

Chemicals

Sephadex G-200 (medium), DEAE-Sephadex (type A-50) and Sepharose 4B were obtained from Pharmacia, Uppsala, Sweden. Heparin (sodium salt; grade II) and monothioglycerol were purchased from Sigma Ltd., Poole, Dorset, U.K. Crosslinked 5% agarose with covalently coupled triazinyl dyes were supplied as Matrix Gels Red A and Blue A by Amicon Corp., Lexington, Mass., U.S.A.; these matrices contained 4.4 mg/ml Procion Red HE3B (Imperial Chemical Industries) and 3.4 mg/ml Cibacron Blue F3GA (Ciba-Geigy), respectively. Purified Sephadex G-75 (Ultradex) and ampholytes (40%, w/v; pH range 5-8) were obtained from LKB, Bromma, Sweden.

Heparin was coupled to CNBr-activated Sepharose 4B as described by Molinari et al. (14); based on the carbazole reaction (2), each ml of matrix contained 1.2 mg of covalently linked heparin. The matrix was stored almost indefinitely at 0° C in 0.25% NaN_3. Each batch of matrix could be used at least three times; after use, it was washed with 1 M-NaCl and then exhaustively washed with 0.25% NaN_3 prior to storage.

Bromo [2-^{14}C]acetic acid (23 mCi/mol) was supplied by the Radiochemical Centre, Amersham, U.K. The radiolabelled material was not diluted with non-radioactive bromoacetic acid prior to use, but otherwise, the synthesis of 17β-[^{14}C]bromoacetoxytestosterone was carried out precisely as described by le Gaillard and Dautrevaux (7). The product of the synthesis was Zimmerman-negative, but could be located on t.l.c. plates by dipping in p-anisaldehyde reagent and heating at 110° C for 10 min (15). Unlike the original authors (7), however, we were unable to obtain good separations of testosterone and [^{14}C]bromoacetoxytestosterone on commercial silica gel plates (Merck; type F254). Reproducible separations were achieved on self-made plates of silica gel (kiesel gel; Merck, type 60) using chloroform : di-ethyl ether, 9 : 1 (v/v) for development. Under these conditions, testosterone and its [^{14}C]bromoacetoxyderivative has R_F values of 0.49 and 0.68, respectively. The specific radioactivity of the [^{14}C] affinity label was approx. 14 mCi/m mol. The radioactive steroid was stored for 1 year at 4° C in toluene : ethanol, 4 : 1 (v/v) without any detectable sign of radiochemical decomposition.

Animals and androgen target organs

Ventral prostate glands were removed from male Wistar rats (350 g body weight) 24 hr after castration and either used immediately or stored in liquid nitrogen for up to 1 week. Kidneys from normal female mice or androgen-insensitive Tfm mice were generously provided by Drs. Mary Lyon and Peter Glenister, Medical Research Council Radiobiology Unit, Harwell, U.K. Kidneys were stockpiled frozen at -20° C for several weeks prior to use.

Analytical procedures

Protein was determined with fluorescamine (Roche, Welwyn Garden City, U.K.), as described by Weigele et al. (23), with bovine serum albumin as reference. Alcohol dehydrogenase and glucose-6-phosphate dehydrogenase activities were determined by specific spectrophotometric analyses (16, 22). Radioactivity was counted in a liquid scintillation spectrometer (Intertechnique; Model SL 300) in a water-miscible phosphor (13). Counting efficiency for ^{14}C was 59% and quenching was assessed by the channels ratio technique. The precipitation and washing of receptor protein-radioactive steroid complexes was accomplished as described by Davies et al. (4).

Preparation of cytosols

Tissue was frozen in liquid nitrogen and pulverized on a metal plate, cooled in acetone-solid CO_2, by a sharp blow from a pre-cooled hammer. Frozen powder was suspended in medium R (25 mM Na_2HPO_4-NaH_2PO_4 buffer, pH 7.4, containing 5 mM monothioglycerol, 1 mM EGTA and 10% w/v glycerol) in the ratio 1 g :4 ml. With careful precautions to maintain operational temperatures as close to 0° C as possible, the tissue suspension was disrupted using a motor-driven, coaxial homogenizer (Silverson Instruments, Chesham, U.K.), at 600 rev/min for 30 sec. Centrifugation at 150 000 g for 20 min yielded a clear supernatant fraction or cytosol, which was carefully aspirated from the sediment to avoid the floating layer of lipid.

RESULTS

Authenticity of the affinity label

Exhaustive tests have been conducted to verify the authenticity and reproducibility of [^{14}C]bromoacetoxytestosterone as an affinity label for human SBG and the androgen receptor from rat prostate (11, 12). Additional proof was derived from a comparison of the binding of [^{14}C] label in kidney cytosols derived from both normal female and Tfm mice; the latter appear to be totally deficient in testosterone-specific receptors, thus explaining their complete insensitivity to androgens (8). As shown in Figure 1 (a and b), we could readily detect a binding protein in normal kidney cytosol but not Tfm cytosol by labelling with [^{14}C]bromoacetoxytestosterone; the binding protein had a sedimentation coefficient of 8S (Fig.1a) and was selectively adsorbed and eluted from columns of heparin-Sepharose 4B (Fig. 1b). From published observations in the literature (8), these are the physicochemical properties of the androgen receptor in mouse kidney. Furthermore, affinity labelling required the native configuration of the receptor protein; structural perturbation with either 4 M urea or 5 mM N-bromosuccimide abolished affinity labelling completely.

Extensive purification of rat prostate receptor

It is essential that all stages be conducted at temperatures as close to 0° C as possible. All apparatus and media were thoroughly cooled before use.

Stage 1
Cytosol (12 ml) was prepared from the pooled prostate glands from 12 rats and labelled for 3 hr in an ice-bath with 200 000 cpm [^{14}C]bromoacetoxytestosterone (approx. 1.2×10^{-6} M). The extent of receptor labelling was estimated either as 8S protein-bound radioactivity by ultracentrifugation (see Fig.1a) or by selective precipitation with protamine sulphate (4), with subsequent washing of the precipitates.

Stage 2
Labelled cytosol was placed directly on a column of heparin-Sepharose 4B (1.4 cm diam x 4.0 cm), equilibrated with medium R. After running in the sample, the column was eluted sequentially as follows: medium R alone, medium R plus 0.10 M NaCl and finally, medium R plus 0.15 M NaCl and 2.5 mg/ml heparin. The flow rate was 0.5 ml/min and 1.25 ml fractions were collected. The peak of radioactivity eluted with heparin (see Fig.1b) was pooled (volume, 10 ml).

Stage 3
The pooled heparin eluate was placed directly on a column of

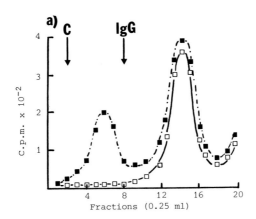

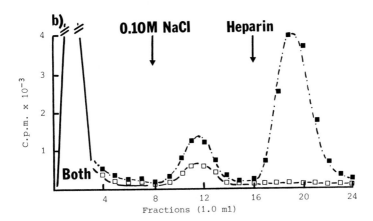

FIG.1. The affinity labelling of mouse kidney cytosols. Kidney
cytosols were labelled for 3 hr at 0° C with 100 000 cpm/ml [^{14}C]
bromoacetoxytestosterone (approx. 0.6x10^{-6}); certain samples
were denatured by the presence of 4 M urea or 5 mM N-bromosuccimide. All were then dialyzed overnight against cold medium R.
(a) Samples (0.1 ml) were separated in 5-20% sucrose gradient (in
medium R), by ultracentrifugation at 100 000 $g_{(av)}$ for 20 hr at
4° C. Sedimentation markers, catalase (C; 11.4S) and γ-globulin
(IgG; 6.7S) were in parallel. (b) Samples (1.0 ml) were separated on heparin-Sepharose columns (1 cm diam x 3 cm), equilibrated
with medium R. The columns were then eluted sequentially with
0.10 M NaCl (in medium R) and 2 mg/ml heparin in medium R. In
both (a) and (b): ■, kidney cytosol from normal female mice; □,
kidney cytosol from Tfm mice or normal mice, labelled in presence
of denaturing agents.

Sephadex G-200 (1.4 cm diam x 33 cm), equilibrated with medium R. Elution was conducted with medium R at a rate of 1.0 ml/min and 1.25 ml fractions were collected. In this standard procedure, the receptor complex eluted as a sharp peak, equivalent to a Stokes radius of 84 Å. The principal fractions were pooled (volume 14 ml).

Stage 4

The pooled G-200 peak was placed directly on a column of immobilized triazinyl dyes (1 cm diam x 4 cm), containing equal volumes of Amicon Gels Red A and Blue A, and equilibrated with medium R. The receptor complex was not retained by this mixed-bed column, but nonetheless, a considerable amount of protein was adsorbed by the matrix and further receptor purification was accomplished. If samples of crude prostate cytosol are processed similarly, with elution of the column by a linear 0.05 - 1.0 M NaCl gradient, a striking separation of alcohol dehydrogenase and glucose-6-phosphate dehydrogenase is achieved. Clearly such mixed-bed columns provide a simple yet efficient method of protein fractionation. The "flow through" peak of radioactivity was pooled (volume, 15 ml).

Stage 5

The labelled receptor preparation was then applied directly to a column of DEAE-Sephadex (1 cm diam x 4 cm) in medium R. The receptor complex is retained by this matrix and resists elution in medium R containing 0.10 M NaCl. However, on raising the ionic strength of the eluant (0.40 M NaCl), the receptor complex is eluted as a sharp peak, in approx. 6 fractions (volume, 1.25 ml each).The pooled peak of radioactivity was dialyzed against 100 ml of 50% (v/v) glycerol, 5 mM monothioglycerol and 0.05% LKB ampholytes (pH range, 5-8) for 5 - 6 hr. Dialysis prepares the sample for isoelectric focusing, but also effects considerable concentration of the labelled receptor (volume, 6 ml).

Stage 6

The last step is isoelectric focusing in a cooled, flat-bed apparatus (LKB; Multiphor). The receptor preparation was mixed with enough 10% glycerol and 1.0% ampholytes, pH range 5-8, to make up a volume of 100 ml. After stirring in 4 g of Ultradex thoroughly, the slurry was poured into the flat-bed and carefully reduced in volume to an even-surfaced gel by evaporation under a cold draught of air. This step was most conveniently conducted by a fan circulator mounted over the flat-bed in a cold room. Gel formation took some 3 hr to achieve. Isoelectric focusing was conducted at an initial voltage of 100 V for 1 hr, then 200 V for

16 hr (overnight). The apparatus was thoroughly cooled by being housed in a cold room and by circulation of ice-cold water through the cooling plattens. The gel was scraped into 30 equal portions, using the septate provided with the apparatus. Each gel sample was then eluted with 3.0 ml of medium R. The labelled receptor, pI 6.3, was recovered in usually 3 fractions (pooled volume, 7.5 ml). Ampholytes seriously interfere with determinations of protein. The labelled receptor was both cleaned up and concentrated by a final absorption and elution cycle from heparin-Sepharose, carried out on one-tenth of the scale described above in stage 1.

General comments

Only the use of affinity labelling is novel here. Much of the purification scheme is based on the protocol of Molinari et al. (14); the efficiency and reproducibility of receptor purification by isoelectric focusing has been amply illustrated by the work of Coffer et al. (3). It is essential that the purification steps are carried out in the order given; in particular, it is critical that the heparin eluate is subjected to gel exclusion chromatography before other fractionation procedures are attempted. In our hands, heparin has a deleterious effect on ion exchange and affinity chromatography.

TABLE 1. The purification of the receptor from rat prostate

STEP	Protein (μg)	D.p.m.[b] x 10^{-4}	Recovery[c]	Specific activity (d.p.m. x 10^{-3}/mg)	Purification[d]
Cytosol[a]	94 000	20	100	2.1	1.0
Heparin 4B	2 670	19	95	71.2	33.9
Sephadex G-200	790	18	90	227.8	108.5
Mixed-bed matrix	210	17	85	809.5	385.5
DEAE-Sephadex	50	15	75	3 000.0	1 428.6
Isoelectric focusing	1-2[e]	14	70	105 000.0	50 000.0

Footnotes: a, based on 8S receptor (sucrose gradients) or protamine precipitation; b, mainly procedural losses, rather than loss of covalent affinity label; c, based on receptor-bound radioactivity; d, based on specific activities; e, these values are only approximate as the assay is difficult at such low protein concentrations.

As reported by others (14), the physicochemical properties of the receptor slowly change during extensive purification. In the present case, this is best seen in sucrose gradients; from 8S in stage 1 and 2, the sedimentation coefficient slowly changes to a lower value of 4S; this conversion is ultimately complete at stage 6.

A typical purification is summarized in Table 1.

DISCUSSION

The present work illustrates the potential importance of affinity labelling in receptor protein purification. The interesting feature of [^{14}C]bromoacetoxytestosterone is its ability to link covalently to the binding site in all androgen receptor proteins, irrespective of their favoured ligand in vivo. In the present paper, the affinity label interacts extensively with mouse kidney and rat prostate receptors, although the androgens normally bound are testosterone and 5α-dihydrotestosterone, respectively. Two pressing aspects remain for work in the immediate future. First, to assess qualitatively, by polyacrylamide gel electrophoresis, the number of proteins present in the purified fractions of receptor. Second, to establish whether receptor associated with the affinity label can be translocated into nuclei in reconstituted, cell-free systems.

REFERENCES

1. Arias, F., Sweet, F., and Warren, J.C. (1972): J. Biol. Chem., 248:5641-5647.
2. Bitter, T., and Muir, H.M. (1962): Analyt. Biochem., 4:330-334.
3. Coffer, A.I., Milton, P.J.D., Pryse-Davies, J., and King, R.J.B. (1977): Molec. Cell Endocrinol., 6:231-246.
4. Davies, P., Thomas, P., and Griffiths, K. (1977): J. Endocr., 74:393-404.
5. Kuhn, R.W., Schrader, W.T., Coty, W.A., Conn, P.M., and O'Malley, B.W. (1977): J. Biol. Chem., 252:308-317.
6. Kuhn, R.W., Schrader, W.T., Smith, R.G., and O'Malley, B.W. (1975): J. Biol. Chem., 250:4220-4228.
7. le Gaillard, F., and Dautrevaux, M. (1977): Biochim. Biophys. Acta, 495:312-323.
8. Mainwaring, W.I.P. (1977): The Mechanism of Action of Androgens. Springer-Verlag, New York.
9. Mainwaring, W.I.P., and Irving, R.A. (1973): Biochem. J., 134:113-127.
10. Mainwaring, W.I.P., and Irving, R.A. (1974): J. Steroid. Biochem., 5:711-716.
11. Mainwaring, W.I.P., and Johnson, A.D. (1980a): Biochem. J., (in press).
12. Mainwaring, W.I.P., and Johnson, A.D. (1980b): Biochem. J., (in press).
13. Mainwaring, W.I.P., Rennie, P.S., and Keen, J. (1976): Biochem. J., 156:253-264.
14. Molinari, A.M., Medici, N., Moncharmont, B., and Puca, G.A.

(1977): Proc. Natl. Acad. Sci. U.S.A., 74:4886-4890.

15. Moore, R.J., and Wilson, J.D. (1976): Methods Enzymol. 36:466-474.

16. Olive, C., and Levy, H.R. (1967): Biochemistry, 6:730-736.

17. Pons, M., Nicholas, J.C., Boussioux, A.M., Descomps, B., and Crastes de Paulet, A. (1973): FEBS Lett., 31:256-260.

18. Sica, V., Parika, I., Nola, E., Puca, G.A., and Cuatrecasas, P. (1973): J. Biol. Chem., 248:6543-6553.

19. Smith, R.G., Iramani, C.A., Buttram, V.C., and O'Malley, B.W. (1975): Nature, 253:271-272.

20. Sweet, F., Arias, F., and Warren, J.C. (1972): J. Biol. Chem., 247:3424-3433.

21. Truong, C., Vignau, M., Torelli, V., Richard-Foy, H., Geynet, C., Secco-Millet, C., Redhuilh, G., and Baulieu, E.E. (1978): J. Biol. Chem.: 8221-8228.

22. Vallee, B.L., and Hoch, F.L. (1955): Proc. Natl. Acad. Sci. U.S.A., 41:327-333.

23. Weigele, M., de Barnardo, S.L., Teng, J.P., and Leningruber, W. (1972): J. Amer. Chem. Soc., 94:5927-5931.

Perspectives in Steroid Receptor Research,
edited by F. Bresciani.
Raven Press, New York © 1980.

Factors That Can Control the Interaction of the Androgen-Receptor Complex with the Genomic Structure in the Rat Prostate

Shutsung Liao, Gian Paolo Rossini, Richard A. Hiipakka, and Chunshing Chen

Ben May Laboratory for Cancer Research and Department of Biochemistry, University of Chicago, Chicago, Illinois 60637, U.S.A.

It is generally believed that the intracellular action of steroid hormones in most target cells is initiated by an interaction of the steroid-receptor complex with chromatin. Although the detailed mechanism is not clear, this interaction appears to cause an increase in the production of certain species of RNA that can play key roles in triggering cellular responses to steroids. (14). If this view is correct, it is important to determine how this interaction can be controlled and what factors regulate this process. We summarize here our study on the effects of steroid structure, energy supply, proteins, RNA, and various drugs on the interaction of the androgen-receptor complex with the genomic structure of the rat ventral prostate.

ANDROGEN STRUCTURE

The affinity of the androgen receptor protein for the prostate nuclear components is markedly enhanced by its binding to a potent androgen such as 5α-dihydrotestosterone (DHT) (7). This is believed to be due to a steroid induced change in the receptor conformation (19). Steroid structure therefore, is important in determining not only the affinity of the steroid for the receptor protein, but also whether the steroid-receptor complex can effectively interact with chromatin and initiate cellular responses. This may be one of the reasons why testosterone, the major testicular androgen in the blood, is not retained by prostate cell nuclei as firmly as its more active metabolite, DHT (2,7), even though the two androgens appear to have similar rates of association with the prostate receptor protein. Because of the structural difference at the A/B ring area, testosterone may not be 'enveloped' (19) by the receptor protein in the same way as DHT and, therefore, may not form a stable androgen-receptor complex or promote a tight association of the receptor protein with the nuclear acceptor molecules.

This essay is dedicated to Elwood V. Jensen, on his sixtieth birthday, whose pioneer work led to the discovery of estrogen receptor and opened a new era in the study of steroid hormone action.

One of the most important functional groups on sex steroid hormones is the 17β-hydroxy group. If this group is removed or replaced by

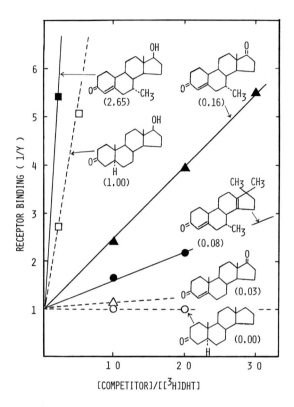

FIG. 1. Relative receptor binding activities of various methyl steroids and steroids having no 17β-hydroxy group. In the receptor binding assay, cytosol from rat ventral prostate and 11 nM 5α-[³H] dihydrotestosterone were incubated with or without nonradioactive competitors, 7α-methyl-19-nortestosterone, 5α-dihydrotestosterone, 7α-methyl-19-norandrost-4-ene-3,17-dione, 7α,17,17-trimethylgona-4,13-dien-3-one, 4-androstenedione, and 17-deoxy-5α-dihydrotestosterone. The amount of the radioactive androgen-receptor complex was estimated from the 3S protein-bound radioactivity after gradient centrifugation. 1/Y is the ratio of the 3S protein-bound radioactivity in the absence of a competitor to the 3S protein-bound radioactivity in the presence of a competitor whose concentration is shown on the abscissa. The numbers in parentheses below the steroid structures are the relative competition indices, which are the ratios of the slope relative to the slope of 5α-dihydrotestosterone. From Chan et al. (5).

a 17α-hydroxy group, the receptor binding affinity and the biological activity of the steroid may be almost completely lost. It is not clear, however, whether the hydroxy group is needed only for high-affinity receptor binding or also for receptor binding to chromatin. As an initial effort in investigating this we have studied the receptor binding activity of several 7α-methyl-19-norandrostenes. Since the 7α-methyl group may help these steroids to bind tightly to the receptor protein (19) even though they lack the 17β-hydroxy group on ring D, it may be possible to analyze whether the 17β-hydroxy group is needed for the receptor complex to bind to the nuclear acceptor and to trigger the hormonal response.

As shown in Fig. 1, the receptor-binding of [^{3}H] DHT was not inhibited by high concentrations of 17-deoxy-DHT. However, 7α,17,17-trimethylgona-4,13-dien-3-one (TMGD), which has no oxygen at ring D, was fairly active in competing with DHT for binding to the receptor protein. According to thin-layer chromatographic analysis, TMGD was not metabolized during the binding assay. The binding activity, therefore, was due to TMGD and not to a metabolite. When it was incubated with the whole-prostate homogenate, TMGD also reduced the nuclear retention of DHT (5). Whether this is due to binding of the TMGD-receptor complex to the nuclear acceptor site has not been determined.

Despite its receptor-binding activity in the cell-free system, we have found TMGD to be neither androgenic nor antiandrogenic. In fact, we have not been able to demonstrate the competitive inhibition of DHT binding to prostate nuclei by TMGD during incubation of minced prostate. It is possible that TMGD is incapable of entering the cell or of being translocated to the intracellular receptor site. Without an oxygen function on ring D, TMGD may behave like a monopolar lipid molecule and intercalate with lipid materials of cellular membranes. This would suggest that one of the important functions for the ring D oxygen is to facilitate the translocation of the steroid to receptor sites by preventing the steroid hormone from being locked into lipid structures.

CELLULAR ENERGY PRODUCTION

About a decade ago, we reported that NaCN or 2,4-dinitrophenol (DNP) can inhibit the nuclear retention of DHT during the incubation of minced prostate with DHT (1,18). These poisons at concentrations below 1 mM and NaN$_3$ at 10 mM can nearly abolish nuclear binding of the DHT-receptor complex.

We found that the amount of androgen-binding receptor as measured by a gradient centrifugation assay was greatly diminished by these inhibitors of cellular energy production during incubation of the minced prostate with [^{3}H] DHT. Since these inhibitors did not affect the stability of the DHT-receptor complex in the cell-free system, these observations suggested that the androgen-binding activity of the

TABLE 1. Energy-dependent steroid binding activity of receptor

Laboratory	Observation	Target	Year	Reference
Munck	Cortisol uptake is dependent on ATP level.	Thymocyte	1968	28,29
Liao	DNP & CN$^-$ inhibit nuclear binding of DHT.	Prostate	1969	1,18
Aronow	Energy-dependent regeneration of GR.	L-cell	1972	13
Liao	ATP enhances receptor binding of DHT.	Prostate	1975	22
Toft	Nucleotides affect PR transformation.	Oviduct	1975	24
Toft	PR interacts with ATP-Sepharose	Oviduct	1975	38
Pratt	Inactivation of GR by alk. phosphatase.	L-cell	1977	30,31
Toft	MoO$_4^-$ blocks PR transformation.	Oviduct	1979	39
Pratt	Reactivation of GR by ATP, DTT, & a heat stable cellular factor.	L-cell & Thymocyte	1979	33,34

GR: glucocorticoid receptor
PR: progestin receptor

receptor protein may be dependent on an energy-requiring receptor activation process.

As summarized in Table 1, the energy-dependent control of receptor binding of steroids has been the concern of several investigators during the last ten years. In 1968, Munck and his associates (28) showed, by adjusting the glucose and oxygen in the culture medium, that the extent of cortisol uptake by thymocytes was correlated with the ATP level in the cells. In 1972, they also suggested that ATP may be involved in the transformation of an inactive receptor protein to the glucocorticoid-binding form (29). Working with L-cells, Ishii et al. (13) reached a similar conclusion.

Subsequently, we were able to show that ATP and GTP at 1-5 mM can enhance the DHT-binding activity of the cytosol receptor fraction prepared from the rat ventral prostate. These nucleoside triphosphates can stabilize the DHT-receptor complex at 20°C and can shift the sedimentation coefficient of the receptor complex (22). Toft et al. (38) also demonstrated that the chick oviduct progesterone-receptor complex, if activated to the nuclear form, can bind to ATP covalently linked to Sepharose. They also found (24) that the rate of activation of the progesterone-bound receptor to the nuclear form is itself inhibited by low concentrations (0.01-1 mM) of various nucleoside triphosphates. At high concentrations, however, these nucleotides stimulated such activation.

More recently, Pratt and his associates (30,31) were able to show that the glucocorticoid receptor from L-cells or thymocytes which were not bound to a glucocorticoid could be inactivated by a mechanism that may involve dephosphorylation. This inactivation could be prevented by a phosphatase inhibitor, such as molybdate. They also succeeded in reactivating the inactive form by incubation with ATP in the presence of DTT and a heat stable factor prepared from the thymocytes, L-cells or liver (33,34). According to Toft, however, molybdate can also inhibit the transformation of the chick progesterone-receptor complex to the form that can be retained by the nuclei (39). These studies strongly support the view that a phosphorylation process is required to maintain the steroid-binding form of the receptor, but that a dephosphorylation process may be needed before the steroid-receptor complex can be retained by the target cell nuclei.

The same mechanism may exist in rat prostate for the androgen receptor. We have been able to use molybdate to stabilize the DHT binding activity of the prostate cytosol receptor and also to inhibit the nuclear retention of DHT-receptor complex in a cell-free system or during incubation of minced prostate (11,32). It should be emphasized that no direct evidence is available at present to show whether the suggested phosphorylation or dephosphorylation process directly involves the receptor proteins or other closely related molecules in the receptor preparations.

INHIBITORS OF RNA SYNTHESIS

We also employed several inhibitors of RNA synthesis to determine whether the interaction of the androgen-receptor complex with nuclei is in any way related to RNA production. As summarized in Table 2, we studied the DHT-binding capacity of the receptor protein and the nuclear retention of the [^{3}H] DHT-receptor complex in a cell-free system and in a minced-tissue incubation system.

As Lohmar and Toft have reported for nuclear retention of the chick oviduct progesterone-receptor complex (25), we have found that rifamycins AF/05 and AF/013 at 30-100 µg/ml can prevent binding of the DHT-receptor complex to the prostate nuclei. Rifampicin was not inhibitory. Prior incubation of the DHT-receptor complex with the active rifamycins can potentiate the inhibitory activity of the drugs. This inhibition could also be seen when receptor binding to purified DNA was analyzed by gradient centrifugation or by DNA-cellulose column chromatography (21).

Actinomycin D at a concentration of 1 µg/ml enhanced the nuclear retention of the radioactive receptor complex by about 30% during the incubation of minced prostate with ^{3}H-DHT. The same level of actinomycin D inhibited [^{3}H]-uridine incorporation into RNA of minced prostate by 80%. The extent of increase in receptor retention by the nuclei was dependent on the concentration of actinomycin D in the incubation medium. At 20 µg/ml, the increase reached a plateau that was more than twice the value seen in the absence of actinomycin D. This enhancement could also be observed when the study was carried out in a cell-free system. Prior incubation of the antibiotic with the nuclei, but not with the receptor complex, enhanced the stimulatory effect of the antibiotic (32).

Actinomycin D can also influence the nuclear retention after the receptor complex has been allowed to bind to the nuclear chromatin. To show this, we incubated radioactive DHT with minced prostate to allow the complex to bind to chromatin. Actinomycin D was then added to the minced tissue and the incubation continued. Finally, nonradioactive DHT was added (to chase the radioactive complex) and the half-life of the radioactive complex determined. In the absence of actinomycin D the half-life of the complex with chromatin at 37° was about 60 minutes; however, the loss was completely prevented, if actinomycin D (1 µg/ml) was present (32).

Chloroquine inhibited the nuclear binding of the DHT-receptor complex. However, once the receptor complex was bound to chromatin, chloroquine acted like actinomycin D and prevented the release of the receptor complex from chromatin. Although rifamycins, actinomycin D, and chloroquine can affect the nuclear retention of the receptor complex, these compounds do not appear to affect the DHT-binding capability of the receptor protein (32).

The fact that only the rifamycins (AF/ 05 and AF/013) which inhibit eukaryotic RNA polymerases, and not rifampicin, which inhibits only the bacterial RNA polymerases, can interfere with the nuclear retention of the progesterone–receptor complex or the DHT–receptor complex indicates that the nuclear steroid receptor complex is in some way involved in the process of RNA synthesis. However, rifamycin can bind nonspecifically to many proteins, and it is not clear whether these antibiotics actually can bind to the receptor protein itself or to other proteins that may be involved in promoting the association of the receptor complex with chromatin or DNA.

The stimulatory effect of actinomycin D on the nuclear retention of the receptor complex is similar to the effect observed by Horwitz and McGuire (12) and by Schoenberg and Clark (35). They reported that the loss of the estradiol–receptor complex from the nuclei of human breast cancer cells (MCF-7 line) and from the rat uterus can be prevented by actinomycin D. McGuire coined the term 'inhibition of the processing of the nuclear receptor', but Clark suggested that actinomycin D may simply prevent the nuclear DNA from degradation by nuclease associated with the nuclear preparations. To check this possibility we used gradient centrifugation to analyze DNA recovered from minced prostate incubated with or without actinomycin D. The results showed that, under the conditions of our study, actinomycin D did not induce

TABLE 2. Effects of various compounds on receptor binding of DHT and nuclear retention of the DHT–receptor complex

Compound tested	Concentration	Receptor binding		Nuclear retention	
		Minced tissue	Cell-free	Minced tissue	Cell-free
KCN	1 mM	–	0	–	0
2,4-DNP	1 mM	–	0	–	0
Rifamycin AF/05	100 μg/ml	ND	0^a	0	–
Rifamycin AF/013	30 μg/ml	ND	0	0	–
Rifampicin	100 μg/ml	0	0	0	0
Actinomycin D	1 μg/ml	ND	0	+	+
Chloroquine	1 mM	0	0	–	+
Cycloheximide	10 μg/ml	ND	0	0	0^b
Na$_2$MoO$_4$	10 mM	0	+	–	–
Pyridoxal-P	1 mM	ND	0^c	ND	–

+: increased; –: decreased; 0: no difference; ND: not determined.
a: some aggregation of the receptor complex.
b: some aggregation of cell nuclei.
c: prevented aggregation of the receptor complex.

gross changes in the size of the DNA in the prostate cell nuclei. It is possible that actinomycin D binding to G in the duplex DNA causes a change in the local DNA protein structure in such a way that the actual receptor binding site is shifted or the binding property altered.

POLYRIBONUCLEOTIDE

Very little is known about the fate of the steroid–receptor complex after it plays its presumed role in promoting the synthesis of RNA. The nuclear receptor or the steroid may be modified in such a way that they do not bind to each other tightly, resulting in the release of the receptor from the genomic structure. In 1969, we suggested that RNA made in the nuclei may bind to the receptor complex and facilitate the release of the complex from the nuclei (Fig. 2). We proposed that the receptor complex, in turn, may play an important role in processing, stabilization, and/or utilization of RNA (18,23). Although direct evidence supporting this idea is still lacking, our studies have shown that both the estrogen- and androgen-receptor complexes can bind to certain ribonucleoprotein particles in the uterus and in the prostate (16,20,40,41).

Since the proposed scheme suggests that certain RNA molecules can promote the release of DHT-receptor complex from DNA or chromatin, we have tested this possibility by using DNA-cellulose column chromatography, gradient centrifugation, and nuclear incubation techniques (21).

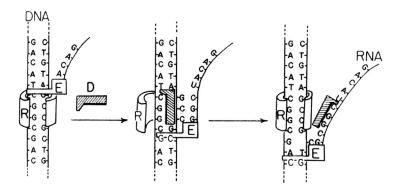

FIG. 2. A hypothetical model of hormone action on gene transcription. R: retarder; E: RNA-polymerase; D: hormone-bound (or modified) protein complex. From Liao and Fang (18).

The results of these investigations have indicated that certain polyribonucleotides can effectively release the DHT-receptor complex from DNA or nuclei. The capacity of the polyribonucleotides to facilitate this release is dependent on the type of nucleotide base and possibly on the size and secondary structure of the polymer. For example, with the DNA-cellulose chromatographic technique poly(G) and poly(U) were reasonably effective at 20 µg/ml, but a similar size of poly(U,G) was far more effective at 3 to 5 µg/ml. Poly(A) and poly(C) were totally inactive, even though they were able to bind to the receptor complex effectively if no other polymer was in the medium to compete with them. Since poly(C) could suppress the activity of poly(G), but not that of poly(U), whereas poly(A) inhibited the action of poly(U), but not that of poly(G), an unpaired base appeared to be needed for the effect. Homopolymers of X, 7-methyl-G, I, and 4-thio-U were as active as poly(U), indicating that the activity is dependent on the presence of an oxygen (or a sulfur atom) at C-6 of purines or C-4 of pyrimidines (21).

Polydeoxyribonucleotides were generally much less active than the ribopolymer counterparts, whereas various mononucleotides or oligo-nucleotides shorter than six base sequences were completely inactive. Except for aurintricarboxylic acid, which can effectively dissociate protein from nucleic acids, other acidic polymers that we have tested, including polyaspartic acid or polyglutamic acid, were far less active than poly(U,G) (U/G = 1,3, or 10) at the same weight concentrations.

We have carried out similar experiments with estrogen-receptor complex from rat uterus and with glucocorticoid-receptor complex from rat liver and found that these steroid-receptor complexes behaved in similar ways as the DHT-receptor complex of rat ventral prostate. Although we have not been able to detect a differential receptor specificity in these experiments, it is conceivable that there are certain natural RNA molecules with the proper nucleotide sequences which are much more effective than poly(U,G) in binding to the steroid-receptor complex and can exhibit high specificity toward different steroid-receptor complexes. In addition, different RNA molecules may contain identical or similar nucleotide sequences, so that more than one RNA species can be selected by the same steroid-receptor complex. Such a scheme may explain the selectivity and multiplicity observed in the induction of different proteins by steroid hormones (21).

PROTEIN

In 1971, we isolated a cytosol protein (named α-protein) from the rat ventral prostate which can interfere with the association of the prostate androgen-receptor complex with cell nuclei or chromatin (8). Subsequently other investigators reported the existence of similar inhibitors in the cytosol of the rat uterus (4), chick oviduct (3), rat liver (27), and rat hepatoma cells (37). In some of these experimental systems, the inhibition was not considered to be a specific phenomenon since bovine serum albumin also shows inhibitory activity. In the prostate (6,36) and hepatic cell system (27,37), however,evidence for specificity has been presented.

The prostate inhibitor, has been purified (6,8, 36). It is a major protein in the cytosol and in the secretory fluid of the prostate and is apparently identical to the "prostatein" of Lea et al. (15), the "prostate-binding protein" of Heyns and DeMoor (10), and the estramustine binding protein of Forsgren et al. (9). The protein binds various sex steroids (androgens, estrogens, and progestins) well, but does not bind glucocorticoids.

To show inhibition a prostate α-protein fraction is mixed with the androgen receptor complex prior to adding prostate cell nuclei. The inhibitor did not appear to cause irreversible destruction of the receptor complex or damage to the nuclear binding site; the nuclei or the receptor complex incubated with the inhibitor had the same binding capacity and ability to respond to inhibitor as did the preparations incubated in the absence of the inhibitor (36).

Besides acting as an inhibitor, α-protein can promote the release of the androgen-receptor complex already attached to chromatin. To show this, we first allowed the radioactive receptor complex to bind to prostate nuclei. The nuclei were then washed to remove the excess receptor complex and were incubated again either with or without the inhibitor. At a low concentration of the inhibitor, a significant loss of radioactivity occurred at 20°C, but not a 0°C. At a high concentration of the inhibitor, the release of radioactivity from the chromatin was evident even at 0°C, but was more obvious at 20°C. Without the inhibitor, there was no temperature-dependent loss of radioactivity from the chromatin. By gradient centrifugation, we found that all radioactivity released from the nuclei was associated with protein that sedimented as 3S (36).

α-Protein has two major subunits, A and B, each with two subcom-ponents. We have found that only the acidic subunit (A) is active at low concentrations. A smaller subcomponent (MW:9000; designated as component I) of subunit A appears to be responsibile for the activity (6). This component has a high acidic amino acid content. The acidic nature of the protein may be, in part, responsible for its modulating action.

Since α-protein, is a secretory protein, and since castration can cause a rapid loss of the membrane structure of the endoplasmic the reticulum of the prostate (18), the androgen-induced increase in the synthesis of this protein may be dependent on the general reconstruc-tion of the cytoplasmic organelles. Such a protein (or one of its components) may be ideal in communicating with the genome about the status of the cytoplasmic reconstruction by acting as a modulator in the interaction of chromatin with the steroid-receptor complex. Although there is no evidence at present to prove that α-protein is a modulator in the intact prostate cell, the possibility that certain protein factors may play such a role should be investigated further.

CONCLUDING REMARKS

Fig. 3 shows our working model for the steps involved in intracellular cycling of the androgen receptor in target cells. In this hypothetical model, the receptor protein (R^0) is activated by an energy-dependent process that is sensitive to respiratory poisons such as CN^-, azide, and DNP. The activated receptor (R) then binds an active androgen (A) such as DHT that may be formed from a precursor like testosterone (A^0). The androgen-receptor complex (AR) is transformed by a temperature-dependent step to the form AR^*, which can be retained tightly by chromatin. The stability of AR (or its transformation) can be affected by ATP and/or MoO_4^{--}. The nuclear retention of AR^* can be inhibited by MoO_4^{--}, pyridoxal phosphate, rifamycins, and chloroquine. The nuclear AR^* appears to have a half life of about 60 to 90 minutes. The release of AR^* may be promoted by certain RNA, but can be inhibited by chloroquine or actinomycin D. Whether the released AR^* is recycled, inactivated, or degraded has not been clearly determined.

The chromatin-receptor interaction presumably causes an increase in the synthesis of certain RNA. The RNA may then be bound and stabilized by the receptor complex, processed, and utilized in the

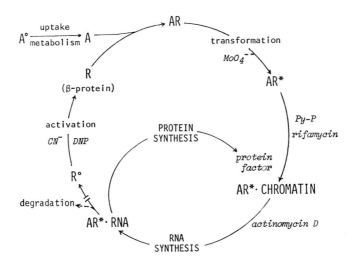

FIG. 3. A hypothetical view of the intracellular pathway of the androgen receptor in the rat ventral prostate. See text for explanation.

synthesis of specific key proteins necessary for the early responses and functions of the target cells (c.f. 17,26). As the hormonal responses of the target cells reach a plateau, certain protein factors produced by the late responses may play a modulatory role by interacting with the receptor protein or chromatin and suppressing the receptor action in the nuclei.

The experimental support for this speculative model is still very fragmentary. For example, it is not clear whether the transformation and changes in binding activities are due to the direct alteration of the receptor protein itself or to other factors that may associate with or act upon the receptor protein. A clear understanding of the phenomena and a more definite delineation of the intracellular pathway of the receptor may be possible only after the functionally definable form of the receptor protein is identified.

ACKNOWLEDGMENTS

We thank Ms. Stephanie Smythe, Ms. Karen Schilling, and Ms. Amy Oberhauser for their skillful technical assistance in carrying out some of the experiments described in this article. We are also grateful to Drs. John C. Babcock and Allan J. Campbell of the Upjohn Company, Michigan, U.S.A. for kindly supplying various synthetic steroids and to Dr. Giancarlo Lancini of Gruppo Lepetit, Milano, Italy for generously sending rifamycins and rifampicin for our studies. The work described in this article was supported by Grant BC-151 from the American Cancer Society, Research Grant AM-09461, and Training Grant CA-09183 from the U.S. National Institutes of Health.

REFERENCES

1. Anderson, K. M. (1969): Thesis, University of Chicago.
2. Anderson, K. M., and Liao, S. (1968): Nature, 219:277-279.
3. Buller, R. E., Schrader, W. T., and O'Malley, B. W. (1975): J. Biol. Chem., 250:809-818.
4. Chamness, G. C., Jennings, A. W., and McGuire, W. L. (1974): Biochemistry, 13:327-331.
5. Chan, K.M.B., Smythe, S., and Liao, S. (1979): J. Steroid Biochem., 11:1193-1196.
6. Chen, C., Hiipakka, R. A., and Liao, S. (1979): J. Steroid Biochemistry, 11:401-405.
7. Fang, S., Anderson, K. M., and Liao, S. (1969): J. Biol. Chem. 244:6584-6595.
8. Fang, S., and Liao, S. (1971): J. Biol. Chem., 246:16-24.
9. Forsgren, B., Bjork, P., Carlstrom, K., Gustafsson, J., Pousette, A., and Hogberg, B. (1979): Proc. Natl. Acad. Sci. U.S.A., 76:3149-3153.
10. Heyns, W., Peeters, B., Mous, J., Rombauts, W., and DeMoor,P. (1978): Eur. J. Biochem., 89:181-186.

11. Hiipakka, R. A., and Liao, S. (in preparation).
12. Howitz, K. B., and McGuire, W. L. (1978): J. Biol. Chem., 253:6319-6322.
13. Ishii, D. N., Pratt, W. B., and Aronow, L. (1972): Biochemistry, 11:3896-3904.
14. Jensen, E. V. (1977): Research on Steroids, 7:1-36.
15. Lea,O. A., Petrusz, P., and French, F. S. (1979): J. Biol. Chem., 254:6196-6202.
16. Liang, T., and Liao, S. (1974): J. Biol. Chem., 249:4671-4678.
17. Liang, T., Mezzetti, G., Chen, C., and Liao, S. (1978): Biochem. Biophys. Acta, 542:430-441.
18. Liao, S., and Fang, S. (1969): Vitam. Horm. (New York), 27:17-90.
19. Liao, S., Liang, T., Fang, S, Castaneda, E., and Shao, T. C. (1973): J. Biol. Chem., 248:6154-6162.
20. Liao, S., Liang, T., and Tymoczko, J. L. (1973): Nature, New Biol., 241:211-213.
21. Liao, S., Smythe, S., Hiipakka, R. A., and Tymoczko, J. L. (in preparation).
22. Liao, S., Tymoczko, J. L., Castaneda, E., and Liang, T. (1975): Vitam. Horm. (New York), 33:297-317.
23. Liao, S., Tymoczko, J. L., Howell, D. K., Lin, A. H., Shao, T. C., and Liang, T. (1972): Proc. 4th Intl. Congr. Endocrinol. Excerpta Medica Int. Congr. Ser. No. 273:404-407.
24. Lohmar, P., and Toft, D. O. (1975): Endocrinology, 96:(Supplement) abstract No. 25.
25. Lohmar, P., and Toft, D. O. (1975): Biochem. Biophys. Res. Commun., 67:8-15.
26. Mezzetti, G., Loor, R., and Liao, S. (1979): Biochem. J. (in press).
27. Milgrom, E., and Atger, M. (1975): J. Steroid Biochem., 6:487-492.
28. Munck, A., and Brinck-Johnsen, T. (1968): J. Biol. Chem., 243:5556-5565.
29. Munck, A., Wira, C., Young, D. A.,Mosher, K. M., Hallahan, C., and Bell, P. A. (1972): J. Steroid Biochem., 3:567-578.
30. Nielsen, C.J., Sando, J. J., and Pratt, W. B. (1977): Proc. Natl. Acad. Sci. U.S.A., 74:1398-1402.
31. Nielsen, C. J., Sando, J. J., Vogel, W. M., and Pratt, W. B. (1977): J. Biol. Chem., 252:7568-7578.
32. Rossini, G. P., and Liao, S. (in preparation).
33. Sando, J. J., Hammond, N. D., Stratford, C. A., and Pratt, W. B. (1979). J. Biol. Chem., 254:4779-4789.
34. Sando, J. J., LaForest, A. C., and Pratt, W. B. (1979): J. Biol. Chem., 254:4772-4778.
35. Schoenberg, D. R., and Clark, J. H. (1979): J. Biol. Chem., 254:8270-8275.
36. Shyr, C., and Liao, S. (1978): Proc. Natl. Acad. Sci. U.S.A., 75:5969-5973.
37. Simons, S. S., Martinez, H. M., Garcea, R. L., Baxter, J. D., and Tomkins, G. M. (1976): J. Biol. Chem., 251:334-343.

38. Toft, D. O., Lohmar, P., Miller, J., and Moudgil, V. (1976): J. Steroid Biochem., 7:1053-1059.
39. Toft, D. O., Roberts, P. E., Nishigori, H., and Moudgil, V.K. (1979): In: Steroid Hormone Receptor Systems (Leavitt, W. W., and Clark, J. H., eds.) Plenum Press.
40. Tymoczko, J. L. (1974): Thesis, University of Chicago.
41. Tymoczko, J. L., and Liao, S. (1971): Biochim. Biophys. Acta, 252:607-611.

Perspectives in Steroid Receptor Research,
edited by F. Bresciani.
Raven Press, New York © 1980.

Activation and DNA Binding of the Glucocorticoid Receptor

Gerald Litwack, *Thomas J. Schmidt, **Radmila D. Marković,
†Howard J. Eisen, ‡Carol A. Barnett, *Denis M. DiSorbo,
and ¶David S. Phelps

*Fels Research Institute and Department of Biochemistry, Temple University School of
Medicine, Philadelphia, Pennsylvania 19140, U.S.A.; and †National Institute of Child
Health and Human Development, National Institutes of Health,
Bethesda, Maryland 20205, U.S.A.*

The concept of an "activation" step in steroid hormone action originated primarily from the results of in vitro studies and until very recently it has been considered as a test tube phenomenon. In these original studies receptors could be extracted from tissues in a form which did not bind to isolated cell nuclei or to DNA. Since this binding capacity could be developed by heating or other treatments, the change in steroid-receptor complexes resulting from these treatments was considered as "activation." Early studies by Jensen and Gorski in 1968 described the in vitro conversion of uterine estrogen receptor complex from a 4S to a 5S form which was thought to be at least part of an activation step (19,22). Our own work in 1963 on the subcellular distribution of radioactive cortisol in the rat actually contained data suggesting nuclear translocation in vivo (32) but we did not appreciate the significance of these results at that time (Fig. 1). Subsequently, a number of laboratories demonstrated that heat, high salt concentration, dilution, gel filtration and specific chemicals (1,2,7,18,20,23,38) could stimulate the rate of activation in vitro. Later, the evidence for nuclear translocation in cell

Supported by Research Grants AM 13531 from the National Institute of Arthritis, Metabolism and Digestive Diseases, AG 00931 from the National Institute of Aging, PCM 78-25767 from the National Science Foundation and CA 12227 from the National Cancer Institute to the Fels Research Institute.

*Trainee on Training Grant T32 AM 07162 from the National Institute of Arthritis, Metabolism and Digestive Diseases to the Department of Biochemistry, Temple University, School of Medicine.

**Present address: Department of Biochemistry and Molecular Biology, University of Belgrade, Yugoslavia.

‡Present address: Department of Biology, San Diego State University, San Diego, California.

¶Graduate student of the Department of Anatomy, Temple University School of Medicine.

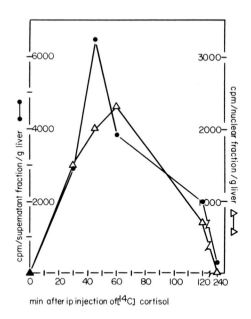

FIG. 1.   Data (1963) recalculated from (32)
showing evidence of nuclear translocation of
cortisol radioactivity.   The peak of nuclear
radioactivity occurs 15 min after the peak of
total cytosolic radioactivity.

cultures was developed without providing much information for an
activation step.   Even until very recently, many investigators
assumed that because receptor complexes are very rapidly activated
in vitro at the temperature of the cell, the only requirement in
the cellular milieu for activation was the availability of the
steroid ligand.   As a consequence of this assumption, activation
did not have to be considered as a discrete step.   Our own decision to study the activation mechanism was made on the basis that
it was a property of receptor complexes amenable to biochemical
analysis; whether there would be physiological significance to
"activation" was uncertain.

    Our experiments concerning activation of glucocorticoid recep-
tors developed rapidly and in several directions.   A small molecule was demonstrated in liver cell cytosol and was called "modulator."   This micromolecule seems to bind to activated receptor
complexes, prevents nuclear translocation and is released by conditions which lead to activation in vitro (6,18,25).   This component and its release from receptor could be implicated as part of
the activation step.   In addition we have approached the nature of
the activated complex, compared to the unactivated complex, using
chemical probes.   These experiments suggest that as a result of activation, certain functional groups which may mediate binding to

DNA emerge on the surface of receptor. After development of a
method to rapidly separate unactivated and activated receptor
complexes (46), the time course of activation in liver and kidney
cytosols either in vitro or following injection of labeled glucocorticoids could be studied. These experiments tell us much about
the molecular forms of glucocorticoid receptors and provide a basis for examining the activities of stimulating and inhibiting
agents which in turn lead to speculations on the molecular mecha-
nism(s) of the activation process. In this communication we summarize these approaches to understanding the mechanism of glucocorticoid receptor activation. Although activation was once considered as primarily an in vitro phenomenon, very recent experiments in Munck's laboratory (40) and in our own (36) indicate that
"activation" actually has physiological significance.

MODULATOR, A MICROMOLECULAR INHIBITOR IN CYTOSOL

The presence of a substance in liver cytosol which inhibited
the translocation of the glucocorticoid receptor to the nucleus
was reported in 1975 (37). Subsequently, indirect evidence from
another laboratory concluded that this inhibitor was a macromolecule, probably a protein (54). Our laboratory was hard at work
on a cytosolic inhibitor of the overall activation process which
was measured by the ability of the activated receptor complex to
bind to DNA or nuclei (6). Gel filtration columns preequilibrated
with buffer were overloaded with cytosol containing the [^{3}H]ster-
oid receptor complex in the unactivated form. In the eluates,
DNA-binding ability was a characteristic of macromolecules which
were the most well-separated from small molecules. As the uniform
concentration of macromolecules moved into contact with small molecules the ability of steroid-receptor complexes to bind to DNA
diminished to zero proportionately to the increased levels of
micromolecules. If the column was first preequilibrated with
small molecules isolated from liver cytosol prior to repeating the
experiment, then subsequently steroid-receptor complexes were in
contact with micromolecules throughout the chromatogram and failed
to bind to DNA (6). In subsequent experiments the low molecular
weight component was shown to be partially heat stable, adsorbed
to DEAE-Sephadex but not to CM-Sephadex, inactive as a substrate
for various peptidases and to be included in various gel filtration media. The last property led to an estimate of a molecular
weight of less than 1500 (6). This low molecular weight factor
was named "modulator." Further experiments with activation by gel
filtration have shown that tris buffer is far more effective than
borate buffer suggesting that tris may compete for the putative
binding between receptor and modulator which may involve formation
of a Schiff base (B.C. Sekula, T.J. Schmidt and G. Litwack, unpublished experiments). Separate experiments in this laboratory
have shown that tris buffer and certain other primary amines increase the rate of activation of the cytosolic glucocorticoid receptor at low temperatures and this activity seems to be related
to the activity of these substances to form Schiff bases (18,45).
Thus it seems possible that amines like tris may compete for

binding of modulator to receptor and make it easier to dislodge
modulator and include it during gel filtration. These earlier
column overload experiments have been repeated and separation of
activated and unactivated receptor complexes by chromatography on
DEAE cellulose has clearly demonstrated that low molecular weight
modulator actually blocks the activation step (B.C. Sekula, unpublished results). This redefined role of modulator clearly distinguishes it from pyridoxal phosphate, which inhibits previously
activated glucocorticoid-receptor complexes (5). The characteristic of Schiff base formation by pyridoxal-P has been used to
probe the appearance of lysine residues following activation. Attempts to measure the binding constant of the interaction of glucocorticoid receptor and pyridoxal-P have yielded values in the
millimolar range (K.P.Dolan, unpublished experiments). Such a
range of values would be inconsistent with the identity of endogenous inhibitor of the activated form and pyridoxal-P since the
total coenzyme is concentrated in liver cytosol to about 40 µM (4).
However, there are some problems inherent in this measurement of
the apparent binding constant. For this measurement cytosolic glucocorticoid receptor complex was used and DNA binding ability of
the activated receptor complex was measured as a function of pyridoxal-P concentration. Virtually all of the pyridoxal-P added exog-
enously appears to be bound in imine form to various proteins having lysine side chains. In consequence the concentration of actual
"free" pyridoxal-P is probably vastly lower than the amount added
and the dissociation of these imine forms must occur to provide a
thermodynamic quantity available for binding to receptor. Thus
within the cell, the binding constant could be much smaller than
has been estimated by in vitro experiments. Not until there are
reactant quantities of native purified activated glucocorticoid
receptor complexes available can the true binding constant be
measured. Attempts are currently underway in this laboratory to
characterize and identify modulator.

The role of pyridoxal-P appears to involve binding exclusively
to the activated form of the glucocorticoid receptor complex. This
conclusion was derived from a study of the inhibition of binding
or receptor complexes to DNA or cell nuclei by pyridoxal-P. The
inhibition of DNA binding by pyridoxal-P was competitive with respect to DNA concentration confirming that the DNA binding site of
the activated receptor complex interacts with pyridoxal-P (5).
These kinetics predict that pyridoxal-P should elute the steroid
receptor complexes bound to DNA, which proved to be the case (14,
25). The elution activity showed the same specificity as the inhibition of DNA binding--namely that the 4-aldehyde group was required (to form a Schiff base) and the presence of a phosphate
group increased the effectiveness of elution (5). Thus one could
speculate that since pyridoxal-P has been shown to occur in the
cell nucleus (4) it could be involved somehow as an off-signal resulting in the detachment of steroid-receptor complex from chromatin (providing receptor actually interacts with DNA). In this
connection, Liao has demonstrated a protein factor which prevents

binding or releases androgen receptor already bound to chromatin (53) and it would be interesting to learn whether this factor is a pyridoxal-P binding protein. Impetus is added to the attractiveness of pyridoxal-P as an endogenous inhibitor by the fact that pyridoxine deficient rats adrenalectomized for 3-6 days yield liver cytosols which are strikingly more efficient in the binding of steroid-receptor complexes to DNA or normal cell nuclei than are similar cytosols prepared from normal controls or deficient animals treated with pyridoxine (11).

The fact that pyridoxal-P interacts with the activated receptor complex and not with the unactivated complex is well supported by experimental evidence (5). In addition, the activated form bound with pyridoxal-P and reduced with sodium borohydride maintains the approximate position of an activated steroid-receptor complex although it is slightly more acidic (Fig. 2). Thus binding of pyridoxal-P does not convert activated receptor-complexes to the unactivated form as determined by elution from DEAE-Sephadex. This

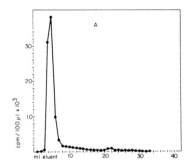
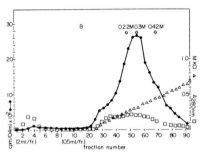

FIG. 2. Effect of pyridoxal-P on activated liver cytosol glucocorticoid receptor after reduction with sodium borohydride. A. Rat liver cytosol was incubated with 30 nM [^{3}H]tramcinolone acetonide (0°, 2 hr); pyridoxal-P (10 mM) is added at pH 7.6 and the mixture activated (25°, 30 min). After cooling to 4°, NaBH$_4$ (5 mM) was incubated (4°, 15 min). This mixture was chromatographed on a Sephadex G-25 column (1.4 x 10 cm) in tris buffer, pH 7.6. B. Macromolecules pooled from fractions of 4 and 5 in A were applied (0.5 ml) to a DEAE-Sephadex A-50 minocolumn (as in Fig. 4) and eluted in 20 mM phosphate buffer, pH 6.8 with a KCl gradient. In similar chromatograms unactivated receptor elutes at 0.4-0.42 M KCl and activated form at 0.22 M (arrows).

more acidic elution position would be expected in view of the fact that one or more ionizable ε-NH$_2$ groups of lysine would be neutralized in the linkage with the coenzyme and an ionizable phosphate group of the coenzyme would either neutralize additional potential positively charged groups on the receptor's surface or would be free to ionize itself. Thus both modulator, which blocks activation, and a potential endogenous inhibitor of the activated complexes regulate the activity of glucocorticoid receptors. It would be very interesting if endogenous inhibitor of activated complexes proves to be pyridoxal-P, since many of the proteins induced by glucocorticoids also contain pyridoxal-P (30,33).

USE OF CHEMICAL PROBES TO STUDY ACTIVATION

In spite of the fact that highly purified glucocorticoid receptor is unavailable in reactant quantities, we decided to test the activities of several chemical probes whose specificities for active groups on protein surfaces are well known. Both specific steroid binding and DNA binding of specifically bound glucocorticoid were measured to determine whether these particular chemical probes blocked either function of the glucocorticoid receptor. Since these measurements were performed with liver cytosol, a change in the activities of the receptor could result by (1) direct interaction of the probe in the active center, (2) direct interaction of the probe at a distant site on the receptor leading to a change in the specific activity by an allosterically induced conformational change, or (3) the probe could have reacted with another molecule which acted secondarily on receptor to produce the observed changes in receptor functions. Even with these alternative or multiple effects, these chemical probes could prove to be useful approaches to begin to explore the nature of the active sites on the surface of the receptor.

We used the following chemical probes: pyridoxal-5'-P for ε amino groups of lysine residues (5), 1,2-cyclohexanedione, for guanidino groups of arginyl residues (12,47) and both ethoxyformic anhydride and photooxidation with rose bengal to probe activity of histidine residues (8,15,60). The actions of pyridoxal-P have been shown to involve Schiff base formation and the structural specificity for this formation with pyridoxal-P analogs has been established. A summary of results in presented in Table 1.

TABLE 1. Summary of effects of specific chemical probes on activities of functional groups of the liver glucocorticoid receptor

Probe	Specificity	Effect on receptor function[a](5,12,13)
Pyridoxal-P (and pyridoxal)	ε Amino groups of lysine residue	Inhibits competitively the binding of activated complexes to DNA. At elevated temperatures increases rate of steroid dissociation
1,2-Cyclo-hexanedione	Guanidino group or arginine residue	Inhibits binding of activated receptor complex to DNA; at 100 mM inhibits ligand binding by 80% which can be prevented by high concentrations of steroid
Ethoxyformic anhydride & photo-oxidation with rose bengal	Histidine residue	Abolishes receptor binding to DNA; neither reagent affects steroid binding

[a]None of the effects reported are due to binding of reagent to DNA.

ACTIVATION MECHANISM STUDIED BY RAPID ION
EXCHANGE CHROMATOGRAPHY

Recently we have discussed a method to separate physically
unactivated and activated forms of the glucocorticoid receptor by
rapid ion exchange on minicolumns of DEAE-Sephadex A-50 (46). In
our previous work liver cytosols were prepared from adrenalectomized male rats 10 min after the intraperitoneal injection of [3H]-
corticosterone. Steroid and steroid metabolites bound to macromolecules were analyzed by long columns of DEAE-Sephadex A-50
requiring about 14 hr. Results of this kind of fractionation allowed the resolution and naming of binding proteins: Binder IA,
ligandin (29); Binder IB, a new receptor-like protein (31), Binder
II, the major liver cytosol glucocorticoid receptor (28); Binder
III, now known to consist of two proteins [IIIA, a new 31,000
molecular weight steroid anion binding protein (56) and IIIB, a
7000 molecular weight polypeptide in the somatomedin fraction (28)]
and IV, containing transcortin (28) (Fig. 3). Tentatively,

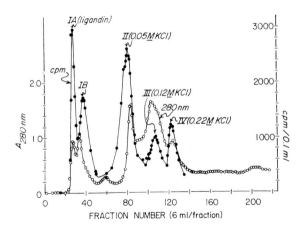

FIG. 3.   DEAE-Sephadex A-50 chromatogram of
[3H]corticosterone bound to macromolecules
10 min after i.p. ·injection of 300 μCi. Column is 3 x 76 cm. Ion exchange elution takes
about 14 hrs at 4°. (Reproduced from (28) by
permission of J. Biol. Chem.

mindful of the reservations cited above, the straightforward interpretation is that a group of positive charges, involved in an
electrostatic interaction with phosphate groups of DNA, emerges on
the surface of the steroid-receptor complex as a result of activation (5). In the case of pyridoxal-P, there is very little inhibition of DNA binding if pyridoxal-P is added to unactivated cytosol followed by reduction with sodium borohydride in the cold, and
the system subsequently activated at 25°. This result shows that
the pyridoxal-P binding site (of receptor) is unavailable for
interaction when receptor is in the unactivated form and becomes

available for interaction upon activation. When the receptor is
in the unactivated form pyridoxal-P must bind to other proteins
in the mixture and these nonspecific complexes are subsequently
reduced by sodium borohydride so that upon elevation of the temperature the coenzyme cannot dissociate from nonspecific protein
complexes and bind to the DNA binding site of the activated receptor. Similar results are obtained if binding to phosphocellulose in place of DNA is measured, leading to the conclusion that
the postulated group of positively charged amino acid residues
interacts with the phosphate groups of DNA. On the other hand,
ethidium bromide sensitive binding occurs with DNA but not with
phosphocellulose, leading to the conclusion that association of
activated receptor complex with DNA is not totally nonspecific
(5). Based on experiments with chemical probes, the group of
positively charged amino acid residues which becomes exposed as a
result of activation is composed minimally of lysine, arginine
and histidine residues. The method which separates unactivated
and activated forms of the glucocorticoid receptor is illustrated
in Figure 4. This minicolumn contains a plug of dextran-coated

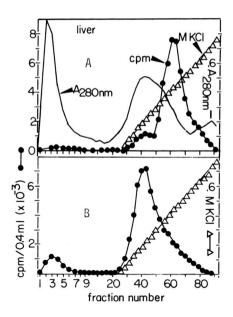

FIG. 4. Separation of unactivated, A, and
activated, B, of liver cytosol using DEAE-
Sephadex A-50 minicolumn (1.4 x 5 cm). All
peaks represent macromolecular bound steroid
because there is a plug of dextran-coated
charcoal at the bottom of the column. Unactivated receptor, A, elutes at 0.4 M KCl while
activated Binder II elutes at 0.2 M KCl and IB
in the buffer (20 mM phosphate buffer, pH 6.8)
as shown in B.

charcoal located at the bottom which removes all free steroid without affecting steroid bound to receptor protein which elutes with other proteins in high enough protein concentration to prevent adsorption (46). Although this procedure works for tissue cytosols, in experiments with cultured cells, where protein concentrations are often too low to use charcoal, charcoal is omitted from the column and macromolecules are prepared first by gel filtration on mini Sephadex G-25 columns. Although this latter procedure separates macromolecular from unbound steroid, it has the disadvantage of being unable to correct for the small amount of steroid dissociation occurring during the subsequent ion exchange process. Consequently, all peaks from tissue cytosols eluted in this procedure represent macromolecularly bound steroid. In the upper figure unactivated liver cytosol is chromatographed and is eluted at 0.4 M KCl. The lower figure shows that heat activation (25°, 30 min) prior to ion exchange chromatography causes the receptor complex to elute at 0.2 M KCl while Binder IB complex appears in the buffer wash (fractions 1-5). The major form has the characteristics of Binder II. Prebinding of activated cytosol to DNA or nuclei causes a pronounced reduction in activated (but not unactivated) peak chromatographed on DEAE-Sephadex. Both Binders II and IB bind to DNA but not all of the IB peak can be removed by this prebinding to DNA. This kind of analysis has been performed using cytosols prepared from several tissues of adrenalectomized rats including kidney (cortex and medulla), thymus, muscle and heart.

Confirmation of ion exchange chromatographic data has been achieved with Sepharose 4-B chromatography to which support anti rat liver Binder II has been attached. This antibody has been prepared in the rabbit to highly purified Binder II (16). Unactivated and activated Binder II are adsorbed by the antibody whereas IB is not. Of particular interest is the observation that the major activated receptor in kidney cortex resembles IB in elution position and Stokes radius (20-25 Å) and does not cross react with anti Binder II either in unactivated or activated form. Cytosolic systems from other tissues appear to resemble liver as summarized in Table 2. It appears that there are two major forms of glucocorticoid receptors. Binder II elutes in the activated form at 0.2 M KCl from DEAE-Sephadex and has a Stokes radius of about 60 Å. In former work (28) employing long ion exchange columns, Binder II was shown to elute at 0.05 M KCl (0.1 M salt if the buffer is included) and had a Stokes radius of 35 Å (26) and a molecular weight of 67,000 (28). The 5.1 S form of the cytosolic major glucocorticoid receptor has a calculated molecular weight of 78,000 (27), which is probably more accurate for Binder II because it is calculated from the Stokes radius and the S value whereas the 67,000 value was estimated directly from gel filtration experiments. The purified Binder II antigen isolated by Eisen (16) also has a molecular weight in the range of 75,000-80,000. Binder IB, which is eluted in the column wash of 20 mM buffer in the rapid ion exchange procedure, is also eluted in the buffer wash on long ion exchange columns just after ligandin

TABLE 2.   DEAE-Sephadex chromatography of activated glucocorticoid receptors recovered in cytosol preparations of various tissues[a]

Tissue cytosol	Binder II (% of total)	Binder IB (% of total)
Liver	90	10
Thymus	95	5
Brain	96	4
Heart	87	13
Kidney medulla	80	20
Muscle	67	33
Kidney cortex	9	91
Whole kidney	5	95

[a]In all of these experiments cytosols were labeled in vitro with 30-50 nM [³H]triamcinolone acetonide for 90 min at 0°. Ion exchange experiments were performed as described in Fig. 4. Pre-binding with DNA causes disappearance of activated Binder II and IB although not all of IB is removed by this procedure.

(pI 9:) (31). It has a Stokes radium of 20-25 Å when eluted in either column procedure. We plan to reisolate Binder IB and pre-pare antibodies directed against it.

The rapid ion exchange minicolumn technique has been em-ployed to study the binding of [³H]triamcinolone acetonide in liver and kidney cytosols from adrenalectomized rats at various times after intraperitoneal injection of 25 μCi (36).   In cytosols from either liver or kidney, unactivated complexes comprised 40-50 percent of the total radioactivity and the acti-vated complexes 30-40 percent in cytosols derived from animals injected 5 min earlier. With time, the percentage of unactivated complexes gradually declined while the activated complexes (IB and II) increased as shown in Table 3. At later times in this table there are sharp declines in the levels of the specific ac-tivated receptors, IB and II, in both tissues and this is assumed to result from translocation to the nucleus. It is to be noted that the unactivated forms of both liver and kidney reach peak concentrations before the activated receptors, IB and II. It is also evident that receptors in the IB position in liver are pres-ent in much greater concentration after injection of the radio-active hormone than after labeling of IB in vitro (see Table 2). In the latter case only about 10 percent of total labeling is in IB and 90% in II.

When unlabeled triamcinolone acetonide in the amount of 100-fold the injected mass was added to the homogenizing medium, sub-sequent analysis by rapid ion exchange chromatography indicated that the data were not altered significantly. This indicated that the level of detectable unactivated receptor was not the result of binding of free radioactive steroid during the preparation of cytosols.

TABLE 3. Time-course of distribution of activated and unactivated receptors in cytosols prepared from adrenalectomized rats injected with [^{3}H]triamcinolone acetonide

Time after injection (min)	Relative amounts of steroid receptors in chromatogram[a]					
	Liver			Kidney		
	Unactivated	Activated		Unactivated	Activated	
		IB	II		IB	II
5	416	182	160	494	42	37
10	1430	1254	589	--	--	--
15	599	2075	930	440	750	159
30	480	1980	2574	180	1352	293
60	5	175	40	74	525	99
120	10	28	40	33	370	29
240	3	16	8	12	275	45

[a]Value of the peak fraction in cpm of a specific receptor form x fractional amount of specific form of receptor (unactivated, IB or II) in chromatogram x 100.

These data indicate that the process of activation is indeed a physiological event. If the conversion of the unactivated to activated forms were an artifact of in vitro manipulation, there should be no time dependence observed, a result contradicted by the information in Table 3. Munck and Foley (40) have shown recently that a time course for the conversion of unactivated to activated receptor, corresponding to Binder II, occurs in thymus cells maintained under tissue culture conditions. In these experiments they used a rapid ion exchange (52) somewhat similar to our own. Our results with the whole animal agree well with the information from experiments in tissue culture and add new information about a second receptor, Binder IB, which has been shown to be a DNA-binding protein (35).

MODIFIERS OF IN VITRO ACTIVATION

Effects of Molybdate on Steroid Binding

Studies dealing with the effects of molybdate on the activation process stem from the original observations by Nielsen et al. (42, 43), concerning the protective effects of molybdate on the rapid inactivation of unbound glucocorticoid receptor in rat liver and L cell 100,000 x g supernatant fractions. These earlier studies indicated that the 100,000 x g particulate material from both rat liver and thymus contains a heat labile component, presumably an enzyme which is capable of inactivating the cytosolic glucocorticoid binding capacity. The observation that the effect of the liver particulate enzyme (0°C) could be blocked by fluoride suggested possible phosphatase activity. A proteolytic mechanism appeared unlikely since the particulate preparations did not rapidly digest radiolabeled protein under the same conditions. The observation that the unbound receptors in the 100,000 x g thymocyte supernatant fraction could be reactivated (50) also argued against a proteolytic mechanism. Although receptor inactivation in these studies was unaffected by a broad spectrum of phosphatase inhibitors, the particulate enzyme was inhibited by 10 mM molybdate, an anion that has been shown to be a potent inhibitor of phosphoprotein phosphatases (44,48) and acid phosphatases (55,58) in a number of systems. Since the action of the thymus particulate inactivating enzyme was not affected by either fluoride or molybdate, it was clear that there was a difference between the nature of the activity in the thymocyte and liver particulate preparations.

The possible inactivation (term used by these investigators to refer to loss of binding capacity) by a dephosphorylation mechanism was supported by subsequent studies by Nielsen et al. (41) which demonstrated that the binding capacity of the high speed supernatant fractions from L cells or rat liver could be inactivated by purified calf intestinal alkaline phosphatase which was devoid of proteolytic activity. Although these data suggested a possible role of a dephosphorylation process in controlling receptor binding, the potential target for this process was not identified. Nielsen et al. (41) hypothesized that either (a) the receptor protein itself could be inactivated by dephosphorylation or (b) a phosphorylated cofactor may be required for binding or (c) that a rather specific protease which is not inhibited by the routinely used inhibitors may be activated (increased activity) by a dephosphorylation mechanism.

However, despite these dramatic results obtained with alkaline phosphatase, several observations suggested that the endogenous receptor-inactivating activity is not due to alkaline phosphatase. First, the level of endogenous phosphatase activity found in the thymus 100,000 x g pellet was more than 3 orders of magnitude less than that required to inactivate the steroid-binding capacity with the calf intestinal enzyme (41). Secondly, the alkaline phosphatase activity, but not the receptor-inactivating effect of the thymus pellet was inhibited by levamisole, which is a potent inhibitor of alkaline phosphatases of non-intestinal origin (57). Finally, alkaline phosphatase was prepared from the rat liver 27,000 x g supernatant fraction. When this was incubated with the 100,000 x g rat liver cytosol no effect was observed, despite the fact that it contained 2.5 times the alkaline phosphatase activity present in the control incubation (which contained a resuspended liver pellet that completely inactivated the glucocorticoid binding capacity).

It is also important to briefly discuss the interaction between ATP, dithiothreitol and molybdate and the effects of the former two compounds on the ability of molybdate to restore (reactivation) glucocorticoid binding capacity. After thorough inactivation of L cell receptors by preincubation of the cytosol at 25°C for 4 hrs and prevention of further inactivation by addition of molybdate, addition of ATP (not ADP. GTP, CTP, UTP, or cyclic nucleotides) results in reactivation of steroid binding capacity

(51). Although maximal reactivation was achieved with 5 to 10 mM ATP, the free concentration of ATP in the presence of molybdate was probably much lower than 5 to 10 mM because of the known ability of molybdate to form phosphomolybdate complexes (44). These results argue against activation via a cyclic nucleotide-independent kinase and support the idea that L cell glucocorticoid receptors can be activated to the steroid binding state by an ATP-dependent phosphorylation mechanism. These same workers (49) have also demonstrated that addition of dithiothreitol to thymocyte receptors inactivated in the presence of molybdate allows total reactivation of the zero time binding capacity. They also found that if the binding capacity was inactivated by preincubation of the cytosol at 25°C, addition of ATP with dithiothreitol enhances the activation obtained with dithiothreitol alone. These data thus suggest that the stabilization and activation of steroid binding capacity in thymocytes requires phosphorylation as well as reduction of the receptor protein itself or some other component which is required for steroid binding.

Possible Role of Dephosphorylation in the In Vitro Activation
of Glucocorticoid Receptor-Complexes

In light of the reported effects of phosphatase inhibitors and exogenous calf intestinal alkaline phosphatase on unbound glucocorticoid receptors, we decided to investigate the effects of these reagents on the subsequent activation of rat liver receptor-complexes. First we studied the effects of several known phosphatase inhibitors on the activation step and employed binding to DNA-cellulose and alteration in elution profiles from DEAE-Sephadex and DEAE-cellulose to measure the extent of activation. Inhibitors such as molybdate (MoO_4) and tungstate (WO_4) were found to block heat (25°C, 30 min) activation as ascertained using the methods mentioned above. Addition of these compounds (10 mM final concentration) to previously heat activated complexes had no effect on the subsequent binding to DNA-cellulose or elution of activated complexes from DEAE-Sephadex or DEAE-cellulose. Unlike MoO_4 and WO_4, other phosphatase inhibitors such as fluoride, arsenate, and levamisole had no demonstrable effect on heat-induced activation of either rat liver or kidney glucocorticoid receptor-complexes. This latter result is not totally unexpected since it is well known that not all phosphatases are blocked by any one inhibitor (57). A third compound, sodium vanadate, which is also a potent phosphatase inhibitor (34) was shown to block the binding of heat activated receptor-complexes to DNA-cellulose while it exhibited no effect on the heat induced conversion of unactivated to activated complexes as chromatographed on DEAE-cellulose. Thus vanadate, which shares common physiochemical properties with molybdate and tungstate, appears to act (like pyridoxal phosphate) at a different step in the pathway of glucocorticoid hormone action.

The precise meshanism(s) by which molybdate (and tungstate) is inhibiting activation of glucocorticoid receptor complexes is at the present unknown. First, molybdate may inhibit directly

$$R^{P?} + S \underset{}{\overset{3}{\rightleftharpoons}} S\cdot R^{P?} \overset{4}{\longrightarrow} S\cdot R' + DNA \overset{5}{\longrightarrow} S\cdot R' - DNA$$

$$2 \Updownarrow 1$$

$$R$$
$$inactive$$

STEP	DEFINITION	COMPOUNDS WHICH AFFECT THIS PARTICULAR STEP	
		stimulate	inhibit
1	inactivation of unbound receptor	theophylline; PNP; PNPP	MoO_4; WO_4
2	reactivation of unbound receptor	ATP: MoO_4	
3	steroid binding to receptor		
4	activation of steroid-receptor complex	theophylline; PNP; PNPP	MoO_4; WO_4
5	binding of activated complexes to DNA		PALP; PAL; VO_3

FIG. 5. Effects of stimulators and inhibitors on glucocorticoid receptor activation: R-P? = putative phosphorylated receptor; S = steroid; R' = activated receptor. Each number corresponds to a discrete step in the mechanism. PNP = p-nitrophenol; PNPP – p-nitrophenylphosphate; PALP = pyridoxal-P and PAL = pyridoxal.

Speculative In Vitro Mechanism of Glucocorticoid Receptor Action

All of the approaches discussed in this manuscript have yielded information which is synthesized into a highly speculative mechanism of glucocorticoid receptor action presented in Figure 6. Starting from the left, free steroid binds to unliganded receptor to form an unactivated steroid-receptor complex. For reasons discussed in the previous section, this form of the receptor may have been phosphorylated in a reactivation step

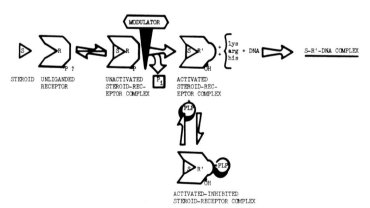

FIG. 6. A diagrammatic representation of a highly speculative activation mechanism. Abbreviations as in Figure 5. The putative role of endogenous modulator is shown.

which would follow release from the nucleus if this mechanism were functioning in the cell. Binding of steroid to receptor may result in a conformational change. If the unactivated receptor is phosphorylated, our evidence (see above) tentatively suggests that dephosphorylation could be the total activation event. This could be accomplished by a phosphoprotein phosphatase intimately associated with receptor or by an enzyme not associated with receptor but available in the cytosol. There is no evidence yet for the existence of such an enzyme. Activation would produce the appropriate conformational change to deliver a group of positively charged amino acid residues to the surface (or, alternatively, the unmasking of such a site without a conformational change) which would be active in electrostatic interaction with phosphate groups of DNA (5). As discussed earlier modulator has been redefined as a low molecular weight component(s) which actually block(s) the activation step. This redefined role of modulator clearly distinguishes this low molecular weight component from pyridoxal phosphate, which, as depicted in Figure 6, inhibits previously activated glucocorticoid-receptor complexes.

REFERENCES

1. Bailly, A., Savouret, J.F., Sallas, N., and Milgrom, E. (1978):Eur. J. Biochem., 88:623-632.
2. Baxter, J.D., Rousseau, G.G., Benson, M.L., Garcea, R.L., Ito, J., and Tomkins, G.M. (1973):Proc.Nat.Acad.Sci.(USA), 69:1892-1896.
3. Bond, J.S., Francis, S.H., and Park, J.H. (1970):J.Biol.Chem., 245:1041-1053.
4. Bosron, W.F., Veitch, R.L., Lumeng, L., and Li, T.-K. (1978): J.Biol.Chem., 253:1488-1492.
5. Cake, M.H., DiSorbo, D.M., and Litwack, G. (1978):J.Biol.Chem. 253:4886-4891.
6. Cake, M.H., Goidl, J.A., Parchman, G.L., and Litwack, G. (1976):Biochem.Biophys.Res.Commun., 71:45-52.
7. Cake, M.H. and Litwack, G. (1978):Eur.J.Biochem., 82:97-103.
8. Chang, G.-G., Hsu, R.Y. (1977):Biochim.Biophys.Acta, 483:228-235.
9. Cox, R.P. and Ponticorvo, G. (1961):Proc.Nat.Acad.Sci. (USA), 47:839-845.
10. Dayan, J. and Wilson, I.B. (1964):Biochim.Biophys.Acta, 81: 620-623.
11. DiSorbo, D.M. and Litwack, G. (1978):Proc.Endoc.Soc., Miami Beach, 60th Meeting, p. 131.

12. DiSorbo, D.M. and Litwack, G. (1978):Proc.Am.Assn.Cancer Res. 19:114.
13. DiSorbo, D.M., Phelps, D.S., and Litwack, G. (1979):Submitted.
14. Dolan, K.P. and Litwack, G. (1978):Proc.Endoc.Soc., Miami Beach, 60th Meeting, p. 308.
15. Ehrlich, R.S. and Colman, R.F. (1978):Eur.J.Biochem., 89: 575-587.
16. Eisen, H. J. (1979):Manuscript in preparation.
17. Fernley, H.N. (1971):In: The Enzymes, edited by P.D. Boyer, 4:417-447, Academic Press, N.Y., 3rd ed.
18. Goidl, J.A., Cake, M.H., Dolan, K.P., Parchman, L.G., and Litwack, G. (1977):Biochemistry, 16:2125-2130.
19. Gorski, J., Toft, D., Shyamala, G., Smith, D., and Notides, A. (1963):Rec.Prog. Horm.Res., 24:45-80.
20. Higgins, S.J., Rousseau, G.G., Baxter, J.D., and Tomkins, G.M. (1973):J.Biol.Chem., 248:5866-5872.
21. Jenner, H.D. and Kay, H.D. (1931):J.Biol.Chem., 93:733-746.
22. Jensen, E.V., Suzuki, T., Kawashima, T., Stumpf, W.E., Jungblut, P.W., and DeSombre, E.R. (1968):Proc.Nat.Acad.Sci. (USA), 59:632-638.
23. Kalimi, M., Colman, P., and Feigelson, P. (1975):J.Biol.Chem., 250:1080-1086.
24. Kato, Y. (1959):Develop.Biol., 1:477-510.
25. Litwack, G. (1979):In: Trends in Biochemical Sciences, in press.
26. Litwack, G. (1975):In: Advances in Enzyme Regulation, edited by G. Weber, 13:151-171, Pergamon Press, Oxford.
27. Litwack, G., Cake, M.H., Filler, R., and Taylor, K. (1978): Biochem.J., 169:445-448.
28. Litwack, G., Filler, R., Rosenfield, S., Lichtash, N., Wishman, C.A., and Singer, S. (1973):J.Biol.Chem., 248: 7481-7486.
29. Litwack, G., Ketterer, B., and Arias, I.M. (1971):Nature, 234:466-467.
30. Litwack, G. and Rosenfield, S.A. (1973):Biochem.Biophys.Res. Commun., 52:181-188.
31. Litwack, G. and Rosenfield, S. (1975):J.Biol.Chem., 250: 6799-6805.
32. Litwack, G., Sears, M.L., and Diamondstone, T.I. (1963): J.Biol.Chem., 238:302-305.
33. Litwack, G. and Singer, S. (1972):In: Biochemical Actions of Hormones, edited by G. Litwack, 2:114-165, Academic Press. New York.
34. Lopez, V., Stevens, T. and Lindquist, R.N. (1976):Arch. Biochem.Biophys., 175:31-38.
35. Markovic, R.D., Eisen, H.J., Parchman, L.G., and Litwack, G. (1979):Submitted.
36. Markovic, R.D. and Litwack, G. (1979):Submitted.
37. Milgrom, E. and Atger, M. (1975):J.Steroid Biochem., 6:487-492.
38. Milgrom, E., Atger, M., and Baulieu, E.E. (1973):Biochemistry, 12:5198-5205.

39. Moog, F. (1959):In: Cells, Organism and Milieu, edited by D. Rudnick, p. 129, Roland Press, N.Y.
40. Munck, A. and Foley, R. (1979):Nature, 278:752-754.
41. Nielsen, C.J., Sando, J.J., and Pratt, W.B. (1977):Proc. Nat. Acad.Sci. (USA), 74:1398-1402.
42. Nielsen, C.J., Sando. J.J., Vogel, M.W., and Pratt, W.B. (1977):J.Biol.Chem., 252:7568-7578.
43. Nielsen, C.J., Vogel, M.W., and Pratt, W.B. (1977):Cancer Res., 37:3420-3426.
44. Paigen, K. (1958):J.Biol.Chem., 233:388-394.
45. Parchman, L.G., Goidl, J.A., and Litwack, G. (1977):FEBS Lett. 79:25-28.
46. Parchman, L.G. and Iitwack, G. (1977):Arch.Biochem.Biophys., 183:374-382.
47. Patthy, L. and Smith, E.L. (1975):J.Biol.Chem., 250:557-564.
48. Roberts, R.M. and Bazar, F.W. (1976):Biochem.Biophys.Res. Comm, 68:450-455.
49. Sando, J.J., Hammond, A.C., Stratford, C.A., and Pratt, W.B. (1979):J.Biol.Chem., 254:4779-4789.
50. Sando, J.J., LaForest, A.C., and Pratt, W.B. (1979):J.Biol. Chem., 254:4772-4778.
51. Sando, J.J., Nielsen, C.J., and Pratt, W.B. (1977):J.Biol. Chem., 252:7579-7582.
52. Sakaue, Y. and Thompson, E.B. (1977):Biochem.Biophys.Res. Commun., 77:533-541.
53. Shyr, C.-I. and Liao, S. (1978):Proc.Nat.Acad.Sci. (USA), 75:5969-5973.
54. Simons, S.S., Jr., Martinez, H.M., Garcea, R.L., Baxter, J.D., and Tomkins, G.M. (1976):J.Biol.Chem., 251:334-343.
55. Spencer, D. (1954):Austral.J.Biol.Chem., 7:151-160.
56. Steeger, J. and Litwack, G. (1978):Fed.Proc., 37:1448.
57. Van Belle, H. (1972):Biochim.Biophys.Acta, 289:158-168.
58. Van Etten, R.L., Waymack, P.P., and Rehkop, D.M. (1974): J.Am.Chem.Soc., 96:6782-6785.
59. Weathers, B.J., Grate, J.H., and Schrauzer, G.N. (1979):J. Am.Chem.Soc., 101:917-924.
60. Westhead, E.W. (1965):Biochemistry, 4:2139-2144.
61. Wilson, I.B., Dayan, J., and Cyr, K. (1964):J.Biol.Chem., 239:4182-4185.
62. Wiseman, A. (1970):In: Handbook of Experimental Pharmacology, Springer-Verlag, N.Y.
63. Zittle, C.A., and Della Monica, E.S. (1950):Arch.Biochem. Biophys., 26:112-122.

Perspectives in Steroid Receptor Research,
edited by F. Bresciani.
Raven Press, New York © 1980.

In Vitro Inactivation of Estrogen Receptor by Nuclei of Estrogen Target Tissues

Ferdinando Auricchio, Antimo Migliaccio, Patrizia Sampaolo, and Andrea Rotondi

Institute of General Pathology, First Faculty of Medicine and Surgery, University of Naples, 80138 Naples, Italy

There is evidence, based mainly on studies with antiestrogens, that nuclear loss of estrogen receptor following its nuclear translocation is a pre-requisite for some hormonal responses, e.g. replenishment of cytosol estrogen-binding activity (1,2) and induction of progesterone receptor (3). This paper describes data on the mechanism responsible for nuclear loss of the receptor, a mechanism presently still unknown.

Using a cell free system we have found that nuclei of mouse uterus and mammary gland are endowed with an activity capable of very rapid inactivation of the 17β-estradiol binding activity of estrogen receptor. This inactivating activity has not been found in the nuclei of muscle and liver. The nuclear localization and the tissue specificity suggest that this activity could have a role in the "in vivo" nuclear turnover of estrogen receptor.

MATERIALS AND METHODS

Reagent grade materials were used in all experiments. Dithiothreitol, egg albumin, calf thymus and 17β-estradiol were obtained from Sigma Chemical Co., St. Louis, MO, U.S.A., Sephadex G-25 (coarse grade) and Blue Dextran were from Pharmacia Fine Chemicals, Uppsala, Sweden. 6,7 [3]H 17β-estradiol (60 Ci/mmol) and 2,4,6,7[^{3}H] 17β-estradiol (85 Ci/mmol) were from the Radiochemical Centre, Amersham, BUCKS, U.K.

BUFFER. The following buffer solutions were used: 10 mM Tris;

HCl, pH 7.4, containing 1 mM-EDTA and 1 mM dithiothreitol (TED-
-buffer) and TED-buffer added with 0.25 M sucrose (TED-sucrose
buffer).

Tissue homogenization and fractionation. Female Swiss mice
of about 30 gm were used. Tissues were mixed with 20 volumes of
cold TED-sucrose buffer and homogenized according to a previously
reported procedure (4). The 750 g pellet was obtained by centrifugation of homogenate at 2°C for 10 min. Cytosol was prepared
either from homogenate or from 750 g supernatant by centrifugation at 150.000 g for 45 min at 2°C in a L2-65 Spinco-Beckman ul-
tracentrifuge using a Ti 50 rotor. Nuclei were purified from the
750 g pellet as follows: the pellet was suspended in TED-sucrose
buffer, layered on top of 2.2 M sucrose and centrifuged at 160.000
g for 75 min at 2°C in a SW 41 Ti rotor. Nuclear extracts were
prepared from nuclei suspended in 2 ml of TED-buffer, slowly shaken at 0°C for 30 min, then sonicated with a 350 G sonifier (PBI
ultrasonics Ltd). Four bursts at power 10, tuning 2, were applied
lasting 15 s each at 1 min intervals. The sonicated sample was
centrifuged at 150.000 g for 10 min at 2°C and the supernatant
(called nuclear extract) utilized.

Preparation of cytosol and nuclear receptors. As estradiol-
-free receptor crude cytosol was used without addition of [3H]
-17β-estradiol. [3H] 17β-estradiol-cytosol receptor complex was
obtained by incubating cytosol with [3H]17β-estradiol (12x10^{-9}M)
alone (high specific activity [3H] 17β-estradiol) and in presence
of a 1000-fold excess of cold estradiol (low specific activity
3H 17β-estradiol) at 0°C for 2 hrs. [3H]17β-estradiol-nuclear
receptor complex was prepared as follows: 10-15 mice were injected intraperitoneally with 2 μg estradiol each and killed 1 hr
later. Uteri were homogenized in TED-sucrose buffer (1:10 by vol),
the 750 g pellet was sedimented and suspended in 2 ml TED-buffer.
The suspension was incubated with high and low specific activity
[3H]17β-estradiol at 0°C for 18 hrs in presence of 0.5 M NaSCN.
This procedure allows extraction of the receptor from the 750 g
pellet and exchange of the cold 17β-estradiol bound to the nuclear receptor with [3H]17β-estradiol (5). The suspension was
centrifuged at 150.000 g for 30 min and the supernatant was filtered through a 20 ml Sephadex G-25 column equilibrated with
TED-buffer to eliminate free hormone and NaSCN. Cold estradiol-
-nuclear receptor complex was prepared in the same way as [3H]17β
-estradiol-nuclear receptor complex, but using cold hormone in-

stead of $[^3H]$17β-estradiol.

Specific estrogen binding activity was determined as the difference between cytosol binding at 0°C for 2 hrs of high and low specific activity $[^3H]$17β-estradiol. Bound estradiol was separated from free hormone by treatment with dextran coated charcoal (1% Norit A, 0,01% T 70 dextran, 0,5% gelatine in TED-buffer).

Receptor inactivating experiments. To study the inactivation of estradiol-free cytosol receptor, samples including uterine homogenates, 750 g supernatants, cytosols, cytosols added with either 750 g pellets, nuclei or nuclear extracts were incubated, unless otherwise specified, at 25°C for the indicated times in absence of $[^3H]$17β-estradiol. The samples were cooled at 0°C immediately after the incubation; then cytosols were prepared from homogenates as well as from 750 g supernatants, or separated by centrifugation at 3200 g for 10 min at 4°C from 750 g pellets and from nuclei. Finally the specific estrogen binding activity of cytosols was assayed.

To study the inactivation of $[^3H]$17β-estradiol-cytosol receptor complex, uterine homogenates and cytosols were previously labelled at 0°C for 2 hrs with high and low specific activity $[^3H]$17β-estradiol. Then, when indicated, cytosols were added at 0°C with either nuclei or nuclear extracts or cold estradiol-nuclear receptor complex. All samples were incubated at 25°C and immediately cooled at 0°C. Then cytosols were prepared from homogenates or separated from nuclei by centrifugation at 3200 g at 4°C for 10 min. Finally cytosols were treated with dextran--coated charcoal and the specific estrogen binding activity measured.

For the study of $[^3H]$17β-estradiol-nuclear receptor complex inactivation, samples of this receptor were incubated at 25°C, then cooled at 0°C and treated with dextran-coated charcoal to measure the estrogen binding activity.

At the beginning of incubation at 25°C, 1×10^{-12} moles of cytosol or 1×10^{-13} moles of nuclear specific estrogen binding sites were present.

Radioactivity was measured in a Beckman liquid scintillation counter by the standard procedures (6), with an efficiency of 40%. Proteins and DNA were measured according to previously reported procedures (7 and 8) using egg albumin and calf thymus

DNA respectively as standards.

RESULTS

<u>Inactivation of estradiol-free cytosol receptor</u>: Fig. 1 shows the loss of specific estrogen binding activity in mouse uterine homogenate and in cytosol incubated at 25°C in TED-sucrose buffer (for details see Materials and Methods). The initial specific binding activity decreases in homogenate at a rate about 8 times faster than in cytosol. After 5 min the residual binding activity is 60 percent in homogenate and 95 percent in cytosol. These results averaged from five different experiments suggest that subcellular particles have a role in the fast inactivation of the receptor in homogenate.

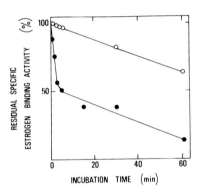

Fig. 1: Time dependent inactivation of estradiol-free receptor in homogenate and in cytosol. Uterus homogenate (●) and cytosol (○) in TED-sucrose buffer were incubated at 25°C for the indicated times, then cooled at 0°C and assayed for cytosol specific estrogen binding activity.

Fig. 2 shows the loss of specific estrogen binding activity of cytosol and homogenate after 5 min of incubation at different temperatures. Again a different behaviour is observed: the loss of activity in cytosol increases with increasing temperature, up to 35°C; in homogenate, the optimum of inactivation is 25°C. Thus, most inactivation in homogenate at 25°C cannot be attributed to heat denaturation; indeed, the optimum at 25°C suggests that an enzymic activity is involved in the inactivation. Therefore we have used 25°C for all subsequent inactivation experiments.

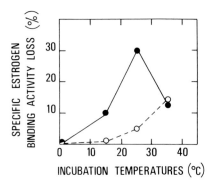

Fig. 2: Temperature dependent inactivation of estradiol-free receptor in cytosol and homogenate. Uterus homogenate (●) and cytosol (○) in TED-sucrose buffer were incubated at the indicated temperatures for 5 min, then cooled at 0°C and assayed for cytosol specific estrogen binding activity.

Fig. 3 shows that after 5 min of incubation at 25°C, the specific estrogen binding activity in the 750 g supernatant (bar B) is as stable as in cytosol (bar A) and much more stable than in homogenate (bar C). These results suggest that the ability of homogenate to inactivate estrogen receptor is in the 750 g pellet. This is reinforced by the finding that 5 min after addition of an equivalent amount of 750 g pellet to cytosol, the residual binding activity is considerably less (bar D) and is similar to that in homogenate (bar C).

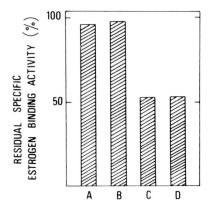

Fig. 3: Inactivation of estradiol-free receptor in: (A) uterus cytosol; (B) 750 g supernatant; (C) homogenate; and (D) cytosol added with an equivalent amount of 750 g pellet. The samples in TED-sucrose buffer were incubated at 25°C for 5 min, then cooled at 0°C and assayed for cytosol specific estrogen binding activity.

Nuclei with a DNA/protein ratio of about 0.4 were prepared from the 750 g pellet. Very little fibrillar contamination of such nuclei was observed under the microscope. Addition of purified nuclei to cytosol increases the inactivation rate of estrogen-free receptor (fig. 4). The nuclear ability to inactivate cytosol receptor can be completely extracted by using the procedure described in Materials and Methods. Indeed, addition of this extract to cytosol inactivates specific estrogen binding activity at a rate identical to that observed after addition of an equivalent amount of nuclei (not shown).

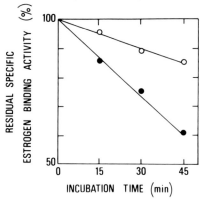

Fig. 4: Time dependent inactivation of estradiol-free receptor in absence and in presence of nuclei. Uterus cytosol in TED-sucrose buffer was incubated at 25°C in absence (O) and in presence (●) of nuclei (about 4 µg DNA/ml of incubation mixture), then cooled at 0°C and assayed for cytosol specific estrogen binding activity.

Inactivation of $[^3H]$ 17β-estradiol-cytosol receptor complex. Cytosols and homogenates were labelled for 2 hrs at 0°C with high and low specific activity $[^3H]$ 17β-estradiol before incubation at 25°C. In analogy with inactivation of estrogen-free receptor (fig. 1) the decrease of initial estrogen binding activity at 25°C is much faster in homogenate than in cytosol (fig. 5).

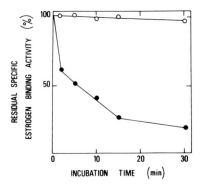

Fig. 5: Time dependent inactivation of $[^3H]$ 17β-estradiol-receptor complex in homogenate and in cytosol. Uterus homogenate (●) and cytosol (O) in TED-sucrose buffer previously labelled at 0°C for 2 hrs with high and low specific activity $[^3H]$17β-estradiol were incubated at 25°C for the indicated times, then cooled at 0°C and assayed for the cytosol specific estrogen binding activity.

The inactivation rate of cytosol specific estradiol binding activity is higher when nuclei are present (fig. 6), like in the case of estrogen-free cytosol receptor (fig. 4).

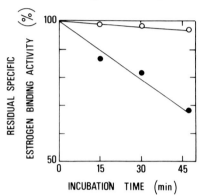

Fig. 6: Time dependent inactivation of $[^3H]$ 17β-estradiol-receptor complex in absence and in presence of nuclei. Uterus cytosol in TED-sucrose buffer previously labelled at 0°C for 2 hrs with high and low specific activity $[^3H]$ 17β-estradiol was incubated at 25°C for the indicated times in absence (○) and in presence (●) of nuclei (about 4 μg DNA/ml of incubation mixture). After cooling at 0°C the cytosol specific estrogen binding activity was assayed.

Table 1 shows the loss of cytosol specific estrogen binding activity after incubation at 25°C in presence of nuclei and nuclear extracts from different tissues. Nuclei from uterus and mammary gland, as well as nuclear extract from uterus, inactivate receptor; on the contrary, nuclei from liver and quadriceps muscle and nuclear extract from liver are totally ineffective.

Inactivation of $[^3H]$ 17β-estradiol-nuclear receptor complex: In the experiment shown in fig. 7, the stability at 25°C of the nuclear $[^3H]$ 17β-estradiol-receptor complex is compared with that of cytosol $[^3H]$ 17β-estradiol-receptor complex. The faster inactivation rate of the $[^3H]$ 17β-estradiol-nuclear receptor complex can be explained by presence of the inactivating system in the preparation of nuclear receptor. In fact, when nuclear receptor in a complex with cold estradiol is added to $[^3H]$ 17β-estradiol-bound cytosol receptor, the inactivation rate of the cytosol receptor increases (fig. 7).

TABLE 1: Inactivation of $[^3H]$ 17β-estradiol-cytosol receptor complex by nuclei and nuclear extracts from different tissues

	DNA/PROTEIN RATIO	DNA IN INCUBATION MIXTURE (μg/ml)	LOSS OF COMPLEX IN CYTOSOL (%)
UTERUS NUCLEI	.39	6.7	30
MAMMARY GLAND NUCLEI	.26	6.1	24
LIVER NUCLEI	.23	5.0	2
QUADRICEPS MUSCLE NUCLEI	.23	7.9	0
UTERUS NUCLEAR EXTRACT	--	--	30
LIVER NUCLEAR EXTRACT	--	--	0

Uterine cytosols were first labelled with high or low specific activity $[^3H]$ 17β-estradiol for 2 hrs at 0°C and then incubated in TED-sucrose buffer (pH 7.4) at 25°C for 20 min in absence (control) and in presence of either nuclei or nuclear extracts from different sources. The extracts were prepared from amounts of nuclei equal to those added as intact nuclei to cytosol. After incubation, cytosols incubated with nuclei were centrifuged at 3200 g to remove nuclei. Thereafter, cytosols were treated with charcoal and the specific estrogen binding activity assessed. A 6% inactivation of control was found and subtracted from the inactivation of cytosols added with nuclei or nuclear extracts. Values in table are averages from three different experiments.

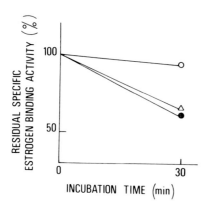

Fig. 7: Inactivation of uterus nuclear and cytosol estradiol receptors at 25°C. [³H]17β-estra- diol-nuclear receptor complex (●) and [³H]17β-estradiol-cytosol re- ceptor complex in absence (○) or in presence (△) of "cold" estra- diol-nuclear receptor complex.

DISCUSSION

A cell-free system for the study of nuclear inactivation of the receptor is now available. Experimentally, such a system of- fers obvious advantages over the intact cell system (1,2,3) and presumably further progress in our understanding of the mechanism of nuclear inactivation of receptor is at hand.

The results presented in this paper show that in this system, as in the case of intact cells, the receptor inactivating activi- ty resides in the nucleus. This analogy suggests that we are pro- bably dealing with the same mechanism in both cases.

This mechanism, furthermore, is shown to be specific in that it is found in nuclei of estrogen target tissues only.

Another promising result of this work is that the receptor inactivating activity can be quantitatively extracted from nuclei, a feature which should make it possible purification and charac- terization of the molecule(s) responsible for this activity. The temperature dependence of the nuclear activity suggests that this molecule is an enzyme(s).

CONCLUSIONS

The 17β-estradiol binding activity of mouse uterus disappears at a much faster rate in total homogenate than in cytosol during incubation at 25°C. Nuclei are responsible for the rapid loss of binding activity observed in homogenate. They inactivate the estrogen-free and estrogen-bound receptor of cytosol, as well as the nuclear receptor. This receptor inactivating activity is present in nuclei and nuclear extracts of estrogen target tissues, but not in nuclei and nuclear extracts of non-target tissues. We suggest that this activity has a role in the "in vivo" nuclear turnover of estrogen receptor.

ACKNOWLEDGMENTS

This research was supported by Progetto Finalizzato "CONTROLLO DELLA CRESCITA NEOPLASTICA" del Consiglio Nazionale delle Ricerche, Roma.

REFERENCES

1. Rochefort, H., Vignon, F. and Capony, F. (1972): Biochem. Biophys. Res. Commun. 47:662-670.
2. Clark, J.H., Anderson, J.N. and Peck, R.J. (1973): Steroids 22:707-718.
3. Horwitz, K.B. and McGuire, W. (1978): J. Biol. Chem. 253:8185-8191.
4. Rotondi, A. and Auricchio, F. (1979): Biochem. J. 178:581-587.
5. Sica, V., Puca, G.A., Molinari, A.M., Buonaguro, F.M. and Bresciani, F. (1980): Biochemistry 19:83-88.
6. Auricchio, F., Rotondi, A. and Bresciani, F. (1976): Molec. Cell. Endocrinol. 4:55-60.
7. Bradford, M.M. (1976): Analytical Biochem. 72:248-254.
8. Giles, K.W. and Meyers, A. (1965): Nature 206:93.

Perspectives in Steroid Receptor Research,
edited by F. Bresciani.
Raven Press, New York © 1980.

Two Binding Sites for Estradiol in Rat Uterine Nuclei: Relationship to Stimulation and Antagonism of Uterine Growth

Barry M. Markaverich, Susan Upchurch, and James H. Clark

Department of Cell Biology, Baylor College of Medicine, Houston, Texas 77030, U.S.A.

INTRODUCTION

A primary event in the mechanism of estrogen action appears to be the interaction of the hormone with receptor sites (type I) in the cytoplasm (16,35). Receptor estrogen complexes are translocated to the nucleus (26,37) where they are probably involved in the regulation of transcriptional events which ultimately result in the stimulation of true uterine growth (18,21,32,35). In addition, we have recently described a second nuclear binding site for estrogen in the rat uterus (16,31). This site, which we have designated as type II, does not appear to be translocated from the cytoplasm, but instead is stimulated or activated by the binding of the receptor estrogen complex in the nucleus (13,16, 31).

Both nuclear estrogen binding sites are readily observed in the adult ovariectomized rat uterus as early as 1 hour following an injection of estradiol (31). Saturation analysis of uterine nuclear fractions from these animals by the [3H]-estradiol exchange assay (Fig. 1A) revealed that these nuclei contained two specific binding components for [3H]-estradiol. The high affinity, low capacity component ($\sim$0.5 pmoles/ml; 1.0 pmole/uterus') represents the type I sites which are translocated from the cytoplasm to the nucleus. Scatchard and Hill analyses of these data, respectively, yielded a Kd $\sim$1nM (Fig. 1B) and a Hill coefficient of 1 for the type I sites (Fig. 1C). In addition, high levels (>2.0 pmoles/ml; >4 pmoles/uterus) of type II sites were also observed (Fig. 1A) with [3H]-estradiol concentrations ranging from 10-40 nM. The sigmoidal nature of the saturation curve at higher concentrations of [3H]-estradiol (Fig. 1A) and a Hill

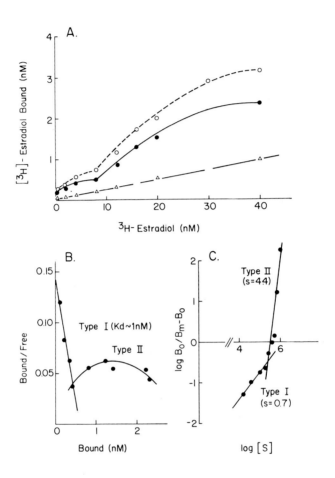

FIG. 1.   Saturation analysis of estrogen binding sites in rat uterine nuclear fractions.   A) The quantity of specifically bound [3H]-estradiol (•)   was determined by incubating nuclei with [3H]-estradiol   (o)   or [3H]-estradiol plus 100-fold molar excess of diethylstilbestrol (Δ) at 37°C for 30 minutes. Mature ovariectomized rats were injected with 10 μg estradiol 1 hour prior to sacrifice.   B) Scatchard analysis of specific binding in Figure 1A.   C) Hill analysis of specific binding in Figure 1A.

coefficient of 4 (Fig. 1C) also suggests that the nuclear type II component may have multiple binding sites for [3H]-estradiol which display positive cooperativity. As predicted from the sigmoidal nature of the saturation curve, a hyperbolic Scatchard plot for the nuclear type II site was obtained (Fig. 1B). Consequently, the Kd for the nuclear type II - [3H]-estradiol complex and the concentration of these sites cannot be accurately obtained by Scatchard analysis. However, the Kd as determined from the concentration of [3H]-estradiol required to half saturate type II sites is in the range of 15-20 nM.

While the physiological significance of the nuclear type II estrogen binding site will be discussed in the subsequent sections of this chapter, it is apparent from the data presented in figure 1A, that nuclear type II sites can interfere with the measurement of estrogen receptors (16). Quantitative resolution of type I and type II sites can be accomplished by temperature or by saturation analysis (16; Fig. 1A) using a wide range of [3H]-estradiol concentrations. The use of single point exchange assays with [3H]-estradiol concentrations in excess of 10 nM has undoubtedly led to erroneous estimates of estrogen receptors in earlier studies by this laboratory and others.

RELATIONSHIP OF TYPE I AND II ESTROGEN BINDING SITES TO UTERINE
GROWTH

We have previously demonstrated that the analysis of different growth response patterns of the uterus to treatment with estradiol or estriol are useful in analyzing important events that control uterine growth (3,4). The results of such analyses are shown in Fig. 2. Estradiol and estriol are of equal potency with respect to all events that occur within the first 3-4 hours after an injection of the hormone. However, after this time the effects of estriol decline rapidly while those of estradiol are sustained for long periods of time. The ability of estradiol to maintain uterotropic responses and to cause uterine growth is correlated with its capacity to cause long-term nuclear retention of the estrogen receptor. Likewise the inability of estriol to cause uterine growth is due to short term residency in the nucleus. These data have important implications with respect to certain concepts which have been proposed to explain the mechanism of action of estrogens, e.g., the cascade hypothesis (6) and the estriol protection theory of breast cancer (43). Such implications have been discussed elsewhere (10) and hence will not be presented here. Instead the differential uterotropic response pattern will be used to ask whether type II sites are also influenced differently by estradiol and estriol.

Mature ovariectomized rats were treated with 10 ug estradiol or estriol and sacrificed at various times following injection. The nuclear levels of type I and II estrogen binding sites were determined by saturation analysis as described in Figure 1A. The data demonstrate that the patterns of nuclear retention of type I sites and elevations of nuclear type II estradiol bind-

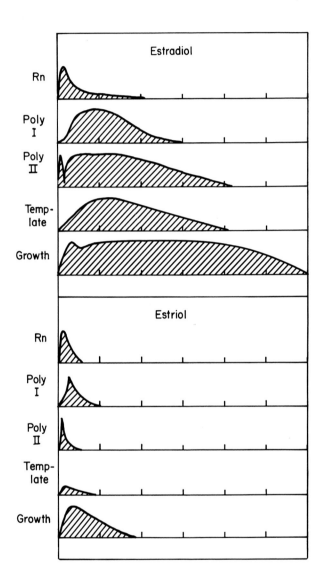

FIG. 2. Effects of estradiol and estriol on several uterotropic responses. Immature rats were injected with 1.0 ug estradiol or estriol and the following responses were measured as a function of time: estrogen receptor in the nucleus (R_n), RNA polymerase I activity (Poly I), RNA polymerase II activity (Poly II), RNA polymerase initiation sites (template) and uterine wet weight (growth).

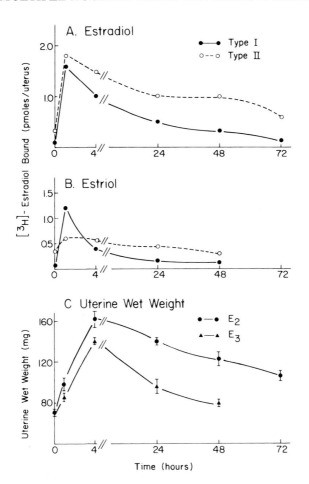

FIG. 3. Temporal effects of estradiol (A) and estriol (B) injection on uterine wet weights (C) and nuclear type I (•) and type II (○) estrogen binding sites. Mature ovariectomized rats were treated with 10 ug of estradiol or estriol and sacrificed at the indicated times following injection. The quantity of specifically bound [³H]-estradiol was determined by saturation analysis of uterine nuclear fractions at 37°C for 30 min.

ing sites are very similar (Fig.3A). Maximal levels of type I and type II sites were reached by one hr after an injection of estradiol. The quantity of type I sites then declined gradually, but was maintained 2-3 fold above controls at 24, 48 and 72 hrs. Estriol treatment also elevated the quantity of type I sites one hr after the injection (compare Fig. 3A + B) and caused a corresponding increase in uterine wet weight at 4 hr (Fig. 3C). However, only estradiol induced long term nuclear retention of the type I site (4-6 hr), sustained elevations of nuclear type II sites (4-48 hr) and stimulated true uterine growth (uterine wet weight at 24-48 hr). Failure of an injection of estriol to stimulate true uterine growth (Fig. 3C) correlated with the inability of this hormone to induce long term (4-6 hr) nuclear retention of type I or to increase the levels of nuclear type II estrogen binding sites above control levels (Fig. 3B).

To examine the relationship between nuclear type II sites and estrogen stimulation of true uterine growth, mature ovariectomized rats were treated with paraffin pellets containing either estradiol or estriol and sacrificed 48 hr following hormone administration. Under these conditions, estriol treatment results in the sustained elevation of nuclear type I sites and the stimulation of true uterine growth in the immature rat (12,33). If elevated levels of nuclear type II sites are related to estrogen stimulation of true uterine growth (either causally or as a secondary response), then increased quantities of this second nuclear estrogen binding component should be observed in animals treated with an estriol implant. The data presented in Figure 4B support this hypothesis and are compared to results obtained by injection (Fig. 4A). Saturation analysis of nuclear fractions by the [^{3}H]-estradiol exchange assay demonstrated that while not as effective as the estradiol implant, the estriol implant resulted in the sustained elevation of occupied type I sites (0.4 pmol/uterus) and a 6-8 fold increase in the number of nuclear type II sites as compared to paraffin controls. Elevation of nuclear type II sites also correlated with the ability of estradiol or estriol to stimulate true uterine growth (Fig. 3 & 4).

These results demonstrate that a positive correlation exists between elevated levels of nuclear type II sites and the stimulation of true uterine growth. This correlation is better than that observed for the classical estrogen receptor (type I site). Type I sites accumulate rapidly in the nucleus after an injection of estradiol; however, they decline to low levels by 24 hrs. In contrast, the level of type II remains elevated for 24-48 hr and true growth of the uterus is observed during this time. An injection of estriol also causes nuclear accumulation of type I, but these sites rapidly disappear from the nucleus and, additionally, neither stimulation of type II sites nor true uterine growth occurs. We have shown previously that a single injection of estradiol stimulated sustained RNA polymerase activity, increased chromatin template activity over long periods of time and elevated DNA synthesis. A single injection of estriol, in contrast, failed to cause these long term uterotropic responses (Fig. 2) (21, 32). We have suggested that these events relate to the ability of estradiol to maintain receptor occupancy in the nucleus for a period of time which is sufficient to stimulate the nuclear mediated events which are obligatory for the production of true growth. One of these obligatory events may be the elevation of type II sites. The failure of an estriol injection to cause true growth results from its inability to maintain type I sites in the nucleus for a sufficient period of time. That

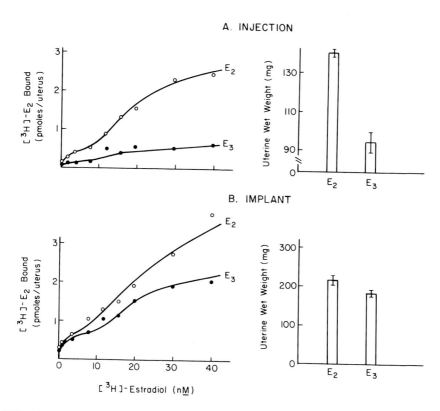

FIG. 4. Saturation analysis of nuclear estrogen binding sites and uterine wet weight response to estradiol (E_2; o) and estriol (E_3; ●) when administered by injection (A) or paraffin implant (B). Mature ovariectomized rats received a single subcutaneous injection (10 ug) of estradiol or estriol, or were implanted with paraffin pellets containing the estrogen (∿2 mg). Animals were sacrificed by cervical dislocation 24 hour following the injection or 48 hours following implant administration. Nuclear fractions were assayed for estrogen binding sites by the [^{3}H]-estradiol exchange assay as described in Fig. 1.

type II sites at least attend, if not cause, true growth appears to be the case since implants of estriol, which sustain occupancy of type I sites, cause the elevation of type II sites and true uterine growth (Fig. 4). Thus, estrogen stimulation of true uterine growth appears to result from nuclear retention of type I sites and to be attended by the rapid and sustained elevation of the level of the nuclear type II estrogen binding site.

In contrast to the above observations, elevations of the nuclear type II site do not correlate with the ability of estradiol or estriol to stimulate early uterotropic responses (1-4 hr) in the rat uterus (Fig. 2 & 3). A single injection of estriol was equivalent to estradiol in stimulating uterine wet weight at 1-4 hr even though estriol treatment failed to elevate nuclear levels of type II sites. We have suggested that early uterotropic events are not obligatory for the stimulation of true growth and that these early responses do not produce a cascade effect which culminates in growth (1, 4, 32). Our present results support this concept. The elevated levels of nuclear type II do not appear to result from a nuclear translocation process as seen for type I sites (12, 26, 37). Type II sites may represent components which are always present in the nuclear compartment and which are activated by estradiol and/or the receptor estradiol complex.

The occurence and stimulation of nuclear type II sites by estrogen is found predominantly in the classical estrogen target organs (Fig. 5A). However small quantities of these sites occur in the spleen and they are elevated by estrogen administration (Fig. 5B). The significance of this observation awaits further study.

The precise requirements for estrogenic stimulation of the nuclear type II site remain to be resolved. The ability of estriol when administered by paraffin implant (Fig. 4) to increase nuclear type II sites and to stimulate true uterine growth suggests that one requirement for the elevation in nuclear type II sites may be sustained nuclear occupancy by receptor hormone complexes. In addition, the specificity of the interaction between receptor hormone complexes and nuclear sites which results in the increase in type II sites must also be considered. This conclusion is supported by the observation that while a single injection of either estradiol or estriol resulted in an equivalent accumulation of receptor hormone complexes at 1-4 hr post-injection, only the receptor estradiol complexes were associated with rapid and sustained elevations of nuclear type II sites between 1 and 48 hr after treatment. Whether the increase in nuclear type II sites in estriol-implanted animals was due to long term nuclear occupancy by receptor estriol complexes or to saturation of specific nuclear binding sites through a lower affinity interaction with receptor estriol complexes remains to be established.

In conclusion, these data indicate that two estrogen binding sites may be involved in the response of the rat uterus to estrogenic hormones. Whereas responses may be mediated through the interaction of estrogen with type I sites, (4, 19, 25, 35) nuclear events associated with true uterine growth (18, 21, 22, 32, 38) may require not only long term nuclear retention of type I sites, but the sustained elevation of the level of nuclear type II sites.

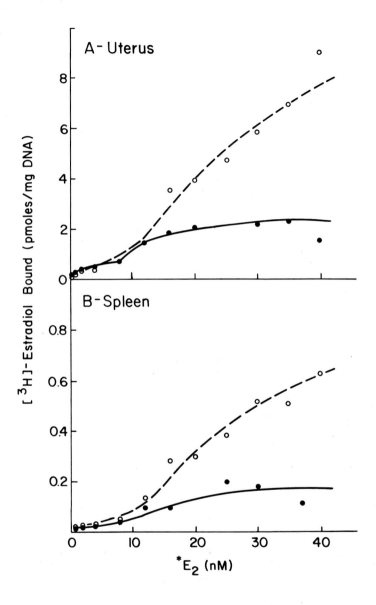

FIG. 5. Saturation analysis of nuclear fractions of uterus (A) and spleen (B) by the [^{3}H]-estradiol exchange assay as described in Figure 1A. Mature ovariectomized rats were injected with saline (●---●) or 10 μg estradiol (o---o) 24 hours prior to sacrifice and specific [^{3}H]-estradiol binding was determined and expressed as pmoles bound per mg DNA.

PROGESTERONE AND DEXAMETHASONE ANTAGONISM OF TYPE II SITES AND
UTERINE GROWTH

As discussed above, the elevation of nuclear type II sites is closely correlated with the stimulation of true uterine growth (31) and therefore, it is conceivable that these sites might be involved in the mechanism by which estrogens cause uterotropic stimulation. One way to test this hypothesis is to block the stimulation of nuclear type II sites and examine the uterotropic response pattern. Since progesterone and glucocorticoids have been used to block uterotropic responses in various ways (7, 11, 24, 30, 39, 70), it seemed possible that these hormones could be used for this purpose.

Mature, ovariectomized rats were given two daily injections of estradiol or a single injection of estradiol on day 1 and an injection of either estradiol plus dexamethasone or estradiol plus progesterone on day 2. All animals were sacrificed 24 hours following the second injection. Pretreatment with estradiol (day 1) was to increase the uterine response to progesterone, presumably by increasing the level of progesterone receptor (29, 34, 42). Saturation analysis of specific nuclear binding sites by the $[^3H]$-estradiol exchange assay shown in Fig. 6A revealed that uterine nuclei from estradiol-treated controls contained approximately 0.2 and 6.0 pmol/uterus of type I and type II sites, respectively. It should be noted that nuclear type II sites are not saturated by 40 nM $[^3H]$-estradiol, and thus the levels of this second estrogen binding component were somwhwat underestimated.

Dexamethasone treatment completely blocked the estrogen stimulated increase in the nuclear type II site (Fig. 6A) and in uterine wet weight (Fig. 6B; $p<.01$) normally observed 24 h following a second injection of estradiol. Nuclear levels of the of the type I site were very similar (0.2 pmol/uterus) in the estradiol and estradiol plus dexamethasone treatment groups suggesting that this antagonist failed to alter nuclear estrogen receptor levels at 24 hours. While not as effective as dexamethasone, administration of progesterone to mature ovariectomized rats reduced levels of the nuclear type II site and decreased ($p < .05$) the uterine wet weight response to estradiol but failed to influence nuclear levels of the type I site.

These results suggest that the antagonistic properties of dexamethasone and progesterone on estradiol-induced uterine growth reside in the ability of these compounds to reduce the numbers of nuclear type II sites while not altering nuclear levels of type I estrogen binding sites. However, these compounds may interfere with nuclear translocation and "processing" of type I sites, thereby reducing the availability of estrogen receptor. To examine this possibility in detail we measured cytoplasmic and nuclear levels of estrogen receptor at 1, 4 and 24 hours following dexamethasone or progesterone administration to mature ovariectomized rats (Fig. 7). The levels of cytoplasmic type I sites were identical in animals treated with estradiol, estradiol plus dexamethasone, or estradiol plus progesterone at 1 and 4 hours post-

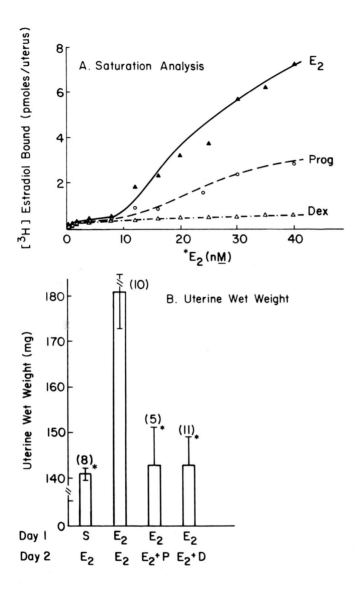

FIG. 6: Saturation analysis of nuclear estrogen binding sites in rat uterine fractions. A) The quantity of specifically bound [^{3}H]-estradiol (pmol/uterus) for each estradiol concentration was determined as described. Mature ovariectomized rats were primed with an injection of estradiol (10 ug) 24 hrs prior to receiving a second injection of estradiol (▲), estradiol + progesterone (o) or estradiol + dexamethasone (△). Animals were sacrificed 24 hrs following the second injection. Estradiol (10 ug), progesterone (2.5 mg) and dexamethsone (5 mg) were

injected subcutaneously in 30% ETOH:0.9% NaCl (v/v). B) Effects of progesterone and dexamethasone on uterine wet weight. Animals received a priming injection of vehicle (30% ETOH in 0.9% saline v/v) or estradiol (10 ug) on Day 1 and a second injection of estradiol, estradiol + progesterone, or estradiol + dexamethasone on Day 2 and were sacrificed 24 hrs later. Values represent the mean $\pm$ SEM for the numbers of observations indicated in parentheses. *significantly different from animals receiving two daily injections of estradiol (p < .01).

injection. By 24 hours, the level of cytoplasmic type I was increased above control (2.0 pmol/uterus) in estradiol (3.6 pmol/uterus) and estradiol plus dexamethasone (3.0 pmol/uterus) treated animals. The lower level of type I sites in the cytosol of progesterone treated rats (2.0 pmol/uterus) as compared to the estradiol treatment group (3.6 pmol/uterus) is consistent with previous reports from this laboratory demonstrating that progesterone blocks the estrogen-induced synthesis of cytoplasmic estrogen receptors 8-24 hours post-injection (23). Apparently dexamethasone treatment does not inhibit this phase of cytoplasmic receptor synthesis (Fig. 7A; compare E_2 vs E_2 + DEX, 24 hr). Similarly, the antagonistic effects of dexamethasone and progesterone on nuclear type II sites and uterine growth do not appear to be the result of alterations in nuclear retention patterns of type I sites since nuclear levels of estrogen receptor were identical at 1, 4 and 24 hours following injection of estradiol, estradiol plus dexamethasone or estradiol plus progesterone (Fig. 7B).

These data suggest that the nature of dexamethasone and progesterone antagonism of uterotrophic responses to estradiol are due to an inhibition of the expression of nuclear type II sites rather than an impedance of receptor/nuclear interactions, "processing" and/or cytoplasmic receptor replenishment. This concept is supported by the observation that a single injection of dexamethasone 24 hrs prior to estradiol administration completely blocks estrogen stimulation of uterine growth and nuclear type II sites (Table I) even though effects on type I sites do not appear to be involved in this inhibition (Fig. 7A & B). Apparently, antagonistic effects of progesterone on nuclear type II sites and uterine growth are dependent upon estrogen pretreatment since progesterone failed to antagonize either of these parameters in the unprimed rat uterus (Table I; compare E_2 vs E_2 + P; primed vs unprimed rats).

Progesterone and dexamethasone were clearly antagonistic when the estrogen was administered acutely (injection). However, antagonism of nuclear type II sites and uterine growth may not be observed if nuclear sites are continually occupied by the receptor estrogen complexes. To examine this possibility, the effects of dexamethasone and progesterone on nuclear type II sites and uterine growth were examined in animals treated with an estradiol-containing paraffin implant. Under these experimental conditions,

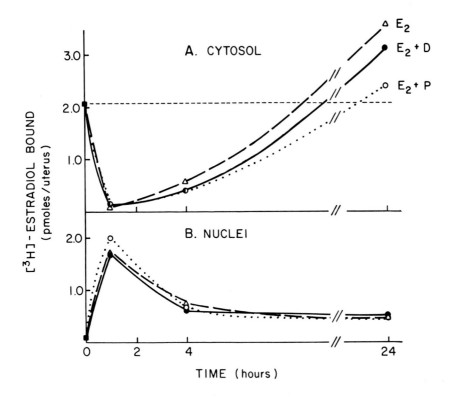

FIG. 7. Temporal effects of progesterone and dexamethasone on cytoplasmic (A) and nuclear (B) levels of nuclear type I sites determined by saturation analysis. Mature ovariectomized rats were treated exactly as described in Fig. 6A and were sacrificed 1, 4 and 24 hrs following the second injection of estradiol (△),estradiol + progesterone (o), or estradiol + dexamethasone (•).

nuclear sites are continually occupied by type I-estradiol complexes (12, 31, 33) and serum levels of estradiol are maintained at 700 pg/ml (data not shown). As is illustrated in Figure 8, an injection of dexamethasone or progesterone in animals with an E_2-implant results in a 4–5 fold reduction in nuclear levels of type II sites 24 hours after injection. These reductions in nuclear type II sites in dexamethasone or progesterone treated rats were accompanied by significant decreases in uterine wet (p < .01) and dry (p < .05) weight (Table II). In fact, under these experimental conditions a single injection of dexamethasone antagonized uterine wet weight and nuclear type II sites for at least 8 days

Table 1.   Progesterone and dexamethasone antagonism of estradiol stimulation of uterine growth in unprimed and estradiol-primed ovariectomized rats

INJECTION[a]			UTERINE WET WEIGHT (mg)	TYPE II SITES (pmoles/uterus)
Day 1 (0900 hr)	Day 2 (0900 hr)			
S	S	$(19)^b$	80 ± 2.6	0.4
S	E_2	(9)	141 ± 5.6^c	2.0
D	$E_2 + D$	(10)	101 ± 4.1	0.5
P	$E_2 + P$	(11)	$154 \pm 41.^c$	1.6
E_2	E_2	(14)	178 ± 7.8	8.0
E_2	$E_2 + D$	(14)	136 ± 5.5^d	1.0
E_2	$E_2 + P$	(9)	142 ± 5.3^d	3.0

a   estradiol (E; 10 ug), dexamethasone (D; 5 mg) and progesterone (P; 2.5 mg) were injected in 30% ethanol:saline vehicle. Animals were sacrificed 24 hours following the second injection

b   number in parenthesis is the number of animals in the treatment group

c   significantly different from saline injected controls ($p < .01$)

d   significantly different from $E_2 + E_2$ treatment group ($p < .01$)

(data not shown) and this response was dose dependent. Doses of dexamethasone ranging from 0.6-5 mg reduced nuclear levels of type II sites (Fig. 9) and uterine wet weight (Fig. 9) in a stepwise fashion with maximum inhibition being achieved with 2.5-5 mg of dexamethasone.

Differential effects of dexamethasone and progesterone were observed on luminal fluid volume (Table II), suggesting that these two antagonists may be acting through separate mechanisms. Whereas progesterone treatment significantly reduced ($p < .01$) fluid imbibition 3-fold below controls, dexamethasone administration did not alter this uterine response to estradiol.

These results clearly indicate that, in addition to the estrogen receptor (type I site), the mature ovariectomized rat uterus contains a second nuclear estrogen binding component which may be

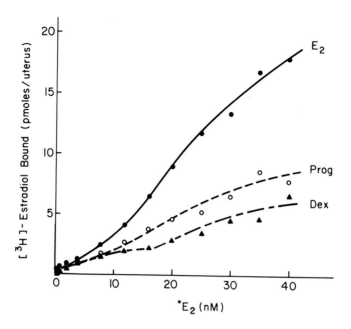

FIG. 8.   Saturation analysis of nuclear estrogen binding sites in
rat uterine fractions. Specific [3H]-estradiol binding is expressed in pmoles bound/uterus and was determined as described in Fig.
1A. Mature ovariectomized rats received a paraffin implant containing estradiol ($\sim$2 mg) 72 hrs prior to an injection of vehicle
(estradiol controls) ($\bullet$), progesterone (o), or dexamethasone
($\blacktriangle$). Hormones were diluted and injected as described in Fig.
6A. Animals were sacrificed 24 hrs following injection.

directly involved in hormone action. As discussed earlier, we
have demonstrated that longterm nuclear retention of a limited
number ($\sim$2000 sites/cell) of the type I sites is necessary for
estrogen stimulation of transcriptional events required for true
uterine growth (1, 2, 8, 21, 32). The results in this section
suggest that elevated levels of nuclear type II site may also be
required for these responses. This concept is supported, but not
proven, by the observation that dexamethasone or progesterone
antagonism of uterine growth was attended by substantial or

Table II. Effects of progesterone and dexamethasone on luminal fluid volume and uterine wet and dry weights in estradiol-implanted rats

Injection[a]	Luminal Fluid Volume (ml)	Uterine Wet Weight (mg)	Uterine Dry Weight (mg)
saline (10)[b]	0.75 ± 0.13	288 ± 8.5	45.4 ± 2.1
progesterone (10)	0.25 ± 0.04[c]	230 ± 7.4[c]	40.0 ± 2.9[d]
dexamethasone (11)	0.66 ± 0.09	219 ± 9.6[c]	40.2 ± 3.0[d]

a   mature ovariectomized rats were implanted with 2 mg estradiol 72 hours prior to receiving an injection of vehicle (30% ethanol in saline), progesterone (2.5 mg) or dexamethasone (5 mg) and sacrificed 24 hours post-injection

b   number in parenthesis is the number of observations in the treatment group

c   significantly different from saline controls ($p < .01$)

d   significantly different from saline controls ($p < .05$)

complete inhibition of nuclear type II sites without measurable effects on nuclear levels of estrogen receptors (Figs. 6 and 8: Tables I and II). In fact, dexamethasone administration 24 hours prior to an injection of estradiol (Table I) completely blocked uterine growth (E_2 vs $D + E_2$) without altering the cytoplasmic depletion/replenishment (Fig. 7A) or nuclear accumulation/retention patterns (Fig. 7B) of type I sites. These findings and previous reports from this laboratory have demonstrated that, in addition to long term nuclear retention of estrogen receptors, the elevation of nuclear type II estrogen binding sites may be required for uterine growth (31).

In contrast to our results which show no significant effect of progesterone or dexamethasone on the total level of the nuclear type I site, it has been suggested that these hormones decrease the quantity of type I receptor sites in rat uterine nuclei (7, 23). These experiments employed one point assays with 10 nM (or greater) [^{3}H]-estradiol and the data were not corrected for the presence of type II sites. Since low levels of type II sites will be measured at this concentration of [^{3}H]-estradiol (Figs. 6 and 8), these results probably reflect the effects of dexamethasone on type II sites. As demonstrated in the present study and in previous reports from this laboratory (16) quantative resolu-

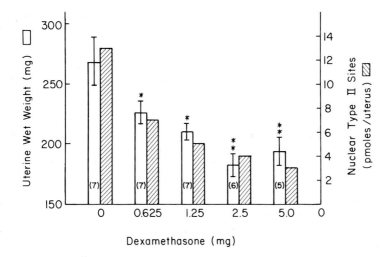

FIG. 9.   Effect of increasing doses of dexamethasone on uterine
wet weight and nuclear levels of type II sites. Mature ovariectomized rats were implanted with paraffin pellets containing
∿2 mg estradiol 72 hrs prior to an injection of vehicle or dexamethasone (0.6–5.0 mg). Uterine wet weights and levels of nuclear type II sites were determined 24 hrs post-injection.
*significantly different from vehicle control (p < .05).
**significantly different from vehicle control (p < .01).

tion of type I and type II sites is difficult and can only be
obtained by saturation analysis (Figs. 6 and 8) using a wide
range of [^{3}H]-estradiol concentrations.
   While the present studies have clearly demonstrated the antagonism of estradiol-induced nuclear type II sites and uterine
growth by dexamethasone and progesterone, the mechanism of this
antagonism remains to be resolved. Cytoplasmic and nuclear receptors for progesterone (41, 42) and the glucocorticoids (36)
have been identified and characterized in the mature ovariectomized rat uterus and these steroid binding proteins are probably involved in the antagonism of nuclear type II-estrogen binding sites
and uterine growth. Although progesterone and naturally-occurring
glucocorticoids are known to interact with both progesterone
and glucocorticoid receptors (17, 27), dexamethasone binds to
the rat uterine progesterone receptor only to a limited extent

through a glucocorticoid receptor. Similarly, although progesterone binds to a limited extent to the glucocorticoid receptor, data presented in these studies suggest that antagonism of uterotrophic responses by progesterone is mediated primarily through the progesterone receptor, not the glucocorticoid receptor. This is suggested by the failure of progesterone, but not dexamethasone, to inhibit estradiol stimulation of nuclear type II sites and uterine growth in the unprimed rat uterus (Table I; compare unprimed vs estradiol primed groups). If progesterone were acting to a significant degree through the glucocorticoid receptor, inhibition of these uterotrophic responses by progestins would not be totally dependent upon estrogen priming. This dependency on estradiol priming probably results from the ability of estradiol to elevate the quantity of progesterone receptors and thus to create a progesterone-responsive uterus (29, 34, 42).

In addition, the ability of progesterone, but not dexamethasone, to decrease the replenishment of the cytoplasmic estrogen receptor (Fig. 7A) and to supress uterine fluid imbibition (Table II) argues for different mechanisms of action. Although dexamethasone (7, 24, 39, 40) and a number of glucocorticoids have been demonstrated to inhibit estrogen stimulation of uterine fluid imbibition (uterine wet weight 3-4 hrs post-injection), apparently this antagonism is not long lasting in the presence of continuous estrogen. This conclusion is supported by the observation that dexamethasone treatment failed to block fluid imbibition in the presence of an estradiol-implant (Table II).

The observed inhibition of nuclear type II sites by dexamethasone and progesterone appears to result from a decrease in the number of sites and not from changes in their estradiol binding properties. Hill coefficients for [3H]-estradiol binding to nuclear type II sites in estradiol-, progesterone- and dexamethasone-treated rats (Fig. 10) were 3.3, 3.2 and 3.3, respectively suggesting that antagonism did not alter the hormone binding characteristics of this second nuclear component for [3H]-estradiol. Furthermore, dexamethasone or progesterone administration did not change the binding specificity of nuclear type II sties for estrogens (Fig. 11). Only diethylstilbestrol, estradiol and estriol, but not progesterone, R5020, cortisol, testosterone or dexamethasone effectively competed with [3H]-estradiol for nuclear type II sites. The level of this competition was not substantially influenced by type I sites since these nuclear preparations were labeled with 40 nM [3H]-estradiol $\pm$ 100-fold excess of competitor and the levels of type I sites (0.5 pmol/uterus) were 10-40 times lower than type II (6-20 pmol/uterus) estrogen binding sites (Fig. 8).

The nature of the interaction of progesterone and dexamethasone with the uterine genome and subsequent inhibition of nuclear type II estrogen binding sites remains to be resolved. However, this effect is long lasting following a single injection of progesterone (>48 hr) and dexamethasone (>8 days) and is not influenced by acute (Fig. 6) or continuous (paraffin implant, Fig. 8) estrogen

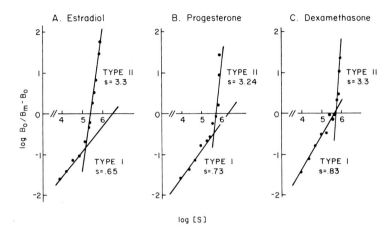

FIG. 10. Hill analysis of specific binding in Fig. 8 for (A) vehicle (estradiol) controls, (B) progesterone- and (C) dexamethasone-treated animals.

(41). Therefore, dexamethasone antagonism of the nuclear type II site and uterine growth is probably a specific event mediated administration. While only indirect, these observations suggest that dexamethasone or progesterone do not block nuclear type II sites by competing with the receptor estradiol complex for identical sites in the nucleus. If this were the case, the continued nuclear residence of type I sites in estradiol implanted animals (31) (Fig. 9) should have diminished the response to dexamethasone or progesterone. This hypothesis is supported in that nuclear retention patterns of the type I site and presumed interactions with nuclear acceptor sites (35) were not altered by dexamethasone or progesterone administration (Fig. 7B).

In summary, these data demonstrate that dexamethasone and progesterone inhibit the ability to elevate nuclear type II estrogen binding sites in the rat uterus and this suppression is correlated with an antagonism of uterine growth. Since nuclear binding and cytoplasmic replenishment of type I receptors are normal under these circumstances, we propose that the estrogen-induced elevation of nuclear type II sites may be involved in the mechanism by which estrogen causes uterine growth.

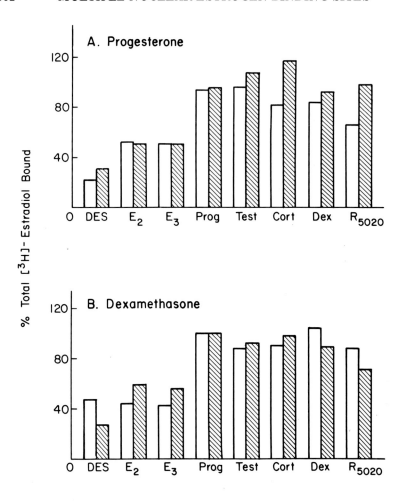

FIG. 11. Hormone specificity of nuclear type II sites following progesterone (A) or dexamethasone (B) administration to mature-ovariectomized rats. Animals pretreated with an estradiol containing paraffin implant (2 mg for 72 hrs) were injected with vehicle (open bars) or 2.5 mg progesterone (A; hatched bars) or 5.0 mg dexamethasone (B; hatched bars) and sacrificed 24 hour post-injection (96 hrs following estradiol implant). Uterine nuclear fractions were incubated with [³H]-estradiol + 100-fold excess diethylstilbestrol (DES), estradiol (E₂), estriol (E₃), progesterone (Prog), testosterone (Test), cortisol (Cort), dexamethasone (Dex) or 17, 21-dimethyl-19-nor-4, 9-pregnadien-3, 20-dione (R5020) as described in Figure 1A. Data are expressed as the percent of total [³H]-estradiol bound in the absence of competitor.

Conclusion

We do not understand the significance of the various forms of estrogen binding sites discussed here; however, suggestions concerning their function may be made. Nuclear type II sites appear to be "stimulated" or "activated" by the translocation of type I sites and remain elevated for 24 hrs or longer in the mature rat. This is much longer than either type I sites or injected [^{3}H]-estradiol remain in the nucleus and correlates well with the time of major stimulation of DNA, RNA and protein synthesis (20). Thus the presence of nuclear type II sites correlates better with uterotrophic stimulation than does the nuclear binding of type I sites. It is possible that this secondary component represents estrogen specific binding sites associated with chromatin that are involved in the control of DNA synthesis and sustained RNA synthesis.

Alternately, type II sites may be a part of the nuclear binding-processing mechanism. We have proposed that the binding of receptor steroid complexes to nuclear sites involves a nuclear retention mechanism and is not a simple function of mass action (9, 15). Type II sites might bind the receptor estrogen complex and form a new complex which would be the functional unit of gene activation and receptor processing. This processing unit could be involved not only in gene activation but also in the recyclling or replenishment of the receptor to the cytoplasm. Thus, it is possible that nuclear type II sites could be precursors of cytosol type I sites. Nuclear processing could also involve the metabolism of the hormone as part of the mechanism by which uterine cells eliminate estrogens from their local environment.

One area which has not been fully explored is the distribution of these specific hormone binding molecules amongst various cell types within target tissues. For instance, we have recently demonstrated that triphenylethylene derivatives primarily stimulate the luminal epithelium of the uterus (14). Likewise, estrogens preferentially cause the growth and differentiation of the tubular gland cells of the chick oviduct over other oviductal cell types (28). This raises the possibility that these classes of specific estrogen binding site might have specific cellular distributions which are important in specific estrogen-induced growth patterns within target tissues.

The ability of progesterone and dexamethasone to decrease the level of nuclear type II sites, while having no effect on the level of nuclear type I sites, implies that the stimulation of these secondary sites may be an intermediate step in the mechanism by which estrogen causes growth. Such cause and effect relationships between the stimulation of nuclear type II sites and growth responses are not proven by these observations, however, and must await futher experimentation.

REFERENCES

1. Anderson, J.N., Clark, J.H., and Peck, E.J., Jr. (1972): Biochem. Biophys. Res. Commun. 48:1460-1468.
2. Anderson, J.N., Peck, E.J., JR., and Clark, J.H. (1973): Endocrinology, 92:1488-1495.
3. Anderson, J.N., Peck, E.J.,Jr., and Clark, J.H. (1974): Endocrinology, 95:174-178.
4. Anderson, J.N., Peck, E.J.,Jr., and Clark, J.H. (1975): Endocrinology, 96:160-167.
5. Barrack, E.R., Hawkins, E.F., Allen, S.L., Hicks, L.L. and Coffey, D.S. (1977): Biochem. Biophy. Res. Comm., 79:829-836.
6. Baulieu, E.E., Wira, C.R., Milgrom, E., and Raynaud-Jammet, C. (1972): In: Karolinska Symposia on Research Methods in Reproductive Endocrinology; Protein Synthesis in Reproductive Tissue, edited by E. Dicsfalusy, pp. 396-419. Karolinska Institutet, Stockholm.
7. Campbell, P.S. (1978): Endocrinology, 103:716-723.
8. Clark, J.H. and Peck, E.J., Jr. (1976): Nature, 260:635-637.
9. Clark, J.H. and Peck, E.J., Jr. (1976): In: Hormone Action and Molecular Endocrinology Workshop, edited by B.W. O'Malley and W.T. Schrader, pp. 1-20, Baylor College of Medicine, Department of Cell Biology, Houston.
10. Clark, J.H. and Peck. E.J., Jr. (1979): In: Female Sex Steroids: Receptors and Function,. Springer-Verlag, Berlin.
11. Clark, J.H., Hseuh, A., and Peck, E.J., Jr. (1977): Annals N.Y. Acad. Sci., 286:161-179.
12. Clark, J.H., Paszko, Z. and Peck, E.J., Jr. (1977): Endocrinology, 100:91-96.
13. Clark, J.H., Hardin, J.W., Upchurch, S., and Eriksson, H. (1978): J. Biol. Chem., 253:7630-7634.
14. Clark, J.H., Hardin, J.W.,McCormack, S.A., and Padykula,H.A. (1978): In: Hormones and Receptors in Breast Cancer, edited by W.L. McGuire, pp. 107-133. Raven Press, New York.
15. Clark, J.H., Peck, E.J., Jr., Hardin, J.W., and Eriksson, H. (1978): In: Receptors and Hormone Action, edited by B.W. O'Malley and L. Birnbaumer, Volume II, pp. 1-31. Academic Press, New York
16. Eriksson, H., Upchurch, S., Hardin, J.W., Peck, E.J., Jr., and Clark, J.H. (1978): Biochem. Biophys. Res. Comm., 81:1-7.
17. Feil, .D., Glasser, S.R., Toft, D.O., and O'Malley, B.W. (1972): Endocrinology, 91:738-746.
18. Glasser, S.R., Chytil, F., and Spelsberg, T.C. (1972): Biochem. J., 130:947-957.
19. Gorski, J., Toft, D., Shyamala, G., Smith,D., and Notides, A. (1968): Rec. Prog. Horm. Res., 24:45-80.
20. Hamilton, T.H. (1968): Science, 161:649-660.
21. Hardin, J.W., Clark, J.H., Glasser, S.R., and Peck, E.J., Jr. (1976): Biochemistry, 15:1370-1374.
22. Harris, J. and Gorski, J. (1978): Endocrinology, 103:240-245.

23. Hseuh, A.J.W., Clark, J.H. and Peck, E.J., Jr. (1976): Endocrinology, 98:438-444.

24. Huggins, C. and Jensen, E.V. (1955): J. Exptl. Med., 102: 335-346.

25. Jensen, E.V. and DeSombre, E.R. (1972): Ann. Rev. Biochem, 41:203-230.

26. Jensen, E.V., Numata, M., Brecher, P.I., and DeSombre, E.R. (1971): In: The Biochemistry of Steroid Action, edited by R.M.S. Smellie, pp. 133-159. Academic Press, London.

27. King, R.J.B. and Mainwaring, W.I.P. (1974) In: Steroid-Cell Interactions, University Park Press, Baltimore.

28. Kohler, P.O., Grimley, P.M., and O'Malley, B.W. (1969): J. Cell Biology, 40:8-27.

29. Leavitt, W.W., Toft, D.O., Strott, C.A., and O'Malley, B.W. (1974): Endocrinology, 94:1041-1053.

30. Lerner, L.J. (1964): Recent Progr. Horm. Res., 20:435-490.

31. Markaverich, B.M. and Clark, J.H. (1979): Endocrinology, (in press).

32. Markaverich, B.M., Clark, J.H., and Hardin, J.W. (1978): Biochemistry, 17:3146-3152.

33. Martucci, C. and Fishman (1977): Endocrinology, 101:1709-1715.

34. Milgrom, E., Thi, L., Atger, M., and Baulieu, E.E. (1973): J. Biol. Chem., 248:6366-6347.

35. O'Malley, B.W., and Means, A.R. (1974): Science, 183:610-620

36. Panko, W.B., Clark, J.H., and Walters, M.R. (1979): Endocrinology, (in press).

37. Shyamala, G. and Gorski, J. (1967): J. Biol. Chem., 244: 1094-1103.

38. Stormshak, F., Leake, R., Wertz, N., and Gorski, J. (1976): Endocrinology, 99:1501-1511.

39. Szego, C.M. and Roberts, S. (1953): Rec. Prog. Horm. Res. 8:419-469.

40. Verlardo, J.T., Hisaw, F.L., and Bever, A.T. (1956): Endocrinology, 59:165-169.

41. Walters, M.R. and Clark, J.H. (1977): J. Steroid Biochem., 8:1137-1144.

42. Walters, M.R. and Clark, J.H. (1978) Endocrinology, 103: 601-609.

43. Wotiz, H.H., Shane, J.A., Vigersky, R., and Brecher, P.I. (1968): In: Prognostic Factors in Breast Cancer, edited by A.P.M. Forest and P.B. Kunkler, pp. 368-376. Livingstone Press, Edinburgh.

Perspectives in Steroid Receptor Research,
edited by F. Bresciani.
Raven Press, New York © 1980.

Specific Uterine Protein Synthesis as a Guide to Understanding the Biologic Significance of the Estrogen–Receptor Interaction

Eugene R. DeSombre and C. Richard Lyttle

Ben May Laboratory for Cancer Research, University of Chicago, Chicago, Illinois 60637, U.S.A.

INTRODUCTION

At the present time, almost 20 years after the first report on the interaction of tritiated estradiol of high specific activity with various tissues in experimental animals (20), we are rapidly approaching the time when we will know the molecular details of how estrogen acts. The keys to the discovery of this knowledge, in the form of the new technology developed by recent advances in purification, analysis, synthesis and amplification of gene products and nucleic acid coding for them, are now at hand and are being applied to analysis of specific steroid regulated proteins such as ovalbumin (6,37,40), tryptophan oxygenase (41), growth hormone (32), mouse mammary tumor virus (39) and uteroglobin (3). Several specific uterine proteins synthesized in response to estrogen, have been studied. Best known is, IP, or the "induced protein," first reported by Notides and Gorski (34). Also, the hormonal regulation of glucose-6-phosphate dehydrogenase has been studied extensively by Barker's laboratory (43). Nonetheless there is need to identify additional, specific estrogen-dependent uterine proteins, to find any which might be absent in the unstimulated uterus and hence most suitable for studying estrogen induction of new gene products.

The past two decades have seen significant advances in our knowledge of the interaction pathway of steroid hormones with their target cells (12,19,25,36). Figure 1 illustrates current knowledge of the estrogen-receptor interaction with its target cell. After entering the cell, probably by a passive diffusion process, the estrogen (E) associates with the extra-nuclear estrogen receptor protein, present in excess amounts over the minute amounts of steroid entering the target cell, an interaction showing the well-documented high affinity and steroid specificity for estrogens. The association of estrogen with its receptor protein endows the complex with a new capability, the ability to undergo a steroid-dependent, energy-requiring activation process. Although the steroid-dependent activation of a cytosol receptor is a common feature of steroid-dependent cells,

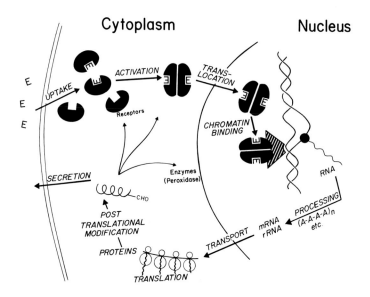

FIG. 1.   Schematic representation of estrogen interaction
with a target cell.

with estrogens the change effected by this activation can be
identified by a characteristic change in sedimentation coefficient
of the complex, from the 4S sedimentation form of the native complex to a 5S form.   As indicated in Fig. 1, data presented by
Notides (35) and also by Jungblut (26) suggest that the steroid-
dependent activation results in a dimerization to the 5S complex.
Most important, activation results in a steroid-receptor complex
with increased affinity for nuclei or, as studied in vitro, DNA
cellulose columns.   It is this property which results in the
binding of the activated complex to various chromatin sites, an
association which apparently leads to the gene transcriptional
events recognized to result from treatment of the target cell with
estrogen.

While major effects on transcription and translation in the
uterus after administration of estrogen to the immature animal
have been characterized, the complex phenomena associated with
estrogen-induced growth of the atrophic uterus makes the study of
this biologic endpoint extremely complicated as a means to eluci-
date the details of the receptor-chromatin interaction related to
gene transcription.   As has been evident from recent studies of
regulation in the oviduct, there is considerable utility to the
study of a specific protein whose concentration is closely regulated by a steroid hormone of interest.   In the uterus such a

protein under control of estrogen is the enzyme peroxidase. Although the estrogen-dependent increase in peroxidase content in the uterus has been known for more than 20 years (27), recent studies in our laboratory (2,9-11,28-30) and elsewhere (5,7,16-18, 23,31,33) have been able to show the dramatic extent of the estrogen stimulation of uterine peroxidase and the sensitivity of this specific uterine protein to hormonal modulation.

This chapter will summarize the present knowledge on the induction and regulation of uterine peroxidase as a specific protein marker and the relationship of changes in peroxidase content with hormonal events involving steroid receptors.

MATERIALS AND METHODS

Animals. Sprague Dawley derived female rats were obtained from ARS/Sprague Dawley, Madison, WI or King Animal Laboratories, Oregon, WI. Female lactating rats, each fostering a litter of ten female pups, were obtained from King Animal Laboratories. The animals arrived in our laboratory at least two days prior to use and each mother and litter was housed in a separate cage. The animals were kept under 12 hour light/dark periods. Immature animals were received at 20 days of age and studied at 21 to 23 days of age. Bilateral ovariectomy was performed using ether anesthesia at least one week prior to use of the animal.

Chemicals. Estradiol, estrone, estriol, diethylstilbesterol, norethindrone, 19-nor-17α-ethynyl-4-androsten-17β-ol-3-one, cycloheximide, 3[2(3,5-dimethyl-2-oxo-cyclohexyl)2-hydroxyethyl] glutarimide, emetine hydrochloride and actinomycin D were obtained from Sigma Chemical Company; progesterone from Schwarz Mann; R5020, 17,21-dimethyl-19-norpregna-4,9,-diene-3,20-dione, and R2858, moxestrol, 11β-methoxy-19-nor-1,3,5(10)-pregnatrien-20-yne-3,17-diol, were obtained by courtesy of Dr. J.P. Raynaud, UCLAF. Parke Davis, CI628, 1-[2-(p[α(p-methoxyphenyl)-β-nitrostyryl] phenoxy)ethyl] pyrolidine monocitrate, was kindly supplied by Dr. Jerry Reel, Parke Davis Company. These substances were dissolved in ethanol followed by dilution in saline to the appropriate concentration for administration. Injection of steroids and hormones was subcutaneous and control animals received vehicle alone. Actinomycin D, cycloheximide and emetine were administered by intraperitoneal injection.

Experimental Procedures. For experiments with neonatal rats the pups in each litter were kept with the foster mother but marked as two groups, providing five animals for the estrogen treated and control groups at each age. After injection the pups were returned to the foster mother until sacrificed by decapitation, 20 hours later. The older animals also were sacrificed by decapitation, four to eight animals per group. The entire uterus from oviduct to cervix was quickly removed, dissected free of fat and connective tissue, nicked, blotted on hard filter paper to excise luminal fluid, and weighed. Each uterus was minced with a scissors into a 12 ml polycarbonate tube with the exception of the uteri of 4 day old animals where groups of 5 uteri were combined

and for the sedimentation analysis studies for estrogen receptor
where five to 20 uteri were pooled prior to homogenization.
Uteri were homogenized in 10 mM Tris-HCl, pH 7.2 buffer (25 mg of
tissue/ml except for sedimentation analysis where 100 mg/ml was
used) for 10 seconds with ice cooling using a polytron PT 10 ST
homogenizer at setting 6. After removal of aliquots for DNA
analysis, the homogenates were centrifuged at 2 C for 45 min at
39,000 x g, or at 250,000 x g in those experiments where cytosols
were to be assayed for estrogen receptor content by sedimentation
analysis. The hypotonic supernatant fraction contains little
peroxidase activity by guaiacol assay. The peroxidase activity
was solubilized by rehomogenizing the sediment with 10 mM Tris-
HCl, pH 7.2 buffer containing 0.5 M $CaCl_2$ as previously reported
(29) and the extract collected by centrifugation for 45 min at
39,000 x g, 2 C.

Peroxidase assays were performed as previously reported (29),
measuring the rate of oxidation of guaiacol at 25°. The assay
mixture contained 13 mM guaiacol and 0.3 mM hydrogen peroxide in
the extraction buffer. The reaction was started by addition of
enzyme and the linear initial rates, measured on a Gilford Model
3401 automated enzyme analyzer, were converted to enzyme units
defined as the amount of enzyme which produced an increase of 1
adsorbence unit per min at 470 nm at 25 C.

For sedimentation analysis of cytosol receptor, the hypotonic
uterine cytosol was incubated at 2° for 30 min with 10 mM Tris,
pH 7.2 buffer containing 500 nM diethylstilbesterol or with buffer
alone. Following this, tritiated estradiol, final concentration
5 nM, was added to each aliquot and after an additional 60 min at
2°, 200μ 1 samples were layered on cold, preformed, 5-20% sucrose
gradients in 10 mM Tris, pH 7.2 buffer. After centrifugation at
250,000 x g for 16 hours, the tubes were punctured at the bottom
and successive 100μ 1 fractions were collected by displacement
with paraffin oil. After addition of a toluene-Triton X-100
scintillation fluid the samples were counted for tritium content
in a Packard Model 3330 scintillation counter at approximately
30% efficiency.

RESULTS AND DISCUSSION

The uterus of the immature or castrate rat has insignificant
peroxidase activity. When a single dose of 1μ g of estradiol is
administered to such an animal, the enzyme is biochemically
detectable by four to six hours, increases for the first twenty
hours and then diminishes, Fig. 2. This dramatic increase in the
amount of uterine peroxidase at 20 hours is elicited by physiologic doses of estrogens but not by other steroids such as progestins, glucocorticoids or androgens. The nonsteroidal estrogen,
diethylstilbesterol, is a potent inducer of uterine peroxidase
(2). Furthermore, as shown in Table 1, when used at a 1 μ g dose
level estrone and estriol are less potent than estradiol in
eliciting the increase in peroxidase at 20 hrs. With these ste-
roidal estrogens, the biologic potency, as measured by induction

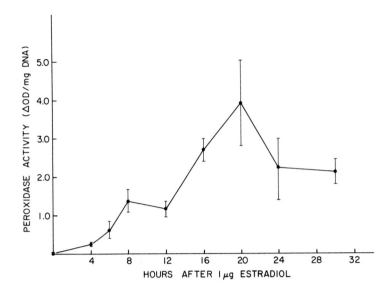

FIG. 2. Time course of estradiol induction of rat uterine
peroxidase. Twenty-one day old female rats were given
1.0 μg estradiol and, at the times indicated, groups of 5
animals were sacrificed. The individual uteri were assayed
for peroxidase as detailed in the Materials and Methods
section. Results are mean values ± S.E.M.

TABLE 1. Uterine peroxidase stimulation by estrone, estradiol and
estriol

	Peroxidase Activity (Units/mg DNA)[a]		
dose	estrone	estradiol	estriol
control	0.19 ± 0.05	0.19 ± 0.05	0.19 ± 0.05
1 μg	0.25 ± 0.09	1.06 ± 0.10	0.45 ± 0.21
10 μg	1.00 ± 0.50	—	0.80 ± 0.42
100 μg	3.63 ± 0.92	—	2.37 ± 0.61

[a]measured in uteri removed 20 hours after administration of
steroid or vehicle as described in the methods, ± S.E.M.

of uterine peroxidase, relates closely with the relative binding
of these estrogens to the estrogen receptor. Clearly at least 10
times more estrone and estriol is required to elicit the same
peroxidase activity as estradiol. With both estrone and estriol,
as we had previously shown for estradiol (29), the induction of
uterine peroxidase is dose dependent. Even though the 20 hr
response to a single dose of estradiol is so dramatic, continued
daily administration of the hormone effects even greater increases
in uterine level of this enzyme (10). The uterine peroxidase content is more than doubled after two days of administration of 1 μg
of estradiol and further dramatically increases at least up to 3
to 4 days of daily treatment. By five to six days of treatment
the uterine peroxidase content and uterine weight seem to have
reached a plateau at levels similar to those observed in the
cycling mature rat at estrus (10). In the cycling rat the peroxidase content of the uterus is lower at metestrus and diestrus
but administration of estradiol can stimulate the uterine peroxidase content to that seen in the rat at estrus (10). Morphologic
studies conducted by Brokelman and Fawcett (5) and Anderson and
co-workers (2,7) show that the peroxidase is localized in the
epithelial elements of the uterus. Thus it would appear that even
though the peroxidase response is elicited only in the endometrium,
its regulation correlates well with growth regulation of the entire uterus. It is also clear, however, that biochemical peroxidase assay results, based on the weight or DNA content of the
entire uterus, underestimate the enzyme concentration as well as
its extent of induction since only a minor portion of the uterus
comprises the peroxidase-positive epithelial elements. The
response of uterine peroxidase following estradiol administration
is not unique to the laboratory rat but, as we have reported
earlier (28), an increase in peroxidase is also seen in the uterus
of the hamster, guinea pig, and mouse after administration of
estradiol. Interestingly, in these four experimental animals, the
sensitivity of the uteri to estrogen-induced increases in weight
correlated closely with their sensitivity to induction of peroxidase, increasing in the order: hamster, guinea pig, rat, and
mouse. Most dramatic, when estradiol was given to the mouse for
two days at a dose of 0.4 μg per 10 g body weight the increase in
peroxidase content of the mouse uterus was more than 1000 fold.
This data would suggest that in addition to being a secretory
product found in luminal fluid (2), the epithelial peroxidase of
the uterus is synthesized as a major cellular product under estrogen control. The intracellular function of this major endometrial
enzyme remains to be elucidated.

Until the reagents necessary for quantitation of specific
messenger for peroxidase are available to definitively show that
following administration of the estrogen there is an increase in
the messenger RNA for this specific marker, the description of the
increase in uterine peroxidase elicited by the hormone as induction must be used with reservation. Especially when assessing
increased enzymatic activity, one must be concerned with possible
activation of pre-existing protein as an alternative possibility

for the apparent stimulation seen. Clearly, although peroxidase
can effect binding and subsequent metabolism of estrogen, there is
no evidence that the hormone is able to directly increase the
uterine content of peroxidase. Moreover, the dramatic estrogen-
dependent increases in uterine peroxidase require prior macromolecular synthesis consistent with de novo synthesis of new protein. As shown in Table 2 actinomycin D, an inhibitor of RNA

TABLE 2. Inhibition of estradiol-dependent increases in uterine
peroxidase by inhibitors of RNA and protein synthesis

Treatment	Peroxidase Activity[a]	
	Units/g	% of E2
Saline	0.05 ± 0.03	0.6
E2 (1 μg)	8.47 ± 3.36	100.0
E2 (1 μg) + Actinomycin D (150 μg)	0.76 ± 0.67	8.9
E2 (1 μg) + Cycloheximide (250 μg)	0.43 ± 0.17	5.0
E2 (1 μg) + Emetine (1.5 mg)	0.51 ± 0.14	6.0

[a]Peroxidase activity by guaiacol assay of $CaCl_2$ extracts of uteri
of rats 20 hours after treatment as shown, $\pm$ S.D.

synthesis, as well as cycloheximide and emetine, inhibitors of
protein synthesis, are effective inhibitors of the estrogen-
dependent increase in uterine peroxidase when given at the same
time as estrogen. Moreover, the temporal relationship of the
actinomycin D and emetine inhibition of estrogen-dependent uterine
peroxidase expression are consistent with a process involving gene
regulation. As reported elsewhere (11) from time course studies
of actinomycin D and emetine inhibition of estrogen-dependent
increases in uterine peroxidase, the requirement for RNA synthesis
for the peroxidase induction precedes by at least 2 hours the
requirement for protein synthesis necessary for the 20 hr response.
Investigations in our laboratory and elsewhere have indicated
that both antiestrogens and progestational compounds can modulate
the estrogen-dependent increases in uterine peroxidase. McNabb
and Jellinck have reported that nafoxidine (U-11100A), when administered along with estradiol, significantly reduced the estradiol-dependent increase in uterine peroxidase activity using the
water soluble product peroxidase assay (33). However these
investigators reported that pretreatment of animals with nafoxidine was less effective than administering both estrogen and antiestrogen concomitantly. We previously reported that the antiestrogen, Parke-Davis CI628, could partially inhibit the estrogen-
dependent increase in uterine peroxidase when administered con-

comitantly with estrogen (29). More recent experiments (9)
clearly show that the CI628 inhibition appears more effective
when given prior to estrogen. Thus when a 40-fold excess of
CI-628 was administered either one hour or 12 hours earlier,
estradiol was found to be incapable of inducing any increase in
peroxidase at 20 hrs. With increasing time, from 24 to 72 hours
after CI628, we observed gradual to complete release of the CI628
inhibition and an increasingly effective estradiol induction of
uterine peroxidase (9). One of the most dramatic effects of long
acting antiestrogens as evident from the reports from the laboratories of Clark (8) and Katzenellenbogen (21) is the prolonged
depletion of cytosol estrogen receptor following antiestrogen
treatment. Studies in our laboratory have shown that following
a 200 μg dose of CI628, the uterine cytosol receptor is completely
absent for at least 12 to 16 hrs, following which it is gradually
restored reaching the control levels by two to three days. Hence
the inhibitory effect of CI628 on the estrogen-dependent increase
in uterine peroxidase correlates very closely with the effect of
CI628 on the availability of cytoplasmic estrogen receptor. At
short times after CI628, when the cytoplasm of the uterine cells
contain insignificant amounts of cytoplasmic receptor, physiologic
doses of estrogen are unable to effect uterine peroxidase induction, consistent with peroxidase induction being an estrogen-
receptor mediated event.

Progesterone has been recognized for some time as an antagonist
of estrogen action (4,24). An earlier report from our laboratory
(1) demonstrated the progesterone antagonism of estrogen-dependent
increases of uterine peroxidase in normal and pregnant adult
female rats, using a histochemical assay for peroxidase. As
shown in Table 3, progesterone and other potent progestins are

TABLE 3.   Progestin inhibition of estrogen induced uterine
peroxidase activity[a]

	Peroxidase Activity (% of E2 alone)		
	100 μg[b]	500 μg[b]	1000 μg[b]
Progesterone	48.4	26.7	19.0
R5020	31.9	9.4	9.6
Norethindrone	31.7	4.2	3.7

[a]Immature rats received 1 μg estradiol (E2) on day one and either
1 μg E2 alone or along with the indicated dose of progestin 24
hours later. Twenty hours after the second injection the animals
were sacrificed and uteri assayed for peroxidase activity by
guaiacol oxidation (29).

[b]Dose of progestin given with E2 on day 2.

also effective inhibitors of estrogen-dependent uterine peroxidase induction in the immature animal. Although studies from a number of laboratories, including our own (1), have confirmed Clark's report (15) that progestin administration decreases the replenishment of the cytosol estrogen receptor complex following administration of estradiol, recent studies in our laboratory suggest that this effect of progesterone is insufficient to explain the inhibitory effect of progesterone on estrogen-dependent uterine peroxidase. Specifically, the data in Table 4 show that

TABLE 4. Time course of progesterone-dependent inhibition of estrogen induction of uterine peroxidase

Treatment time[a] (hours after E2)	Peroxidase Activity[c]	
	Units/g	% of E2 alone
Control[b]	11.95 ± 4.8	100.0
0	4.14 ± 1.6	34.6
1	2.02 ± 1.9	16.9
2	0.70 ± 0.4	5.9
4	1.03 ± 0.5	8.6
6	4.62 ± 2.3	38.7
11	11.57 ± 3.6	96.0

[a]Treatment time is the time, in hours, after 1 μg estradiol (E2) that 500 μg progesterone was administered. In each case all animals were sacrificed 20 hours after E2 for assay of uterine peroxidase.

[b]Control animals received no progesterone.

[c]Peroxidase activities given as mean values of 5 uteri per group $\pm$ S.E.M.

progesterone, given up to several hours following estradiol, is still able to effect inhibition of the 20 hr response in uterine peroxidase due to estrogen. Clearly by one to two hours after estradiol treatment the estrogen receptor complex has already left the cytosol and is localized in the nucleus. Therefore it will be important to determine whether the progesterone receptor complex can effect release of estrogen-receptor complex from the nucleus. Our preliminary studies with progesterone are consistent with a block of the estrogen-dependent peroxidase induction occurring prior to RNA synthesis since the timing of the progesterone effect, Table 4, is similar to the timing of the inhibition of the estrogen dependent peroxidase induction by actinomycin D (11). In any event it is apparent that studies of the molecular mechanism of the antagonistic effect of progestin relative to estrogen-dependent marker synthesis can be a powerful tool to help clarify the nature of this important biologic phenomenon.

The final example of the usefulness of studies relating uterine peroxidase regulation with estrogen receptor–mediated processes relate to the ontogeny of estrogen sensitivity of the developing uterus. Studies of the estrogen sensitivity of the postnatal rat uterus have consistently shown that this tissue is able to respond to hormone significantly before puberty. Most parameters of response which have been studied, however, show no significant estrogen stimulation before day 10 but are generally responsive by 15 days of age. An exception to this is the specific protein IP, first reported by Notides and Gorski (34), and found by both Katzenellenbogen and Greger (22) and Walker et al. (44) to be stimulated by estrogen in the five day old rat. As shown in Fig. 3, the uterus of the untreated four to 22 day old rat does not

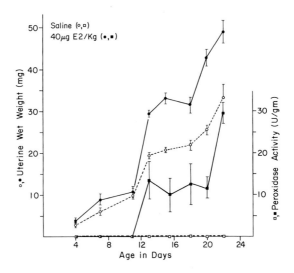

FIG. 3. Effect of estradiol on uterine weight and uterine peroxidase concentration in the postnatal female rat. Estradiol (40 μg /Kg body weight, closed symbols and solid lines) or saline (open symbols, dashed lines) was administered subcutaneously to 5 pups each from the same foster mother fed litter and the pups were sacrificed 20 hr later for assay of uterine weight (circles) and uterine peroxidase (squares). Values given as means $\pm$ S.E.M.

contain any endogenous peroxidase. Treatment of 4,7 and 11 day
old animals with a significant dose of estradiol (40 µg/Kg) is
unable to elicit any measurable peroxidase in this tissue. It is
also important to note that in these animals estradiol has no
significant affect on uterine weight. However the 13 day old rat
showed a significant sensitivity to estradiol, seen both in the
significant increase in uterine wet weight and the dramatic
increase in uterine peroxidase content following a single injection of the same amount of estradiol on a body weight basis.
Clearly after 13 days of age estrogen is able to effect significant increases in both uterine weight and peroxidase of the developing animals. Although, as shown by Raynaud (38), the early
postnatal rat contains high concentrations of the estradiol binding protein, α-fetoprotein, it appears that the ability of α-
fetoprotein to decrease the amount of circulating estrogen is not
the explanation for the delayed uterine sensitivity to estradiol
after birth. In particular as shown in Fig. 4, when similar

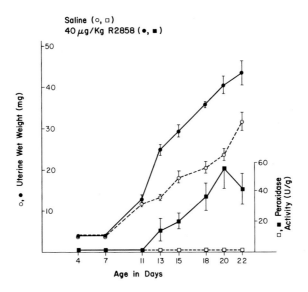

FIG. 4. Effect of R2858 on uterine wet weight and uterine
peroxidase concentration in the postnatal female rat.
Protocol, symbols and procedures detailed in Figure 3.

experiments were conducted with the synthetic estrogen, R2858, an
estrogen which does not show appreciable affinity for α-fetoprotein, the same pattern of estrogen sensitivity during develop-

ment was seen. Again in this experiment estrogen elicited no
response in either uterine wet weight or peroxidase induction in
the 4,7 and 11 day old rats. While the uterus grew significantly
between 7 and 11 days, estrogen could not stimulate further
growth. The R2858 stimulated increases in uterine weight and
uterine peroxidase in all rats 13 days or older but none younger
than 13 days. The potent non-steroidal estrogen, diethylstilbesterol, also an estrogen with little affinity for α-fetoprotein, is
similarly ineffective in stimulating uterine growth or uterine
peroxidase in animals younger than 11 days old but, like estradiol
and R2858, is a very active estrogen in older pups as we have
recently reported (30). Furthermore, we observe progesterone
inhibition of the estrogen-dependent stimulation of uterine peroxidase in the developing animal occurs at about the same time, 11
to 14 days of age (30). Hence these results indicate that the
estrogen inducibility of uterine peroxidase in the postnatal rat
correlates very well with the estrogen stimulation of uterine
weight and that peroxidase appears to be a good marker for the
sensitivity of the uterus to estrogen.

Obviously of great interest in this regard is the relationship
of the ontogeny of estrogen receptor to the estrogen sensitivity
of the developing uterus. As shown in Figure 5, the estrogen
receptor content of the 5 and 7 day rat uterus is detectable but
low. Between 7 and 9 days of age there appears to be significant
increase in estrogen receptor since the level of cytoplasmic 8S
receptor in the nine day old rat uterus is about the same as that
seen in the 21 day old animal, even though the latter but not the
former uterus is fully responsive to estrogen. The data presented
in Figure 5 correspond only to 8S receptor complex from sedimentation analysis. As noted by others (42), uterine cytosol of
early postnatal rats also contains appreciable amounts of an
estradiol binding 4S component. Since the binding of tritiated
estradiol to this 4S component is inhibited by preincubation with
excess estradiol, but not diethylstilbestrol, it is most probable
that the binding is due to α-fetoprotein. However quantitation of
"estradiol-receptor" data where specificity is shown using inhibition by non-radioactive estradiol itself, as is common practice in
the field, gives erroneous results due to the presence of α-fetoprotein. Our results, Figure 5, agree with those of Somjen, Kaye
and Lindner (42) who also used sedimentation methods. Because of
the large amounts of α-fetoprotein in cytosols of early postnatal
rat uteri it is difficult to determine whether small amounts of
specific 4S cytosol estrogen receptor may also be present. More
important however is whether the cytosol receptor found in uteri
of these young rats transmigrates to the nucleus. Recent studies
in our laboratory have shown that when exposed to estrogen in vivo
or in vitro the uterine cytosol receptor of the nine or ten day
old animal is fully capable of nuclear transmigration and shows
the same physical characteristics of the estrogen receptor in the
21 day old, fully responsive uterus. Hence the nine or ten day
old rat uterus, which contains estrogen receptor but does not
appear to be estrogen responsive, is an important model for deter-

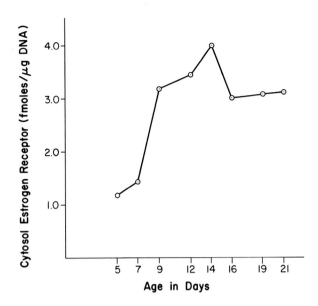

FIG. 5. Cytosol estrogen receptor content of postnatal
female rat uteri. Hypotonic uterine cytosols were analyzed
by sedimentation methods as described in Materials and
Methods. Diethylstilbesterol inhibitable binding of tritiated estradiol in 8S and aggregate regions of the sucrose
gradients were added to obtain the amount of cytosol estrogen receptor in the uteri of the untreated rats.

mination of biologically important interactions of the estrogen
receptor complex.

Recent efforts in our laboratory have been directed to the
purification to homogeniety of uterine peroxidase for characterization and preparation of antibody. These efforts have resulted
in an approximate 6000 fold purification of the enzyme from estradiol stimulated adult rat uterus, providing material which by SDS
electrophoresis shows greater than 90% of the protein staining
material in a single band. Current efforts in our laboratory are
directed to production of antibodies to rat uterine peroxidase.
With such antibodies we will have the tools necessary to detect
hormone-dependent changes in marker protein content and relate
this to changes in amount of messenger RNA for this marker protein
under conditions of estrogen treatment and other hormonal modulation. Although the biologic function of peroxidase in the uterus
is unknown, studies of the regulation of this porphyrin containing,
complex glycoprotein can provide important information to eluci-
date the macromolecular details of the estrogen receptor inter-

action and particularly its relation to gene transcription. With
new technology based on antibody to estrogen receptor (13,14)
providing the means to characterize chromatin binding sites for
receptor protein, independent of labelled steroid, along with the
evolving capability to identify and quantitate nucleic acid for a
specific protein response dependent upon the estrogen–receptor
interaction, one can predict that the coming years should allow
major advances in our understanding of estrogen receptor mediated
gene regulation in complex mammalian target organs like the uterus.

ACKNOWLEDGEMENTS

These investigations were supported by grants from the American
Cancer Society, BC–279, and the National Cancer Institute DHEW,
CA 21525. We are indebted to Richard Garay, Peter Chioros,
Restituto Dizon, Jeffrey Wheat and Leighton Toney for valuable
technical assistance.

REFERENCES

1. Anderson, W.A., DeSombre, E.R. and Kang, Y–H. (1977): Biol.
    Reprod., 16:409–419.
2. Anderson, W.A., Kang, Y–H. and DeSombre, E.R. (1975): J. Cell
    Biol., 64:668–681.
3. Beato, M., editor (1980): Steroid Induced Uterine Proteins,
    Elsevier/North Holland Biomedical Press, in press, Amsterdam.
4. Brenner, R.M. (1969): In: The Mammalian Oviduct, edited by
    E.S.E. Hafez and R.J. Blandau, pp 203–229, Univ. Chicago
    Press, Chicago.
5. Brokelmann, J. and Fawcett, D. (1969): Biol. Reprod., 1: 59–
    71.
6. Chan, L. and O'Malley, B.W. (1978): Ann. Internal Med., 89:
    694–701.
7. Churg, A. and Anderson, W.A. (1974): J. Cell Biol., 62: 449–
    459.
8. Clark, J.H., Hardin, J.W., McCormack, S.A. and Padykula, H.A.
    (1978): In: Hormones, Receptors and Breast Cancer, edited by
    W.L. McGuire, pp 107–133, Raven Press, N.Y.
9. DeSombre, E.R. and Lyttle, C.R. (1978): In: Hormones,
    Receptors, and Breast Cancer, edited by W.L. McGuire, pp 181–
    197, Raven Press, N.Y.
10. DeSombre, E.R. and Lyttle, C.R. (1979): In: Steroid Hormone
    Receptor Systems, edited by W.W. Leavitt and J.H. Clark,
    pp 157–171, Plenum Publishing Corp., N.Y.
11. DeSombre, E.R. and Lyttle, C.R. (1980): In: Steroid Induced
    Uterine Proteins, edited by M. Beato, in press, Elsevier/
    North Holland Biomedical Press, Amsterdam.
12. Gorski, J. and Gannon, F. (1976): Annu. Rev. Physiol., 38:
    425–450.
13. Greene, G.L., Closs, L.E., DeSombre, E.R. and Jensen, E.V.
    (1979): J. Steroid Biochem., 11:333–341.

14. Greene, G.L., Closs, L.E., Fleming, H., DeSombre, E.R. and Jensen, E.V. (1977): Proc. Natl. Acad. Sci. U.S.A., 74:3681-3685.
15. Hsueh, A.J.W., Peck, E.J. and Clark, J.H. (1975): Nature, 254:337-339.
16. Jellinck, P.H. and Lyttle, C.R. (1972): Adv. Enzyme Reg., 11:17-33.
17. Jellinck, P.H., McNabb, T., Cleveland, S. and Lyttle, C.R. (1976): Adv. Enzyme Reg., 14:447-465.
18. Jellinck, P.H. and Newcombe, A. (1978): J. Steroid Biochem., 8:1193-1195.
19. Jensen, E.V. and DeSombre, E.R. (1973): Science, 182:126-134.
20. Jensen, E.V. and Jacobson, H.I. (1960): In: Biological Activities of Steroids in Relation to Cancer, edited by G. Pincus and E.P. Vollmer, pp 161-178, Academic Press, N.Y.
21. Katzenellenbogen, B.S. (1978): In: Hormones, Receptors and Breast Cancer, edited by W.L. McGuire, pp 135-154, Raven Press, N.Y.
22. Katzenellenbogen, B.S. and Greger, N.G. (1974): Mol. Cell. Endocr., 2:31-42.
23. Keeping, H.S. and Jellinck, P.H. (1978): J. Steroid Biochem., 9:1049-1054.
24. Lerner, L.J. (1964): Rec. Prog. Hormone Res., 20:435-490.
25. Liao, S. (1975): Int. Rev. Cytol., 41:87-172.
26. Little, M. Szendro, P., Teran, C., Hughes, A. and Jungblut, P.W. (1975): J. Steroid Biochem., 6: 493-500.
27. Lucas, F.V., Neufeld, H.A., Utterback, J.G., Martin, A.P. and Stotz, E. (1955): J. Biol. Chem., 214:775-780.
28. Lyttle, C.R. and DeSombre, E.R. (1977): Nature, 268:337-339.
29. Lyttle, C.R. and DeSombre, E.R. (1977): Proc. Natl. Acad. Sci. U.S.A., 74:3162-3166.
30. Lyttle, C.R., Garay, R.V. and DeSombre, E.R. (1979): J. Steroid Biochem., 10:359-363.
31. Lyttle, C.R. and Jellinck, P.H. (1972): Biochem. J., 127:481-487.
32. Martial, J.A., Baxter, J.D., Goodman, H.M. and Seeburg, P.H. (1977): Proc. Natl. Acad. Sci. U.S.A., 74:1816-1820.
33. McNabb, T. and Jellinck, P.H. (1976): Steroids, 27:681-689.
34. Notides, A. and Gorski, J. (1966): Proc. Natl. Acad. Sci. U.S.A., 56:230-235.
35. Notides, A., Hamilton, D.E. and Auer, H.E. (1975): J. Biol. Chem., 250:3945-3950.
36. O'Malley, B.W. and Means, A.R. (1974): Science, 183:610-620.
37. Palmiter, R.D., Mulvihill, E.R., McKnight, G.S. and Senear, A.W. (1978): Cold Spring Harbor Symp. Quant. Biol., 42:639-647.
38. Raynaud, J. (1973): Steroids, 21:249-258.
39. Ringold, G.M., Yamamoto, K.R., Tomkins, G.M., Bishop, J.M. and Varmus, H.E. (1975): Cell, 6:299-305.
40. Robins, D.M. and Schimke, R.T. (1978): J. Biol. Chem., 253:8925-8934.

41. Schultz, G. Beato, M. and Feigelson, P. (1973): Proc. Natl. Acad. Sci. U.S.A., 70:1218-1221.
42. Somjen, G.J., Kaye, A.M. and Lindner, H.R. (1974): Mol. Cell. Endocr., 1:341-353.
43. Smith, E.R. and Barker, K.L. (1977): J. Biol. Chem., 252: 3709-3714.
44. Walker, M.D., Gozes, I., Kaye, A.M., Reiss, N. and Littauer, U.Z. (1976): J. Steroid Biochem., 7:1083-1085.

Perspectives in Steroid Receptor Research,
edited by F. Bresciani.
Raven Press, New York © 1980.

Estrogens, Estrogen Receptors, and Progesterone Receptors in Fetal and Newborn Guinea Pigs— A Model for the Study of the Biological Effect of Estrogens

J. R. Pasqualini, C. Sumida, B. L. Nguyen, A. Gulino, and C. Gelly

C.N.R.S. Steroid Hormone Research Unit, Foundation for Hormone Research, 75014 Paris, France

INTRODUCTION

Estrogen receptors appear in the fetal compartment at an early age of gestation (at least from 30 days) in the different fetal tissues of guinea pig (uterus, testis, lung, kidney, brain) (11). These specific binding sites are present in the cytosol and nuclear fractions and their concentration increases with fetal evolution and decreases after birth (11,13,14). In this paper, we summarize recent data concerning the concentration of estrogens and progesterone in the different compartments of the pregnant guinea pig, the number of occupied and unoccupied specific estrogen binding sites in fetal uterus and the biological action of estradiol on the progesterone receptor protein in fetal and newborn guinea pigs.

1) Concentration of estradiol, estrone and progesterone in the different compartments of pregnant guinea pigs

Table 1 indicates the concentration of estradiol, estrone and progesterone in the fetal and maternal plasma and in the amniotic fluid and of estrogens in the fetal uterus. The concentrations of estrogens are relatively low in the different biological fluids but its concentration is very high in uterine tissue.

2) Estrogen receptors in the different fetal tissues of guinea pig

Studies on the physico-chemical properties of the macromolecules which specifically bind estradiol (dissociation constants, sedimentation coefficients, isoelectric points) show the same values in the different fetal tissues, suggesting that the same receptor protein is present in the different fetal tissues, but the number of sites (n) is 20-60 times higher in the fetal uterus than in the other fetal tissues (Table 2).

TABLE 1.   Concentration of estradiol, estrone and progesterone in pregnant guinea pigs (55-65 days of gestation)

	Fetal plasma	Maternal plasma	Amniotic fluid	Fetal uterine tissue pg/g
Estradiol pg/ml	9 - 11	20 - 30	20 - 40	770 - 1100
Estrone pg/ml	95 - 105	90 - 100	40 - 60	850 - 1200
Progesterone ng/ml	0.2 - 2.0	130 - 200	0.4 - 0.6	-*

Determination carried out by radioimmunoassay
-* not evaluated

TABLE 2.   Characteristics of the specific binding of ^{3}H-estradiol to macromolecules in the different fetal tissues of guinea pig (55-60 days of gestation)

Fetal tissues	Kd 4°C M x 10^{-10}	n (fmoles/mg protein)	S	pI
Uterus	2 - 5	70 - 88	8	6.1 - 6.2
Lung	4 - 8	2 - 3.7	8	6.1 - 6.2
Kidney	2.5 - 4	1.1 - 4.5	8	6.1 - 6.2
Brain	5 - 8	1.5 - 5.0	7 - 8	6.1 - 6.2

Kd : Dissociation constant (4°C)
n : number of specific binding sites
S : Sedimentation coefficient
pI : Isoelectric point

3)   Evaluation of the occupied and unoccupied estradiol binding sites in fetal and newborn uterus and effect of estradiol on the translocation of cytoplasmic receptor into the nucleus

Using the exchange assay (2,16) the concentrations of the occupied and unoccupied binding sites of estradiol were determined in protamine sulfate precipitates of the cytosol and of the 0.6M KCl nuclear extract of the uterus. As indicated in Table 3, the total number of sites is very high (19 pmoles/mg DNA or 80 pmoles/g tissue) and is 4-5 times higher than the values found in the uterus of immature or castrated rats (3,16). The concentration of occupied sites in the cytosol and nuclear fractions of fetal uterus (9 pmoles/g tissue) corresponds approximately to the concentration of endogenous estradiol plus estrone (7 pmoles/g tissue) (14) in the tissue. It is interesting to note that the number of occupied binding sites (∿10000 binding sites per cell) is in the range of values of total estradiol receptor concentrations in immature or adult rat uterus (1).

As indicated in Table 3, the incubation of fetal uterus with estradiol translocates only 50 % of the cytosol receptor into the nucleus. Furthermore, the total number of specific sites decreases 40-50 % when compared with values in fetal uterus which was not exposed to estradiol.

TABLE 3. Occupied and unoccupied estradiol binding sites in the fetal and newborn guinea pig. Effect of estradiol on the translocation of the cytoplasmic estradiol receptors. (pmoles/mg DNA) (13)

	Controls			$+E_2$ (5 x 10^{-8}M)
	Fetal uterus (55-65 days)	Newborns	Immature rats	Fetal uterus
Rc	15.43 ± 2.35	7.71 ± 1.41	4.65 ± 0.42	0.65 ± 0.24
RcE_2	2.42 ± 0.93	0.13 ± 0.09	0	6.26 ± 0.90
Rn	1.27 ± 0.57	0.50 ± 0.14	0.34 ± 0.02	1.01 ± 0.53
RnE_2	0.02 ± 0.02	0	0	4.93 ± 1.21
R Total	19.13 ± 3.24	8.34 ± 1.98	4.99 ± 0.43	12.85 ± 1.91

Specific binding of ^{3}H-estradiol was determined in protamine sulfate precipitates of cytosol and nuclear extract after incubation with 1 x 10^{-8}M ^{3}H-estradiol (with and without a 100-fold molar excess of unlabelled estradiol) at 4°C overnight for unoccupied cytosol (Rc) and nuclear (Rn) binding sites and at 30°C or 37°C for occupied binding sites (RcE_2 and RnE_2).

4) Progesterone receptors in the fetal uterus of guinea pig
Specific binding sites for progesterone are found in the cytosol and in the nuclei of fetal uterus of guinea pig at the end of gestation (9). As is indicated in Table 4, these specific binding sites are not a contamination of fetal plasma protein which also binds progesterone with an affinity similar to that of the receptor (8), however, the other physico-chemical properties (pI, thermolability, binding to the synthetic progestagen R-5020) are very different.

5) Relationship of estradiol and progesterone receptors in the fetal uterus of guinea pig during fetal development
Comparative studies on the determination of estradiol and progesterone receptors in the fetal uterus show that the estradiol receptor appears at an early age of gestation but the progesterone receptor is absent until 45-50 days (Table 5). At that period, the progesterone receptor appears and increases throughout fetal evolution. This data suggests the possibility that estrogens and probably estrogen receptors are involved in the biosynthesis of the progesterone receptor protein in the fetal uterus.

TABLE 4.   Comparative physico-chemical properties of the specific binding of ^{3}H-progesterone (^{3}H-P) and ^{3}H-R-5020 in fetal uterine cytosol and plasma of guinea pig (8,9)

	Fetal uterus		Fetal plasma	
	^{3}H-P	^{3}H-R-5020	^{3}H-P	^{3}H-R-5020
Dissociation constant K_D 4°C ($\times 10^{-9}$M)	3.3 ± 1.7	0.7 ± 0.3	0.88 ± 0.35	No specific binding
Coefficient of sedimentation (S)	6-7 ; 4	6-7 ; 4	4.6	-
Isoelectric point (pI)	5 - 5.5	-	< 3	-
Temperature * effect	Thermo labile	Thermo labile	Thermo-resistant	No specific binding

* Aliquots of fetal uterine cytosol fraction or diluted fetal plasma (1/10 - 1/50 ^{V}/v) were pre-heated for 1h at 37°C in the absence of the hormone and then reincubated with ^{3}H-progesterone or ^{3}H-R-5020 (4 x 10^{-9}M) with or without a 100-fold excess of the unlabelled steroids to measure the number of specific binding sites after adsorbing the unbound radioactive steroids with dextran charcoal.

6)   Induction and stimulation of progesterone receptors by estrogens in the fetal and newborn uterus of guinea pig

Preliminary experiments showed that after subcutaneous injection of 40 µCi of ^{3}H-estradiol to the mother, 0.8-1 % of the total radioactivity injected reached the fetuses. From this result, the dose of 1mg/kg/day injected to the mother for 3 days was chosen and the progesterone receptors were evaluated on day 4 in the fetal uterus. The newborn animals were treated s.c. with 10-100 µg of estradiol for 2 days and the progesterone receptor evaluated on day 3. Figure 1 indicates a 7 to 10-fold stimulation of progesterone receptors over control values during fetal development. It is observed that after birth this stimulatory effect diminishes very significantly (12).

7)   Effect of the estradiol dose injected to the mother on the progesterone and estrogen receptors of the fetal uterus

Different quantities of estradiol were injected (0.1 to 5 mg) to the pregnant guinea pig and the effect on progesterone and estradiol receptors was analysed in the fetal uterus 24h after administration of the hormone. As is indicated in Figure 2, the maximal stimulation of the progesterone receptor was obtained with a dose of estradiol of 1mg/kg. A drastic decrease in the total number of specific estradiol binding sites (cytosol + nuclei,   occupied and unoccupied) can also be observed. There is as yet no clear explanation for this phenomenon, but it is possible that estradiol, in this fetal tissue, controls the synthesis of its own receptor. It is interesting to remark that similar data were found in vitro, after culture of the MCF-7 cell line of human breast cancer (6).

TABLE 5. Concentration of specific binding sites for estradiol (E_2-R) and for progesterone (P-R) in the cytosol of the uterus of guinea pig during development (11,12)

Days of gestation	E_2-R fmoles/mg protein	P-R fmoles/mg protein
34 - 35	85 - 95	N.D.
36 - 37	140 - 200	N.D.
44 - 45	300 - 490	N.D.
50 - 54	550 - 680	30 - 45
55 - 65	580 - 880	70 - 140
Newborns		
< 24h	380 - 450	160 - 220
2-3 days	340 - 420	200 - 250
7-8 days	300 - 400	200 - 230

N.D. : Not detectable
E_2-R : Estrogen receptors
P-R : Progesterone receptors

Cytosol fractions of uteri of fetal and newborn guinea pigs were incubated with 4×10^{-9}M ^{3}H-estradiol or ^{3}H-progesterone (with or without a 100-fold molar excess of unlabelled steroid) for 4h at 4°C. Bound and unbound steroids were separated by adsorption with dextran-coated charcoal. The values represent the extremes of 4-5 determinations.

8) Prolonged effect of estradiol on the fetal uterine progesterone receptor

As the effect of estradiol on the progesterone receptor is very intense and maximal stimulation was observed 16h after the administration of the estrogen to the mother, it was interesting to investigate the duration of this effect. Estradiol was injected to the mother, 1mg/kg/day, for 3 days and the progesterone receptor in the fetal uterus was evaluated 2 and 4 days after the last administration of estradiol. As is indicated in Table 6, the values of the progesterone receptor are still very high at least 4 days after the last injection, indicating that this biological response is of long duration in the fetal uterus. This observation is in contrast to the response in the uterus of the immature guinea pig in which the progesterone receptor concentration diminished by 80 % 24h after the last administration of diethylstilbestrol (5).

TABLE 6. Prolonged effect of estradiol (E_2) on the ^{3}H-progeste-
rone (R-P) and ^{3}H-R-5020 (R-R-5020) specific binding
sites in the cytosol of fetal guinea pig (55-64 days of
gestation) (12)
(fmoles/mg protein)

Treatment Days 1,2,3 Evaluation	(P-R)		R-R-5020	
	Control	+E_2	Control	+E_2
Day 4	70 - 120	500 - 700	130 - 220	1100 - 1300
Day 8	70 - 120	400 - 600	130 - 220	850 - 1050

Pregnant guinea pigs were injected (s.c.) with 1mg estradiol/kg/
day for 3 days. On day 4 and day 8 the fetuses were removed by
laparotomy and the fetal uteri were excised. The cytosol fraction
of fetal uterus was incubated with 4 x 10^{-9}M ^{3}H-progesterone or
^{3}H-R-5020 (with or without a 100-fold excess of unlabelled steroids) at 4°C for 4h. The values are the extremes of 3-4 determinations.

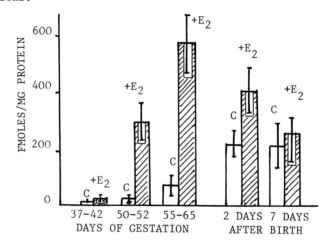

FIGURE 1.   EFFECT OF ESTRADIOL TREATMENT ON SPECIFIC BINDING OF
^{3}H-PROGESTERONE IN UTERINE CYTOSOL DURING DEVELOPMENT

Pregnant guinea pigs were injected subcutaneously with 1mg/kg/day
of estradiol (E_2 treated animals) or 40 % ethanol-saline vehicle
(control animals) for 3 days. On day 4, the animals were anesthe-
tized, the fetuses separated and the fetal uterus removed and
cytosol fraction prepared. The newborn animals were injected
subcutaneously for 1 day with 1 to 100 µg of estradiol in 40 %
ethanol-saline. Animals were sacrificed on day 2 and uterine
cytosol isolated. Cytosols were incubated with 3-4 x 10^{-9}M ^{3}H-
progesterone with or without a 100-fold molar excess of unlabelled progesterone for 4 to 18h at 4°C.

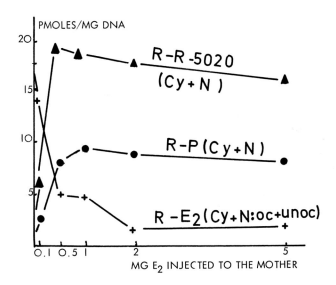

FIGURE 2.   DOSE RESPONSE CURVE OF ESTRADIOL TREATMENT ON PROGESTERONE, R-5020 AND ESTRADIOL RECEPTORS IN THE FETAL UTERUS OF GUINEA PIG

Pregnant guinea pigs were injected with 0.1, 0.5, 1, 2 or 5 mg estradiol/kg. 1 day later, the animals were sacrificed, fetuses were separated and fetal uteri were excised. Specific binding of ^{3}H-R-5020 was determined in the cytosol and 0.6M KCl nuclear extract of fetal uterus after incubation with 4×10^{-9}M ^{3}H-progesterone or ^{3}H-R-5020 with or without a 100-fold molar excess of unlabelled steroid at 4°C overnight. Specific estradiol binding was determined in protamine sulfate precipitates of cytosol and nuclear extract (1×10^{-8}M ^{3}H-estradiol with and without a 100-fold molar excess of unlabelled estradiol) under conditions of exchange. The values represent the concentrations of total receptors in cytosol and nucleus.

9) Action of estriol on the fetal uterine progesterone
                              receptor
     It is well known that estriol is quantitatively the most
important estrogen produced during human pregnancy, particularly
at the end of gestation. Studies carried out on the biological
effect of this estrogen on the uterus of immature animals showed
that its action (uterotrophic effect) is 1/10 that of estradiol
and it has been suggested that this weak effect is due to the
short retention time of estriol in the nucleus (4). In this
connection, the biological action of estriol was compared with
estradiol after injection of 1mg/kg/day for 3 days to pregnant
guinea pigs. The data shown in Table 7 indicate that both estrogens had an equal effect on the stimulation of progesterone
receptors in the fetal uterus.

TABLE 7.   Comparative effect of estradiol (E_2) and estriol (E_3)
           on the progesterone (P-R) and R-5020 receptors in
                 the fetal uterus of guinea pig
                    (55-65 days of gestation)

	P-R		R-R-5020	
	C	N	C	N
Control (Non treated)	0.9	0.03	2	0.15
+Estradiol	10.5	0.5	15.5	0.9
+Estriol	9.0	0.4	18.0	2.0

     Pregnant guinea pigs were injected (s.c.) with 1mg estradiol
or estriol/kg/day for 3 days. On day 4 the fetuses were removed
and fetal uteri were excised. Specific binding of ^{3}H-progeste-
rone and ^{3}H-R-5020 was determined in the cytosol fraction (C)
and 0.6M KCl nuclear extract (N) of fetal uterus by incubating
with 4 x 10^{-9}M ^{3}H-progesterone or ^{3}H-R-5020 (with and without a
100-fold excess of unlabelled steroid) at 4°C overnight.

DISCUSSION AND CONCLUSION

     The present data show that in fetal life, estrogens can elicit
a biological effect by increasing the number of progesterone
receptors in the fetal uterus. The estrogens are capable of inducing these receptors at an early stage of gestation (37-42 days)
when the progesterone receptor is not yet detectable. At the end
of gestation, estradiol treatment stimulates the progesterone
receptor 7-10 times in relation to the non-treated animals. On
the other hand, this stimulatory effect diminishes in the new-
borns ; there is a 2-fold stimulation in the 2-day-old animals
and 1.2-fold at 7 days. It is interesting to mention that the
stimulatory effect on the progesterone receptor is observed also
in the fetal ovary, but not in other fetal tissues or in the
placenta (unpublished observations).

As indicated in Table 1, the concentration of estradiol in the fetal plasma of guinea pig is relatively low but its concentration in fetal uterine tissue is 30-50 times that in the plasma. This selective uptake and concentration of the hormone could imply that the endogenous estrogens have a biological activity in the fetus, as it is well known that selective retention occurs for all steroid hormones in target tissues in extra-uterine life. The biological action could also be explained by the very high concentration of estradiol receptor sites which are occupied by the endogenous hormone (2.7 pmol/mg DNA).

The low concentration of the hormone in the plasma could also be the result of a defense mechanism which controls the biological action of the hormone in the fetus. This control can be carried out by the intense metabolism of the hormone in the fetal compartment, mainly to the formation of sulfates (10).

Another aspect of this data is the drastic decrease of the total specific binding sites for estradiol (cytosol + nuclei : occupied and unoccupied) in the fetal uterus after injection of the hormone to the mother. This decrease is 70-80 % in relation to the non-treated animals. This is not due to the possible presence of salt-resistant sites in the nucleus because 92-96 % of the total radioactivity in the nucleus is found in the 0.6M KCl nuclear extract. This decrease, which is not found in immature rats (7), could be explained by a control of the biosynthesis of the estradiol receptor protein by the hormone itself. This argument is supported by the prolonged effect of estradiol on the stimulation of the progesterone receptor as indicated in Table 7. The high concentration of progesterone receptor in the fetal uterus 4 days after the last dose of E_2 is the same as that obtained after 24h. It is interesting to remark that estradiol has a similar effect on the decrease of estradiol receptor which has recently been observed in breast carcinoma cells of the MCF-7 line (6), and in normal mammary tissue (Shyamala, personal communication).

Finally, it is observed that the action of estriol on the stimulation of the progesterone receptor in the fetal uterus is of the same intensity as that of estradiol. This is an important finding since it is well known that the production rate of estriol increases very significantly at the end of human pregnancy (40-60 mg/24h). This effect is different from that obtained in the uterus of immature rats in which it was demonstrated that estriol has a uterotrophic effect of only 1/10-1/6 that of equimolar quantities of estradiol and a shorter nuclear retention time (4). The fact that the biological effect is similar for the two estrogens in the fetal uterus could be explained by a regulation of the plasma concentration of estriol in the fetus through the placenta.

In conclusion, the fetal guinea pig is a useful model for the study of the biological effect of estrogens. At present, two effects are well established : an early effect on the stimulation of the progesterone receptor and a later effect on the growth of the uterus.

REFERENCES

1. Anderson,J.N., Clark,J.H. and Peck,E.J. Jr. (1972) : Biochem. J., 126:561-567.
2. Chamness,G.C., Huff,K. and McGuire,W.L. (1975) : Steroids, 25:627-635.
3. Clark,J.H., Anderson,J. and Peck,E.J. Jr. (1972) : Science, 176:528-530.
4. Clark,J.H., Paszko,Z. and Peck,E.J. Jr. (1977) : Endocrinology 100:91-96.
5. Freifeld,M.L., Feil,P.D. and Bardin,C.W. (1974) : Steroids, 23:93-103.
6. Horwitz,K.B. and McGuire,W.L. (1978) : J. biol. Chem.,253: 2223-2228.
7. Katzenellenbogen,B.S. and Ferguson,E.R. (1975) : Endocrinology 97:1-12.
8. Millet,A. and Pasqualini,J.R. (1978) : C.R. Acad. Sc. Paris (Serie D), 287:1429-1432.
9. Pasqualini J.R. and Nguyen B.L. (1979) J. Endocr., 81:144P-145P.
10. Pasqualini,J.R., Sumida,C. and Gelly,C. (1976) : Acta Endocrinologica, 83:811-828.
11. Pasqualini,J.R., Sumida,C., Gelly,C. and Nguyen,B.L. (1976) : J. Steroid Biochem., 7:1031-1038.
12. Pasqualini,J.R., Sumida,C., Nguyen,B.L., Tardy,J. and Gelly C. (1979) J. Steroid Biochem., 11:(in press).
13. Sumida,C. and Pasqualini,J.R. (1979) : Endocrinology, 105: 406-413.
14. Sumida,C. and Pasqualini,J.R. (1979) : J. Steroid Biochem., 11:267-272.
15. Sumida,C., Gelly,C. and Pasqualini,J.R. (1978) : Biol. Reprod., 19:338-345.
16. Zava,D.T., Harrington,N.Y. and McGuire,W.L. (1976) Biochemistry, 15:4292-4297.

Perspectives in Steroid Receptor Research,
edited by F. Bresciani.
Raven Press, New York © 1980.

Estrogen and Progesterone Receptors in Normal Mammary Gland During Different Functional States

G. Shyamala and S. Z. Haslam

Lady Davis Institute for Medical Research, Sir Mortimer B. Davis Jewish General Hospital, Montreal, Quebec H3T 1E2, Canada

INTRODUCTION

Studies on a variety of target tissues for progesterone have demonstrated specific cytoplasmic progesterone receptors (1-8). In rodents, progesterone is known to be an important hormone for mammary gland cell proliferation and differentiation (9-11); progesterone is also an antagonist of lactogenesis (12-15) and can inhibit molecular events leading to casein synthesis (16). In rats, progesterone can enhance the induction of mammary tumors by DMBA (17), and at certain doses cause tumor regression (18,19). Similar to other target tissues for estrogen in normal and neoplastic mammary glands, estrogen receptors (ER) and progesterone receptors (PgR) are present and the PgR levels are augmented with estradiol treatment (20-29). However, it has also been demonstrated that in the absence of estradiol physiological doses of progesterone do not sustain the growth of established mammary tumors despite the initial presence of PgR (24). Thus, it is not clear whether the presence of progesterone receptors in mammary tissues is an indication of it being sensitive to progesterone or being sensitive to estrogen. Therefore, it is necessary to delineate the role of PgR in mediating progesterone regulated events and distinguish between its use as a marker for estrogen action in mammary tissues. Since the effect of estrogen and progesterone in normal mammary glands can vary according to the developmental state of the tissue, any understanding of the role of estradiol, ER and/or PgR will have to take into consideration that particular developmental state of the tissue. To this extent, the present studies were undertaken in an attempt to delineate the mechanism(s) by which these receptor levels are modulated and the ability of these receptors to mediate hormonal effects under different developmental states.

MATERIALS AND METHODS

Animals

Female Balb/c mice were used at 2-5 months of age and were from our own colony. Intact or ovariectomized virgin, pregnant or lactating mice were obtained and used as described previously (28,29). Unilateral thelectomy was accomplished by nipple cauterization prior to mating.

Isotopes

The synthetic progestin [^{3}H]R5020 (17,21-dimethyl-19-nor-4,9-pregnadiene-3,20-dione) (specific activity: 86.0 Ci/mmole) and estradiol (2,4,6,7-^{3}H) (specific activity: 90-115 Ci/mmole) were purchased from New England Nuclear Corp., Boston, MA.

Hormones

All hormones used for injections were purchased from Sigma Chemical Company, St. Louis, MO. Unlabelled R5020 was purchased from New England Nuclear Corp., Boston, MA. The hormones were administered by subcutaneous injection. Steroid hormones were administered as a solution in 1% ethanol in saline or in sesame oil, prolactin was administered in saline, pH 8.5.

Steroid Receptor Assays

Tissue homogenates were prepared in a phosphate-glycerol buffer (5 mM sodium phosphate, 10 mM thioglycerol, 10% glycerol, pH 7.4) and centrifuged at 12,350 x g for 1 hr. Unless otherwise specified, the supernatants designated as cytoplasmic extracts were used for steroid receptor assays. For measurements of PgR, aliquots of cytoplasmic extracts were incubated with either 20 nM (mammary glands) or 50 nM (uterus) of [^{3}H]R5020 alone or in the presence of a 100-fold excess of unlabelled R5020. For measurements of ER, aliquots of cytoplasmic extracts were incubated with 7.5 nM (mammary gland) or 20 nM (uterus) of [^{3}H]estradiol either alone or in the presence of a 100-fold excess of unlabelled estradiol. All incubations were done in ice for 4 hours prior to assay. The bound radioactive steroid in all the incubations was estimated using the dextran coated charcoal (DCC) assay of Korenman (30) as described previously (29,31) for mammary glands.

At this point, it is necessary to make some comments on the estimation of PgR in mammary glands using R5020 as the ligand in binding studies. Previously, we have reported that dexamethasone can significantly compete for certain specific R5020 binding sites in mammary gland; these binding sites did not appear to be high affinity PgR (29,31). Subsequent studies revealed that inclusion of dithiothreitol (DTT) in the buffer augmented the degree of competition by dexamethasone to specific R5020 binding

sites which was consistent with recent observations in our laboratory that the glucocorticoid binding sites in mammary tissues
were stabilized by DTT (McBlain and Shyamala, unpublished observations). Therefore, in the present studies DTT was not included
in the homogenizing buffer and the specific binding data reported
in these studies do not include any correction for competition by
dexamethasone to specific R5020 binding sites.

α-Lactalbumin Measurement

α-Lactalbumin activity was assayed by the method of Ip and Dao
(32) with modifications as follows. Mammary tissue was homogenized with two 15 sec bursts of a Polytron PT 10-ST (Brinkmann
Instruments, Inc., Westbury, NY). Homogenates were not centrifuged but used after filtration through organza. The reaction
mixture contained either 20 or 50 μl of homogenate, 2 μmol Tris-
HCl buffer (pH 7.4), 1 μmol $MnCl_2$, 60 nmol UDP-galactose
[supplemented with approximately 15,000 cpm UDP-[^{14}C]galactose
(New England Nuclear Corp., Boston, MA)]. The total volume of
the reaction mixture was 100 μl. α-Lactalbumin activity was estimated in the presence of excess bovine milk galactosyltransferase
(5 milliunits; Sigma) and 2 μmol of D-glucose acceptor to form
[^{14}C]lactose. A standard curve was generated with increasing
amounts of bovine α-lactalbumin to ensure that the reaction was
in the linear portion of the curve with respect to α-lactalbumin
concentration. To correct for the production of [^{14}C]galactose
resulting from endogenous hydrolysis of UDP-[^{14}C]galactose, a
control reaction was included for each sample in the absence of
acceptor. The incubations of the reaction mixture were done at
37°C for 30 min and the reaction was stopped by cooling in ice
and subsequently adding 100 μl of cold water. The content of
each tube was quickly passed through a column (0.5 x 4 cm) of
Bio-Rad AG 1-X2 anion exchange resin in the chloride cycle. Reaction tubes were washed with 0.5 ml of water that was then
transferred to the columns. Neutral sugars on the column were
eluted with another 1 ml of water directly into scintillation
vials. Radioactivity in the eluate was measured with 10 ml of
formula 950A (New England Nuclear, Boston, MA) by liquid scintillation counting. Recovery of neutral sugars from the column
was over 80% with no elution of UDP-galactose. For histological
studies to determine degree of lobuloalveolar differentiation
mammary tissue samples were prepared as described previously (29).
DNA content of tissues was estimated according to Cerriotti (33)
and protein concentration was assayed according to Lowry (34).

RESULTS AND DISCUSSION

Relationship Between the Levels of Progesterone Receptors (PgR) and the Developmental Stages of the Mammary Gland

To assess the relationship between development and PgR levels, mammary cytoplasmic extracts of virgin, pregnant and postpartum mice were assayed for PgR and, as shown in Fig. 1, the receptors were present in the cytosols of virgin and pregnant mice; however, binding had decreased at mid-pregnancy by ∿3.5 fold, by day 1 of lactation by 10 fold and was totally undetectable during established lactation (days 2-15). Between 16 and 25 days post-partum, PgR were occasionally, but not consistently, detected (data not shown). At 28 days postpartum, PgR were consistently detected in mammary cytoplasmic extracts. It was possible that the observed modulations in the level of cytoplasmic PgR might have resulted from changes in cell number as a function of development; however, this did not appear to be the case since as also shown in Fig. 1, the differences in the levels of PgR were also apparent when the data was expressed on the basis of DNA.

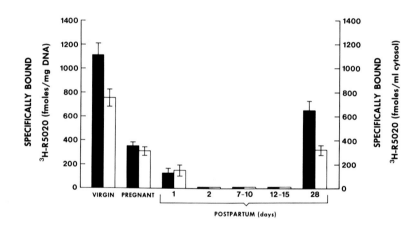

FIG. 1. The relationship between cytoplasmic progesterone receptor levels in mammary glands and different stages of mammary gland development. (■) Data expressed on the basis of DNA. (□) Data expressed on the basis of ml cytoplasmic extract which is equivalent to one gram tissue. Each bar represents the mean ± S.E.M. of 4-8 separate experiments. Virgin = adult non-ovariectomized; pregnant = 12-14 days of pregnancy. Reproduced from Haslam and Shyamala (1979b).

In order to ensure that the observed lack of PgR in the cyto-sol of lactating mammary tissue was not due to cellular factors which might have interfered with the assay conditions, experiments were performed with combined cytoplasmic extracts of mamm-ary glands and uteri which were known to contain PgR. The mixed cytoplasmic extracts were obtained either by combining the

individual cytosols or cohomogenizing the uteri with mammary
glands and then centrifuging the cohomogenate. As shown in
Table 1, mixing the uterine cytosol with lactating mammary cytosol either directly or by cohomogenization failed materially to
decrease the expected number of progesterone receptor sites
contributed by the uterine cytosol. Thus the observed lack of
progesterone receptors in the lactating mammary cytosol could
not have resulted from interference with the assay by factors
present in the cytosol.

TABLE 1. Binding of $[^3H]$R5020 in uterine and mammary cytosol

(a) Incubation	Specifically bound $[^3H]$R5020 (fmol/ml)	Protein concentration (mg/ml)
Mammary cytosol + buffer (1:1,v/v)	none	20.1
Uterine cytosol + buffer (1:1,v/v)	5473	4.1
Mammary cytosol + uterine cytosol (1:1,v/v)	5533	-
(b) Incubation	Expt. 1	Expt. 2
Uterine cytosol	3945	17001
Mammary cytosol	none	none
Mixed cytosol from cohomogenates	1844	9548

In all experiments 1.0 ml of mammary cytosol was equivalent to
1 g of tissue and 1.0 ml of uterine cytosol was equivalent to
five uteri. (a) Mixed cytosols were incubated at 0°C for 4 hr
with 50 nM $[^3H]$R5020 either alone or in the presence of 100 fold
excess of unlabelled R5020. (b) In Expt. 1, 7.6 nM $[^3H]$R5020
was used with 100 fold excess of unlabelled R5020. In Expt. 2,
50 nM $[^3H]$R5020 was used with 100 fold excess of unlabelled
R5020. Adapted from Shyamala and McBlain (1979).

The Effect of Estradiol on Progesterone Receptors and its Relationship to Mammary Gland Development

Since it is known that in certain target tissues for estrogen
including certain mammary tumors, estradiol can stimulate the
synthesis of PgR, the effect of estradiol on PgR levels in
mammary glands was examined. As shown in Fig. 2, estradiol significantly increased the level of cytoplasmic PgR in castrated
virgin mice; the K_d of the progesterone-receptor complex of
mammary tissues of estradiol treated animals (0.97 nM) was similar to that of the saline treated animals (1.5 nM) and both

values are similar to the previously reported Kd values for
progesterone-receptor complexes in various target tissues (6).

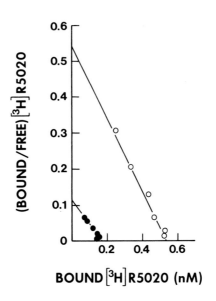

FIG. 2. Saturation analysis of specific binding of
[³H]R5020 in cytoplasmic extracts of mammary glands
of castrated virgin mice. Portions of cytoplasmic
extracts from 0.9% NaCl- (•) or estradiol-treated
(○) mice were incubated for 4 hr at 4°C with various
concentrations of [³H]R5020 either alone or in the
presence of a 500 fold excess of unlabelled R5020.
Bound [³H]R5020 was determined on duplicate portions.
The results represent specific binding per g of
mammary tissue. Reproduced from Haslam and Shyamala
(1979a).

In contrast to the mammary gland of virgin mice, both in control and estradiol treated lactators, mammary tissue did not have
detectable levels of PgR whereas the uteri of the same animals
had PgR; furthermore uterine PgR was significantly stimulated by
estradiol administration (Fig. 3). In experiments where lactating mice received two doses of estradiol spaced 24 hr apart,
there was still no detectable level of PgR in mammary tissues
(data not shown). The results of similar experiments performed
with castrated lactators are shown in Fig. 4. As may be seen,
ovariectomy did not result in the appearance of PgR in mammary

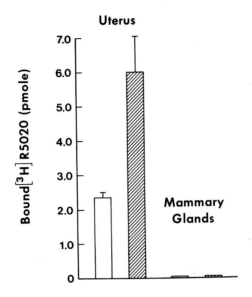

FIG. 3. Effect of estradiol on the amounts of cytoplasmic
PgR in the uterus and mammary glands of lactating mice.
Two groups of lactating mice between day 7 and day 10 of
lactation were given a single injection of either 0.9%
NaCl (□) or 3 μg of estradiol (▨). The results are
expressed as means ± S.E.M. for four experiments and
represent the binding per g of mammary tissue or per
uterus. Reproduced from Haslam and Shyamala (1979a).

tissue of lactators and also did not significantly affect the
level of PgR in the uterus as compared to intact lactators.
However, in estradiol treated castrated animals, the uterine PgR
levels were significantly higher than control and in contrast to
the uteri, estradiol once again failed to stimulate PgR synthesis
in mammary glands. Measurement of progesterone levels in the
plasma revealed a significant reduction in the levels present in
castrated lactators as compared to intact lactators (Murphy,
B.E.P. and Shyamala, G., unpublished observations).

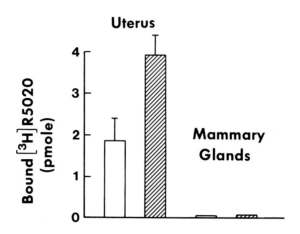

FIG. 4. Effect of estradiol on the amounts of cytoplasmic PgR in the uterus and mammary glands of castrated lactating mice. Mice were castrated at day 2 of lactation, a single injection of 0.9% NaCl (□) or 3 μg of estradiol (▨) were given on day 9 and tissues were assayed at day 10. The results are expressed as means ± S.E.M. for five experiments and represent binding per g of mammary tissue or per uterus. Reproduced from Haslam and Shyamala (1979a).

From studies on rats, it is known that lactation is accompanied by a pseudopregnant state characterized by an inhibition of gonadotropin secretion, an increase in prolactin secretion and maintenance of corpus luteum function: this pseudopregnant state is associated with very low serum levels of estradiol during early lactation and a high serum concentration of progesterone (37). Since studies on uterus have demonstrated that both low levels of estrogen (7,35,36) and high levels of progesterone (38,39) can lead to decreased levels of PgR the hormonal milieu of lactation may be expected to adversely affect the levels of PgR. The PgR levels in the uterine tissue of lactators is low as compared to nonlactators but can be elevated with the administration of estradiol. Thus, lack of an adequate estrogenic environment may be one aspect of the hormonal milieu of lactation which contributes to decreased levels of PgR in the uterus. However, in the case of mammary glands, the lack of detectable levels of PgR during lactation and the inability of these tissues to synthesize PgR under the influence of estradiol in both intact and castrated states indicated that the hormonal milieu of lactation alone could not have been responsible for the absence of PgR in these mammary glands.

Identification of the Hormone(s) Responsible for Progesterone Receptor Modulation during Mammary Gland Development and Differentiation

In view of the observed pattern of PgR modulation vis a vis pregnancy and lactation, it was important to determine whether this modulation was directly related to mammary gland differentiation or resulted indirectly due to changes in the hormonal milieu during pregnancy and lactation. It is known that in rodents in the absence of ovaries, mammary growth similar to that observed during pregnancy can be experimentally induced by administration of estradiol and progesterone; the mammary growth under these conditions is characterized by complex epithelial network with numerous ducts, ductal branches and alveoli (9,10). Therefore in the following studies mammary growth was experimentally induced by administration of estradiol (E) and progesterone (P) for 14 days and the effect of these hormones on PgR levels was examined. The results of these experiments are shown in Table 2. Administration of E.alone resulted approximately in a 4-5 fold increase in PgR over the basal level in ovariectomized control mice. Progesterone had no effect on PgR when administered alone but in combination with E inhibited the E-mediated increase in PgR by approximately 20%. The data on the uterus confirmed earlier observations that estradiol augmented the synthesis of PgR while progesterone antagonized this estradiol-mediated effect.

It is well established that lactogenic hormones are present in high levels during pregnancy and are necessary for the initiation and maintenance of lactation (40). To this extent, it was decided to examine the role of prolactin (Prl) in the modulation of PgR in mammary tissue. Since the primary aim of this study was to identify the hormonal basis for the decrease of PgR observed between pregnancy and lactation, the effect of Prl was studied in animals which had been pretreated with exogenous E and P such that the mammary gland had attained a developmental state comparable to that observed in mid-pregnancy. The results of these experiments as shown in Table 3 revealed the following. (1) In the absence of any exogenous hormones, mammary PgR decayed rapidly to the basal level similar to that observed in ovariectomized controls which did not receive any hormonal treatment. (2) E augmented the synthesis of PgR. (3) Prl had no significant effect on PgR either alone or in combination with other hormones.

TABLE 2. Effect of estradiol and progesterone on cytoplasmic progesterone receptor levels in mammary gland and uterus of ovariectomized virgin mice

Specific binding of $[^3H]$R5020

Treatment	Mammary gland		Uterus	
	fmoles/ml cytosol	fmoles/mg protein	fmoles/uterus	fmoles/mg protein
Oil	195 ± 30	11.5 ± 1.8	455 ± 162	386 ± 137
E	962 ± 32	46.0 ± 1.5	8369 ± 676	1435 ± 116
P	262 ± 31	15.0 ± 1.8	533 ± 19	249 ± 8.9
E+P	769 ± 37a	37.3 ± 1.8	2644 ± 338	518 ± 66

ap = .01 E alone > E+P (T-test).
As indicated ovariectomized mice were given 14 daily injections of various hormones or oil and tissues were assayed 24 hr later. The results are expressed as mean ± S.E.M. of three to four experiments. One ml of mammary cytosol is equivalent to one gram tissue. E = estradiol, 1 µg; P = progesterone, 1 mg.

TABLE 3. Effect of prolactin either alone or in various combinations on the cytoplasmic progesterone receptor levels in the mammary gland and uterus of ovariectomized virgin mice pretreated with estradiol and progesterone

Specific binding of [^{3}H]R5020

Treatment	Mammary gland		Uterus	
	fmoles/ml cytosol	fmoles/mg protein	fmoles/uterus	fmoles/mg protein
Oil	231 ± 11	16.5 ± 0.8	3082 ± 143	822 ± 38
Prl	380 ± 72	19.4 ± 3.7	2835 ± 134	764 ± 36
E	1352 ± 130	75.5 ± 7.3	11980 ± 283	1770 ± 42
E+Prl	1380 ± 52	70.9 ± 2.7	12697 ± 310	1720 ± 42
E+P	803 ± 98	33.4 ± 4.1	3309 ± 371	614 ± 69
E+P+Prl	662 ± 79	31.2 ± 3.7	3382 ± 246	599 ± 44
P	183 ± 40	10.3 ± 2.3	861 ± 149	215 ± 37
P+Prl	122 ± 19	6.8 ± 1.1	1187 ± 146	302 ± 37

Ovariectomized virgin mice were pretreated with 14 daily injections of E (1 μg) and P (1 mg) prior to five daily administrations of either oil or hormones as indicated; tissues were assayed 24 hr later. The results are expressed as means ± S.E.M. of four experiments. One ml of mammary cytosol is equivalent to one gram tissue. E = estradiol (1 μg); P = progesterone (1 mg); Prl = prolactin (1 mg).

(4) P reduced the PgR levels either when administered alone or in combination with other hormones. However, it was possible that the reduced cytoplasmic PgR levels due to P administration were the result of partial translocation of the PgR to the nucleus and not due to a true decrease in the cellular PgR. The effect of all the hormonal combinations on uterine PgR appear to be similar to that of mammary PgR as discussed above. Taken together the data in Tables 2 and 3 indicated that hormones of pregnancy could modulate PgR levels; but since the modulations were essentially similar in both mammary glands and uterus this could not account for the total absence of PgR during lactation. Thus it seemed probable that in addition to the hormonal milieu, the state of differentiation of the mammary tissue itself might contribute to the loss of PgR.

The Influence of Mammary Gland Differentiation on Progesterone Receptor Levels

(a) Relationship between the state of differentiation and PgR levels.

There are a number of morphological and biochemical criteria by which the differentiated mammary gland can be distinguished from the quiescent virgin mammary gland. In the present studies designed to evaluate the relationship between mammary gland differentiation and PgR modulation one morphological and one bio-chemical criterion was used; these were the degree of lobuloal-veolar development (LAD) and the concentration of enzymatically α-lactalbumin enzyme activity, respectively.   The relation-ship between PgR levels and mammary gland differentiation as it exists normally is illustrated in Table 4. As may be seen there was an inverse relationship between the PgR levels and mammary gland differentiation; the highest level of α-lactalbumin activity and LAD was detected during postpartum at which time there was a total loss of PgR in mammary tissue. However, it was noteworthy that even with maximum LAD such as that seen during late pregnancy there was only a submaximal concentration of α-lactalbumin acti-vity and PgR was still present in the mammary tissue. It was only during lactation a maximal concentration of α-lactalbumin activity was present with a total loss of PgR. It is believed that the increase in α-lactalbumin activity seen during lactation is due to the changes in the hormonal milieu associated with parturition and lactation (12-15). However, as stated earlier, the hormonal milieu in itself could not account for the total loss of PgR ob-served during lactation and as such these results revealed a possible independent role of the lactating cell in the modulation of PgR. Therefore the studies were designed such that the in-fluence of the hormones of lactation could be dissociated from the secretory state of the gland so that the separate influence of each of these components on PgR level could be examined.

TABLE 4. Relationship between mammary gland differentiation and cytoplasmic progesterone receptor levels

Developmental state	Degree of LADa	α-Lactalbumin activity nmol lactose formed/30 min/mg protein	Specific binding of [3H]R5020 fmoles/mg protein
Virgin	none	none	45.8 ± 4.9
Pregnancy:			
14 days	++	2.47 ± 0.19	19.2 ± 3.7
16 days	+++	8.01 ± 3.77	10.8 ± 0.9
19 days	++++	33.8 ± 0.05	9.36 ± 2.4
Lactation:			
7-15 days	++++	61.8 ± 14.7	none

Intact mice at specified states of development were used. The results are expressed as means ± S.E.M. of two to five experiments. aLAD was assessed histologically as previously described (29); ++ = mammary tissue composed of 50% lobuloalveolar epithelial cells and 50% adipose cells; ++++ = 100% of mammary tissue composed of lobuloalveolar epithelial cells with no visible adipose cells.

(b) Effect of unilateral thelectomy on PgR levels.

It is well known (40) that in addition to an appropriate hormonal milieu, initiation and maintenance of copious milk secretion requires the physical removal of milk; this is accomplished in nature by suckling. By preventing suckling on one side of a lactating mouse, using the technique of unilateral thelectomy (nipple removal), it is possible to obtain fully lactating mammary tissue on the intact side and nonlactating mammary tissue on the thelectomized side in the same animal without altering the hormonal milieu of lactation. Thelectomy alone had no effect on mammary or uterine PgR levels in virgin and pregnant animals, i.e. PgR levels in the intact and the thelectomized glands were virtually identical and uterine PgR levels were not different from those obtained in intact non-thelectomized mice (Tables 4 and 5). Furthermore, thelectomy did not prevent the decrease in PgR levels observed during pregnancy. However, a significant departure in the PgR levels between thelectomized and intact glands became apparent in lactating animals. PgR were detectable in thelectomized, nonlactating glands but were absent in intact lactating glands and the uterine PgR values were virtually identical to intact non-thelectomized mice thus demonstrating the mammary gland specific effect of thelectomy and hence lactation on PgR. Furthermore, exogenous administration of estradiol augmented the PgR levels in the thelectomized, non-lactating mammary tissue and in the uterus, while in the lactating non-thelectomized glands there was still no PgR (Fig. 5). Thus these results conclusively establish that while hormones do influence PgR levels it is a functionally lactational state which is responsible for mammary gland specific absence of PgR and insensitivity to estrogenic stimulation.

(c) Effect of lactational involution on PgR levels in mammary glands.

Just as the initiation and maintenance of lactation in mammary tissue is accomplished by suckling, lactation can be terminated by the removal of pups. Natural lactational involution is generally completed by 28 days postpartum at which time the pups are weaned and PgR are present in mammary tissue (Fig. 1). Prior to 28 days postpartum, lactational involution can be experimentally induced by the premature withdrawal of pups. Since lactational secretion seemed to be primarily responsible for the total absence of PgR, it was of interest to study the reappearance of PgR as a function of involution and to identify the basis for this reappearance. The data illustrating the relationship of lactational involution and PgR is shown in Table 6. As may be seen, as a function of time after involution, PgR levels in mammary gland increased; however, as may be noted both with natural involution (28 days postpartum; Fig. 1) and lactational involution (Table 6), the levels of PgR that were obtained were lower than that seen in virgin mammary gland. To see whether this lower level of PgR during involution might have resulted from

TABLE 5. Effect of thelectomy on cytoplasmic progesterone receptor levels in mammary gland and uterus

A. MAMMARY GLANDS

Specific binding of [3H]R5020 (fmoles/mg protein)

Developmental state	Intact mammary glands	Thelectomized mammary glands
Virgin	42 ± 4.9	57 ± 7.6
Pregnancy - 14 days	21 ± 3.1	29 ± 3.1
Lactation - 7 days	0	10.2 ± 2.7

Animals were unilaterally thelectomized prior to mating. The results are expressed as mean ± S.E.M. and represent data from 3-4 experiments.

B. UTERUS

Specific binding of [3H]R5020 (fmoles/mg protein)

Developmental state	Intact animals	Thelectomized animals
Virgin	1000 ± 157	955 ± 291
Lactation - 7 days	443 ± 33	344 ± 98

The results are expressed as mean ± S.E.M. and represent data from 3-4 experiments.

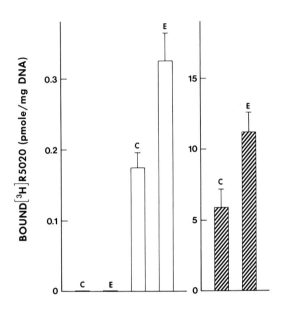

FIG. 5. Effect of estradiol on cytoplasmic PgR of mammary glands and uterus of unilaterally thelectomized lactators. Two groups of unilaterally thelectomized lactating mice were given a single injection of either saline (C) or 3 µg of estradiol (E) for 24 hr prior to tissue removal. The binding represents specific binding only and is mean ± S.E.M. of 3-4 experiments.(■)Non-thelectomized lactating mammary glands. (□)Thelectomized non-lactating mammary gland.   (▨)Uterus.

an inadequate estrogenic milieu, the effect of estradiol on PgR levels in these tissues was examined. As illustrated in Fig. 6 and 7, although PgR were present in naturally and experimentally involuted mammary gland, estradiol was without any effect in augmenting the levels of PgR. Thus it would appear that while the basal levels of PgR were restored in mammary tissue by 28 days postpartum or after pup removal the "inhibitory" effect of lactation and non-responsiveness of mammary tissue to estrogen was still present. This "inhibitory" influence imparted during lactation was further suggested by the results of experiments described below (Table 7). Animals were thelectomized prior to mating and were kept with their pups until 28 days postpartum. PgR were measured at that time. In thelectomized mammary tissue, which never experienced lactation, PgR levels were similar to

TABLE 6. Cytoplasmic progesterone receptor levels in mammary
tissues during experimentally-induced lactational involution

No. of days without pups	Specifically bound [3H]R5020 fmoles/g tissue	fmoles/mg DNA
1	0	0
2	0	0
3	0	0
4	68 ± 37	62 ± 34
5	148 ± 17	125 ± 14
8[a]	260 ± 20	306 ± 23

[a]Day 8 is equivalent to day 15 postpartum; cytoplasmic extracts of mammary tissues of day 15 postpartum animals kept with
their pups contained no detectable PgR (see Fig. 1). Reproduced
from Haslam and Shyamala (1979b).

virgin levels and 2 fold higher than that present in the contra-
lateral intact mammary gland which had lactated; the uterine PgR
values were not different from control values (intact 28 days
postpartum) or virgin uterine PgR values, again demonstrating
mammary tissue specific inhibitory effect of lactation. This
maximal uterine PgR level in animals undergoing lactational involution comparable to that of intact virgin animals was also
presumably the reason for the lack of an estradiol mediated aug-
mentation of uterine PgR in experiments described in Fig. 6 and
7.

Modulation of Cytoplasmic Estrogen Receptor Levels as a Function of Development and Differentiation

It is generally believed that the lack or reduced ability of a
target tissue to respond to estradiol may be due to an absence or
reduced level of cytoplasmic ER in the tissue. Since estradiol
could augment the levels of PgR in mammary tissues, it was likely
that this effect of estradiol was mediated through ER. Thus it
was possible that the modulation of PgR in mammary tissues was
the result of varying levels of ER. To this extent, the ER
levels in mammary tissues of varying developmental states were
measured. As shown in Table 8, the ER levels were also modulated
in mammary tissue as a function of development and the striking
observation was the increased levels of ER during established
lactation. These results confirmed earlier observations reported
by others (41-44). It might be argued that the differences in
the ER level between different developmental states might have
resulted from varying amounts of endogenously bound ER. However,
this did not appear to be the case since (a) the uterine ER
levels remained fairly constant during all the different states

fully differentiated mammary glands such as the lactating mammary glands. Therefore, a resolution of the molecular basis for the "refractoriness" of lactating mammary tissue to estrogen in experimental systems may provide a plausible model for the elucidation of the hormonal regulation of mammary neoplasia.

ACKNOWLEDGMENTS

Tyra Bresciani was a woman of outstanding courage and optimism and this article is affectionately dedicated to her memory by one of us (G.S.).

These studies were supported by a grant from the National Cancer Institute of Canada. S.Z. Haslam is a recipient of the National Institutes of Health National Research Service Award 5F32CA06098-02 from the National Cancer Institute, U.S.A. The authors thank Mary Dowdall, Jamilah Hafiz, Louise Leonard and Terry Smith for technical assistance, Ms. S. Fraiberg for secretarial assistance and Ms. C. Lalonde and Mr. D. Saxe for preparation of illustrations.

REFERENCES

1. Sherman, M.R., Corrol, P.L., and O'Malley, B.W. (1970): J. Biol. Chem. 245: 6085-6096.
2. Milgrom, E., and Baulieu, E.-C. (1970): Endocrinology 87: 276-287.
3. McGuire, W.L., and Bariso, C.D. (1972): Endocrinology 90: 496-506.
4. Feil, P.D., Glasser, S.R., Toft, D.O., and O'Malley, B.W. (1972): Endocrinology 91: 738-746.
5. Milgrom, E., Perrot, M., Atger, M., and Baulieu, E.-E. (1972): Endocrinology 90: 1064-1070.
6. Philibert, D., Ojasoo, J., and Raynaud, J.-P. (1977): Endocrinology 101: 1850-1861.
7. Leavitt, W.W., Chen, T.J., Allen, T.C., and O'Neal Johnston, J. (1977): Ann. N.Y. Acad. Sci. 286: 210-225.
8. Kawashima, M., Kamiyoshi, M., and Tanaka, K. (1978): Endocrinology 102: 1207-1213.
9. Lyons, W.R., Li, C.H., and Johnson, R.E. (1958): Rec. Progr. Horm. Res. 14: 219-248.
10. Nandi, S. (1959): Univ. Calif. Publ. Zool. 65: 1-128.
11. Bresciani, F. (1965): Exp. Cell Res. 38: 13-32.
12. Kuhn, N.J. (1969): J. Endocrinol. 44: 39-54.
13. Davis, J.W., Wilkman-Coffelt, J., and Eddington, C.L. (1972): Endocrinology 91: 1011-1019.
14. Denamur, R., and DeLouis, C. (1972): Acta Endocrinol. 70: 603-618.
15. Murphy, G., Sriyanayagam, A.D., and Kuhn, N.J. (1973): Biochem. J. 136: 1105-1116.
16. Rosen, J.M., O'Neal, D.L., McHugh, J.E., and Comstock, J.P. (1978): Biochemistry 17: 290-297.
17. Higgins, C., and Yang, N.C. (1962): Science 137: 257-262.
18. McCormick, G.M., and Moon, R.C. (1967): Cancer Res. 27:626-631.

19. Stoll, B.A. (1967): Brit. Med. J. 3: 338-341.
20. Puca, G.A., and Bresciani, F. (1969) Endocrinology 85: 1-10.
21. Shyamala, G., and Nandi, S. (1972) Endocrinology 91: 861-869.
22. McGuire, W.L., Carbone, P.P., Sears, M.E., and Escher, G.C. (1975): In: Estrogen Receptors in Human Breast Cancer, edited by W.L. McGuire, P.P. Carbone and E.P. Vollmer, Raven Press, New York.
23. Asselin, J., Labrie, F., Kelly, P.A., Philibert, D., and Raynaud, J.-P. (1976): Steroids 27: 395-404.
24. Horowitz, K.B., and McGuire, W.L. (1977): Cancer Res. 37: 1733-1738.
25. Markland, F.S., and Hutchins, T.W. (1977): Prog. Cancer Res. Therapy 4: 23-38.
26. Koenders, A.J.M., Ceurts-Mespot, A., Zolinger, S.J., and Benraad, Th.J. (1977): Prog. Cancer Res. Therapy 4: 71-84.
27. McGuire, W.L., and Horowitz, K.B. (1978): Prog. Cancer Res. Therapy 10: 31-42.
28. Haslam, S.Z., and Shyamala, G. (1979a):Biochem. J. 182: 127-131.
29. Haslam, S.Z., and Shyamala, G. (1979b):Endocrinology 105: 786-795.
30. Korenman, S.G. (1968): J. Clin. Endocrinol. Metab. 28: 127.
31. Shyamala, G., and McBlain, W.A. (1979): Biochem. J. 178: 345-352.
32. Ip, C., and Dao, T.L. (1978) Cancer Res. 38: 2077-2083.
33. Ceriotti, G. (1952): J. Biol. Chem. 198: 297-303.
34. Lowry, O.H., Rosebrough, N.J., Farr, A.L., and Randall, R.J. (1951): J. Biol. Chem. 193: 265-275.
35. Toft, D.O., and O'Malley, B.W. (1972): Endocrinology 90: 1041-1045.
36. Rao, B.R., and Weist, W.G. (1973) Endocrinology 92: 1229-1240.
37. Smith, M.S., and Neill, J.D. (1977) Biol. Reprod. 17: 255-261.
38. Milgrom, E.L., Atger, T.M., and Baulieu, E.-E. (1973): J. Biol. Chem. 248: 6366-6374.
39. Vu Hai, M.T., Logeat, F., Warembourg, M., and Milgrom, E. (1977): Ann. N.Y. Acad. Sci. 286: 199-209.
40. Cowie, A.T., and Tindall, J.S. (1971): In: The Physiology of Lactation, edited by H. Darson, A.D.M. Greenfield, R. Whittman and G.S. Brindley, pp. 84-135. Edward Arnold (Publ.), London.
41. Hseuh, A.J.W., Peck, E.J., Jr., and Clark, J.H. (1973): J. Endocrinol. 58: 1-9.
42. Gardner, D.G., and Wittliff, J.L. (1973): Biochemistry 12: 3090-3096.
43. Leung, B.S., Jack, W.M., and Reiney, C.C. (1976): J. Steroid Biochem. 7: 89-95.
44. Hunt, M.E., and Muldoon, T.G. (1977): J. Steroid Biochem. 8: 181-186.
45. Ho, R.J., and Sutherland, E.W. (1971): J. Biol. Chem. 246: 6822-6827.

46. Stormshak, F., Leake, R., Wertz, N., and Gorski, J. (1976): Endocrinology 99: 1501-1511.
47. Nunez, J., Plas, C., and Correze, C. (1977): In: European Symposium on Hormones and Cell Regulation, edited by J. Dumont and J. Nunez, pp. 119-135. North Holland Publishing Company, Amsterdam.
48. McGuire, W.L., Pearson, O.H., and Segaloff, A. (1976) In: Estrogen Receptors in Human Breast Cancer, edited by W.L. McGuire, P.P. Carbone and E.P. Vollmer, Raven Press, New York.

Perspectives in Steroid Receptor Research,
edited by F. Bresciani.
Raven Press, New York © 1980.

Steroid Receptor Analyses and Endocrine Therapy of Breast Cancer

Marc E. Lippman

Medical Breast Cancer Section, Medicine Branch, Division of Cancer Treatment, National Cancer Institute, National Institutes of Health, Bethesda, Maryland 20205, U.S.A.

Introduction

Since the pioneering work of George Beatson (1) who induced tumor regressions in patients with advanced breast cancer by oophorectomy, it has been appreciated that some human breast cancers will respond to endocrine manipulations. It is established that patients who respond to such endocrine therapies not only may have significant regressions of tumor deposits but have 2-3 fold longer survivals when compared with non-responders. Unfortunately, no more than about one-third of unselected patients with metastatic disease will experience objective tumor regressions. Thus, if such therapies are applied universally, the majority of patients will be needlessly exposed to the morbidity and mortality associated with these treatments. While most clinicians would agree that endocrine therapies are generally better tolerated than cytotoxic chemotherapy, the higher response rates to systemic drug therapy combined with the hazards of ineffective endocrine therapy have strongly encouraged a search for more rational means of patient selection for different treatment modalities.

Until recently, the only available biochemical or clinical means of differentiating patients who respond from those who do not respond to endocrine therapy have been insufficiently reliable for general adoption. Enormous progress in the understanding of the mechanisms by which hormones interact with specific target issues has profoundly altered this situation (2). Studies from many laboratories have revealed that the initial step in hormone action is the binding of the hormone to highly specialized receptor proteins. On the basis of this premise, Jensen (3) and Terenius (4) independently demonstrated specific binding of radioactive estrogen to some human breast-cancer specimens and correlated the presence of this binding activity with clinical endocrine responsiveness. Numerous subsequent investigators have confirmed and amplified these pioneering investigations, and several reviews adequately document the usefulness of this assay (5,6).

In this review, an effort will be made to summarize some of our work with respect to steroid receptor analyses and human breast cancer. Studies reviewed here will concentrate on five areas. First, steroid receptor analyses in benign breast disease; second, quantitive analyses of steroid receptors in breast cancer; third, correlations between clinical parameters and endocrine therapy for breast cancer; fourth, sequential and multiple steroid receptor analyses; and fifth, steroid receptor analyses in male breast cancer.

Complete descriptions of all methodologic considerations have been previously published (7). These assay methods have been validated against unknown standards provided by The National Surgical Adjuvant Breast Project.

Benign Breast Disease

Biopsies from 55 female patients with benign breast disease were analyzed for estrogen receptor (ER). Thirty-one specimens were classified as fibroadenoma; 16 as fibrocystic disease and 8 as other miscellaneous benign lesions such as lipoma, papilloma, etc. Table 1 shows the results of the ER assay as a function of tumor histology. Overall, 21 of 55 (38%) patients with benign breast disease had a positive ER assay. Fifty-five percent of fibroadenomas were positive for ER compared to 17% for other benign lesions (4 patients with fibrocystic disease). The proportion of fibroadenomas containing ER is significantly greater (p less than 0.01) than that for the other benign lesions; however, there is no significant difference when receptor positivity is compared between fibroadenomas and fibrocystic disease.

Table 1. Estrogen Receptor Status as a Function of Tumor Histology

Tumor Histology	Estrogen Receptor Positive	Estrogen Receptor Negative
Fibroadenoma N=31	17 (55%)	14 (45%)
Fibrocystic disease N=16	4 (25%)	12 (75%)
Other benign	0 (0%)	8 (100%)

The mean age of patients with ER positive tumors was 26.9 years compared to 36.4 years for patients with ER negative tumors (p less than 0.01). Also, all of the ER positive tumors were in premenopausal patients, 21/47 (44%), compared to 0 of 8 in postmenopausal patients (p less than 0.05). In Table 2, ER status is shown as a function of laterality of the tumor and location and size of the largest tumor nodule. No correlation was found between ER status and these parameters, though data were available in only half of the patients concerning tumor location. There is a trend, however, for the frequency of ER positivity to decrease as tumor size increases (p equals 0.07).

Table 2. Estrogen Receptor Status as a Function of Laterality of the Tumor and Location and Size of the Largest Nodule

	N	ER Positive	ER Negative
Laterality of tumor			
Left	18	37%	63%
Right	27	37%	63%
Bilateral	7	17%	83%
Unknown	3	67%	33%
Location of largest primary nodule			
Upper-outer	18	28%	72%
Upper-inner	2	50%	50%
Lower-outer	3	0%	100%
Lower-inner	3	67%	33%
Areolar	1	100%	0%
Unknown	28	43%	57%
Size of largest nodule			
0-2 cm	17	47%	53%
2-5 cm	27	30%	70%
greater than 5 cm	4	0%	100%
Fixed to skin	0	–	0
Unknown	7	71%	29%

Estrogen receptor has been reported to be present in significant amounts in the normal mammary gland. It has long been appreciated that benign breast pathology is associated with a significantly increased risk of developing breast cancer. On the other hand, little evidence has been advanced to suggest that fibroadenomata are premalignant. Normal breast cells are ER positive as well as the majority of post-menopausal breast cancers while postmenopausal benign lesions have a very low incidence of ER positivity. The lower frequency of receptor positivity in benign tumors as compared to malignant tumors is strong evidence against a continuous gradation from normal tissue to benign breast disease to cancer and a point against believing that benign breast disease is generally a direct precursor of malignancy.

Finally, all of the receptor positive tumors were found in premenopausal patients, and patients with receptor positive tumors were younger than those patients with ER negative tumors. It is also known that there is a decreased incidence of benign breast disease in women using oral contraceptives. One may speculate whether the pharmacologic doses of estrogen contained in oral contraceptives are modulating the growth of benign breast tumors via interaction with the ER much the same way pharmacologic concentrations of estrogens may lead to regressions of some metastatic breast cancer deposits. This concept also suggests a possible role for antiestrogens such as tamoxifen in the treatment of benign breast disease.

Table 3. Characteristics of the patients whose tumors were assayed for steroid hormone receptors.

Number of patients	329	
Age of patients	<40	15%
	40-49	22%
	50-59	38%
	60-69	16%
	>70	9%
	Median	52.5 years
Menopausal status	Pre	27%
	Post	73%
Nodal status at diagnosis	0	45%
	1-3	26%
	>4	29%
Location of primary tumor	Left Breast	48%
	Right Breast	49%
	Bilateral	3%
Location of the largest primary tumor nodule	Upper-outer	47%
	Upper-inner	13%
	Lower-outer	15%
	Lower-inner	5%
	Areolar	21%
Size of the largest tumor nodule	0-2 cm	42%
	2-5 cm	39%
	>5 cm	17%
	Fixed	2%
Disease status	NED	52%
	Local	3%
	Metastatic	45%

Quantitative Steroid Receptor Analyses in Breast Cancer
Turning next to breast cancer, three hundred and twenty-nine

patients with breast cancer had one or more steroid hormone receptor assays performed on tissue from either their primary tumor or from a metastasis. The characteristics of these patients are shown in Table 3. The median age of the patients was 52.5 years. Twenty-seven percent were premenopausal and 73% were postmenopausal. Nodal status, location of the primary tumor, and location and size of the largest primary tumor nodule are listed. Fifty-two percent of the patients had no evidence of macroscopic disease after their mastectomy was performed; 45% had metastatic disease at the time of the assay, and the final 3% had locally unresectable disease.

The frequency distributions of the estrogen, progesterone, androgen and glucocorticoid receptors are unimodal. There is a progressive increase in proportion of patients possing lower values.

In analyzing our data, results were expressed as either fmols/mg cytoplasmic protein or fmols/mg breast tumor. There is a strong correlation between steroid hormone receptor values expressed in either manner. For estrogen receptor the Kendall rank correlation coefficient is 0.80 and this correlation is significant at the p less than 0.001 level. This same correlation exists for the progesterone, androgen and glucocorticoid receptor and data for all three receptors have Kendall rank correlation coefficient greater than 0.80 when receptor values expressed as fmols/mg cytoplasmic protein are plotted against receptors values expressed as fmols/mg breast tumor. This indicates that expression of data in either manner is equivalent and, most importantly, that the manner of expression of the data does not significantly influence the classification of tumors as positive or negative.

Table 4.   The frequency of steroid hormone receptor positivity in patients with breast cancer

	Number of Assays	% Positive
ER	328	53
PR	176	38
GR	187	52
AR	208	31

Table 4 lists the incidence of steroid hormone receptor positivity among our patients with breast cancer using the cutoff values defined in Reference #7. The ER was positive in 53% of the tumors and the progesterone receptor (PR) in 38%. Fifty-two percent of the tumors were positive for glucocorticoid receptor (GR) and 31% for androgen receptor (AR).

Table 5. Steroid hormone receptor positivity as a function of laterality of the primary tumor.

| | Percent Positive | | | |
	ER	PR	AR	GR
Left breast	77/151 (51%)	35/80 (44%)	32/99 (32%)	41/80 (51%)
Right breast	85/157 (54%)	28/36 (33%)	27/100 (27%)	50/99 (51%)
Bilateral	7/9 (78%)	2/3 (67%)	3/4 (75%)	4/4 (100%)

Table 6. Steroid hormone receptor positivity as a function of location of the largest primary tumor nodule.

| | Percent Positive | | | |
Breast Quadrant	ER	PR	AR	GR
Upper-outer	34/68 (50%)	7/25 (29%)	12/41 (29%)	16/39 (41%)
Upper-inner	10/18 (56%)	4/10 (40%)	4/14 (29%)	4/12 (33%)
Lower-outer	9/21 (43%)	3/11 (27%)	3/13 (23%)	9/12 (75%)
Lower-inner	5/7 (71%)	3/4 (75%)	2/4 (50%)	4/4 (100%)
Areolar	18/30 (60%)	8/19 (42%)	8/22 (36%)	11/19 (58%)

In Tables 6 and 7, steroid hormone receptor positivity is presented as a function of location and size of the largest primary tumor nodule. No correlation was found between the presence or absence of any steroid hormone receptor and either location or size of the primary tumor.

Table 7. Steroid hormone receptor positivity as a function of the size of the largest tumor nodule

| | Percent Positive | | | |
Size of primary tumor	ER	PR	AR	GR
0-2 cm	43/84 (51%)	11/39 (28%)	17/55 (31%)	22/48 (46%)
2-5 cm	46/78 (59%)	22/45 (49%)	13/53 (25%)	25/48 (52%)
>5 cm	17/34 (50%)	7/14 (50%)	7/20 (35%)	7/16 (44%)
Fixed tumor	2/4 (50%)	1/3 (33%)	2/2 (100%)	2/2 (100%)

In Table 8, steroid hormone receptor positivity is analyzed as a function of extent of disease. Fifty-six percent of patients with no evidence of disease after their mastectomy was performed had a positive ER compared to 47% of patients who had the assay performed on a metastasis. This trend toward a lower frequency of ER positivity in metastatic tumor was not statistically significant. This trend was not evident for the other 3 steroid hormone receptors.

Table 8. Steroid hormone receptor positvity as function of extent of disease

| | Percent Positive | | | |
Extent of Disease	ER	PR	AR	GR
No evidence of disease	96/172 (56%)	34/93 (37%)	38/120 (32%)	54/112 (48%)
Metastatic disease	68/145 (47%)	30/80 (38%)	23/83 (28%)	40/72 (56%)

Table 9 lists the frequency of the steroid hormone receptors as a function of the type of tissue assayed. Breast, skin, node or soft tissue containing metastatic breast cancer appeared to have an equal frequency of receptor positivity. Unfortunately, we have at the present time, too few specimens from sites such as lung, liver or bone marrow to be able to comment on the frequency of receptor positivity at these sites.

Table 9. Steroid hormone receptor positivity as a function of type of tissue assayed

Tissue assayed	Percent Positive			
	ER	PR	AR	GR
Breast	109/202 (54%)	39/109 (36%)	45/144 (31%)	65/132 (49%)
Skin-soft tissue	34/74 (46%)	16/36 (44%)	12/35 (34%)	15/27 (56%)
Node	17/35 (49%)	8/21 (38%)	7/22 (32%)	15/23 (65%)
Other	7/17 (41%)	2/10 (20%)	0/7 (0%)	2/5 (40%)

Table 10 shows analysis of each of the receptors as a function of age. No correlation with age existed for progesterone, androgen or glucocorticoid receptor but there appeared to be a significant association between ER and age. The ER was positive in 44% of patients less than 40 years and in 69% greater than age 70.

Table 10. Steroid hormone receptor positivity as a function of age

Age	Percent Positive			
	ER	PR	AR	GR
less than 40	22/40 (44%)	8/26 (31%)	13/37 (35%)	14/30 (47%)
40-49	34/71 (48%)	12/33 (36%)	10/44 (23%)	20/36 (56%)
50-59	66/124 (53%)	28/67 (42%)	23/75 (31%)	34/66 (52%)
60-69	31/53 (58%)	12/33 (36%)	11/33 (33%)	16/34 (47%)
greater than 70	18/26 (69%)	4/14 (29%)	6/15 (40%)	11/17 (65%)

The median estrogen receptor value is significantly higher in postmenopausal patients compared with the premenopausal patients (p less tha 0.02). However, when patients are separated into premenopausal and postmenopausal subsets, receptor values no

longer correlate significantly with age. This suggests that ER
is actually correlating with menopausal status and that menopausal
status correlates with age.

Table 11 lists the percent of patient tumor samples positive
for each of the steroid hormone receptors as a function of menopausal status. There are no statistically significant associa-
tions between either progesterone, androgen or glucocorticoid
receptor and menopausal status, though the trends are all toward
postmenopausal patients having higher values.

Table 11. Steroid hormone receptor positivity as a function of
menopausal status.

Menopausal status	Percent Positive			
	ER	PR	AR	GR
Pre	36/80 (45%)	12/44 (27%)	14/52 (27%)	21/46 (46%)
Post	122/214 (57%)	44/116 (38%)	43/131 (33%)	66/119 (56%)

Table 12 shows the analysis of ER as a function of axillary
nodal status. All ER assays were performed on tissue at the time
of mastectomy. Patients with ER positive tumors have a more
favorable axillary nodal status at the time of mastectomy. The ER
positive group contains a greater proportion of node negative patients. The Wilcoxon rank test (adjusted for time and continuity)
was used to compare the distributions, and the distributions do
differ significantly (p less than 0.05). There was no association
between the other steroid hormone receptors and axillary nodal
status.

Table 12. Estrogen receptor status as a function of axillary nodal
status

Number of positive axillary nodes	ER Positive	ER Negative
0	52 (61%)	30 (41%)
1-3	13 (15%)	23 (31%)
4-10	10 (12%)	13 (18%)
greater than 10	10 (12%)	8 (11%)

We next examined some of the relationships between steroid
receptor status and response to endocrine therapy in metastatic
breast cancer. Eighty-five patients with metastatic breast cancer
had an estrogen receptor assay performed immediately prior to the
institution of an endocrine therapy regimen. Of the 85 patients,

52 possessed tumors which were ER positive and 33 had ER negative tumors. The mean ER value in the ER positive group was 80.6 fmols/mg cytoplasmic protein and the mean ER value in the ER negative group was 1.4 fmols/mg cytoplasmic protein. The ER positive and negative groups were essentially identical with respect to age, menopausal status, Karnofsky performance index, disease free interval, number of sites involved with metastatic tumor and prior therapy. A wide variety of endocrine therapies were employed in both groups. The proportion of patients in each group receiving a specific therapy was similar and any given therapy was administered equivalently in ER positive and negative patients. These data are summarized in Table 13.

Table 13. Characteristics of patients receiving endocrine therapy

	ER Positive	ER Negative
Number of patients	52	33
Mean ER (fmols/mg cytoplasmic protein)	80.6	1.4
Age (mean $\pm$ S.E.M.)	49 $\pm$ 7	52 $\pm$ 7
Menopausal status		
Pre	25%	24%
Post	75%	76%
Karnofsky index (mean $\pm$ S.E.M.)	91.3 $\pm$ 7	85.4 $\pm$ 9
Disease free interval (mean (mo))	44	36
Number of sites involved		
1	13	7
2	16	7
greater than 3	23	19
Prior therapy	27/52 (51%)	21/33 (63%)
Endocrine	15/52 (28%)	6/33 (18%)
Chemotherapy	21/52 (40%)	19/33 (57%)

Overall, 34 of 52 patients (65%) whose tumors were ER positive achieved an objective response compared to 3 of 33 patients (9%) in the ER negative group (p less than 0.0001). Furthermore, as shown in Table 14, as the amount of ER increased, the likelihood of response also appeared to increase. The response rate between

Table 14. Response rate to endocrine therapy as a function of ER concentration

ER (fmols/mg cytoplasmic protein)	Response Rate
$0 \leq ER < 10$	3/33 (9%)
$10 \leq ER \leq 20$	3/10 (30%) p greater than .05
$20 < ER \leq 50$	7/11 (63%) p less than 0.001
$ER \geq 50$	24/31 (77%) p less than 0.00001

0 and 10 fmols (ER negative group) is only 9%. This increases to 30% between 10 and 20 fmols. Between 20 and 50 fmols, 63% of patients have an objective response and 77% of patients whose tumors contained greater than 50 fmols of ER/mg cytoplasmic protein responded. Also in the ER positive group, the distribution of ER vales for responders was significantly different from non-responders (p less than 0.05).

Table 15. Response rate to endocrine therapy as a function of site of involvement and ER status

	ER Positive	ER Negative	P Value ER+ vs ER−
Skin	19/36 (52%)	1/20 (5%)	p < 0.01
Soft Tissue	11/19 (57%)	1/14 (7%)	p < 0.01
Node	13/21 (61%)	0/14 (0%)	p < 0.01
Lung	10/16 (62%)	2/11 (18%)	p < 0.05
Pleura	0/1 (0%)	0/6 (0%)	—
Ascites	—	0/4 (0%)	—
Brain	0/1 (0%)	0/1 (0%)	—
Liver	5/9 (55%)	0/10 (0%)	p < 0.01
Bone	15/30 (50%)	2/19 (10%)	p < 0.01
Bone Marrow	4/6 (67%)	0/6 (0%)	p < 0.05

Since response rate to endocrine therapy was associated with the quantitative amount of ER, we next examined the probability of an association between the amount of ER and response duration. The patients were divided into two groups. One group was composed of all patients with tumors containing greater than 50 fmols of ER. No significant correlation was found between the duration of remission and the amount of ER. Also without regard to this arbitrary cutoff of 50 fmols, there was no correlation between the amount of ER and response duration.

We further analyzed responses to endocrine therapy as a function of both ER status and site of metastasis. Results are summarized in Table 15. In general, metastatic tumors were more likely to respond to endocrine therapy in patients whose tumors were ER positive regardless of disease site. Although not all of these sites were biopsied, it appears that the estrogen receptor value at any site predicts with a high degree of probability response at other sites of involvement. Metastatic disease in the liver and the lung which was ER positive responded at a rate in excess of 60% which was equal to the response rate in "good prognosis" sites such as skin and soft tissue disease. Patients with visceral tumor involvement had a somewhat lower percentage of ER positive tumors as compared to patients without visceral metastases (53% versus 69%). These data imply that the lower response rates of these sites are more likely due to more frequency involvement by ER negative tumors than to intrinsic hormone unresponsiveness.

The overall frequency of ER positivity in the 85 patients treated with endocrine therapy in this study was 52 of 85 (61%). This does not differ significantly from our previously published frequency of 52% ER positivity in a breast cancer population (19). Finally, we examined the effect of prior therapy on endocrine responsiveness. Forty of 85 patients had received prior chemotherapy. Twenty-one of 40 (52.5%) were ER positive. Of the 45 patients who did not receive prior therapy, 69% were ER positive but this difference does not approach statistical significance. Furthermore, the mean ER value in patients who received prior chemotherapy is 51.5 fmols versus 46.1 fmols in patients who had not received prior chemotherapy (p less than 0.10). Of the 21 patients in the ER positive group who received prior chemotherapy, 14 had an objective response to endocrine therapy (67%) compared to a response rate of 20 of 31 (64%) in those ER positive patients who had not received prior treatment with chemotherapy. Prior treatment with chemotherapy did not alter the low response rate in ER negative tumors. Thus, prior chemotherapy did not significantly alter the concentration of ER or the predictive value of the test, though there was trend towards a reduced incidence of ER positivity.

With respect to prior endocrine therapy, 15 patients in the ER positive group and 6 patients in the ER negative group had received prior treatment. Of the 15 patients in the ER positive group, 8 (53%) responded to prior therapy while only 1 of 6 in the ER negative group responded to prior endocrine therapy. In the present trial, of the 8 patients in the ER positive group who responded to prior therapy, 6 responded to subsequent endocrine therapy. Of the 7 non-responders to prior therapy in the ER positive group, 2 responded in this trial. Although 2 of 7 is not significantly different from the 3 of 33 rate in our ER negative

group in this trial, there may be a trend towards a higher response rate in ER positive tumors which have failed prior endocrine therapy than in ER negative patients overall. This suggests
that failure to respond to endocrine therapy may in some cases be
a function of the type of endocrine treatment; that is, the receptor positivity does predict endocrine dependence but the therapy
employed does not adequately alter hormone levels. Overall, 8 of
the 15 ER positive patients who had received prior endocrine therapy responded and none of the 6 ER negative patients responded to
endocrine therapy. The response rate of this subset of patients
who had received prior therapy is not different from the response
rates of the group of patients with prior endocrine therapy.
Thus, prior endocrine therapy did not significantly alter the predictive value of the ER assay.

   Thus, estrogen receptor analysis plays a major role in predicting response to endocrine therapy in metastatic breast cancer.
It has also been suggested that the presence of both the estrogen
receptor and the progesterone receptor in a tumor will further increase the response rate to endocrine manipulation (8). Many
human breast cancers also possess an androgen receptor (4,9,10,11)
and both androgens and anti-androgens are effective endocrine
therapies in some breast cancer patients (12). A specific gluco-

Table 16. Characteristics of the patients treated with endocrine
          therapy as a function of progesterone receptor status.

	PR positive	PR negative	p value PR+ vs PR-
Number of patients	18	26	
Mean PR value (fmols/mg cytoplasmic protein)	74	4	
Menopausal status			
Pre	33%	27%	$p > 0.1$
Post	67%	73%	
Karnofsky index (mean $\pm$ 1 S.D.)	89 $\pm$ 12	92 $\pm$ 12	$p > 0.1$
Disease free interval (median) (mo)	14	18	$p > 0.1$
Visceral disease	5/8	9/26	$p > 0.1$
Number of sites involved with metastatic tumor			
1	4/18	6/26	
2	8/18	9/26	$p > 0.1$
$\geq$3	6/18	11/26	

corticoid receptor is found in many normal human tissues and in over 50% of human breast cancer specimens (7,13). The studies summarized below describe response rates to endocrine therapy as a function of progesterone, androgen, and glucocorticoid receptor status in a series of patients with metastatic breast cancer. Of the 85 patients who responded to endocrine therapy, variable subsets had additional analysis for progesterone and androgen and glucocorticoid receptors. Of these patients, 44 had a progesterone receptor (PR) assay performed; 54 had an androgen receptor (AR) assay performed and 44 had a glucocorticoid receptor (GR) assay performed. Fewer patients had receptors assessed for hormones other than estrogen because of sample size limitations and the higher priority given to the estrogen receptor.

Of the 44 patients who had a PR assay performed on their tumor, 18 were PR positive and 26 were PR negative. The characteristics of these two groups are listed in Table 16. The PR positive and negative groups are similar with respect to age, menopausal status, Karnofsky performance index, disease free interval, number of sites involved with metastatic disease, and proportion of patients with visceral involvement with tumor.

Both groups of patients received standard endocrine therapy. Possible therapies employed in these patients consisted of estrogens, anti-estrogens, androgens, oophorectomy, and medical and surgical adrenalectomy. Various endocrine therapies were distributed equally between the two groups. In addition, a given therapy was administered using a common set of guidelines independent of receptor status.

Eleven of 18 patients (61%) whose tumors contained PR in excess of 20 fmols/mg cytoplasmic protein responded objectively to endocrine therapy whereas 8 of 26 patients (35%) whose tumors contained less than 20 fmols (p equals 0.09) responded. It is important to note, however, that in this study, although the 20 fmol value appears useful in predicting response to therapy, the distribution of PR concentration among responders and patients who did not respond is not significantly different when analyzed by Wilcoxon rank-sum analysis. Table 17 lists objective response rates to endocrine therapy as a function of both ER and PR status. Eleven of 14 patients (79%) whose tumors contained both ER and PR responded compared to 8 of 14 (57%) whose tumors contained ER but lacked PR. This difference is not statistically significant (p greater than 0.1). None of the 4 patients whose tumors lacked ER but contained PR responded to endocrine therapy.

Table 17. Objective response rate to endocrine therapy as a function of estrogen and progesterone receptor status

	ER positive		ER negative	
	PR positive	PR negative	PR positive	PR negative
Response rate	11/14	8/14	0/4	0/12

The ability of the PR to increase the predictive index of the ER is better demonstrated if we analyze only patients who have not received prior therapy. These data are illustrated in Table 18. In this small subset of patients, 6 of 7 (86%) responded if their tumors contained both receptors compared to a response rate of 3 of 9 (33%) in those patients whose tumors contained ER but lacked PR. Thus, in patients who have received no prior therapy, the PR does appear to increase the predictive index of the ER.

Table 18. Objective response rate to endocrine therapy as a func- of progesterone receptor status in patients who are estrogen receptor positive and who have received no prior therapy

	Response rate	
ER positive - PR positive	6/7 (86%)	
		p = 0.11
ER positive - PR negative	3/9 (33%)	

We wondered why the presence of PR might appear to correlate less well with endocrine response in patients with prior therapy. We therefore examined the dependence of PR on ER. If we analyze all the patients on whose tumors ER and PR assays were performed in our laboratory over the past 3 years (175 patients), the Kendall rank correlation coefficient is a positive 0.22 with a p value less than 0.0001. This analysis demonstrates that as ER values increase, there is a corresponding increase in PR values.

In this small series of patients analyzed in this endocrine therapy trial in which 50% have received prior therapy, no significant quantitative relationship between ER and PR can be demonstrated. When those patients who received prior therapy are compared with those patients who did not receive prior therapy, we find a stronger correlation between ER and PR values among the group of patients not receiving prior therapy. The Kendall rank correlation coefficient of (log (ER) + 1) versus (log (PR) + 1) for the 25 patients receiving endocrine therapy who had prior treatment is 0.09. It is not significantly different from zero (p equals 0.54). For the 19 non-previously treated patients currently receiving endocrine therapy, the Kendall rank correlation coefficient is 0.17, but is also not significantly different from zero (p equals 0.33). There is a trend toward a stronger quantitative relationship between ER values and PR values in the subset of patients who received no prior therapy. These data suggest that the lack of a quantitative relationship between ER and PR in patients having received prior therapy may indicate that progesterone receptor levels are no longer an estrogen dependent function and may explain the failure of the PR to increase the predictive index in this group of patients as compared to patients who have not received prior therapy.

Quantitative ER determinations may be of more value than PR in predicting response to endocrine therapy for several reasons.

First, prior therapy does not affect the predictive index of ER. Second, all 4 of our patients who were PR positive but ER negative failed to respond to endocrine therapy. Third, Pollow et al. (14) have recently shown that PR concentration in normal mammary cytosol of premenopausal women depended on the day of the menstrual cycle and that the binding of progesterone was highest around the time of ovulation.

Of the 54 patients who had an androgen receptor assay performed on their tumor, 19 were AR positive and 35 were AR negative. The two groups were similar with regard to age, menopausal status, Karnofsky performance index, disease free interval and proportion of patients with visceral involvement.

In Table 19, we analyze the relationship between response to endocrine therapy and both estrogen and androgen receptor status. As seen in this table, although presence of AR is able to predict response to therapy, the concentration of ER has an overwhelming influence on response rate. No differences were observed between AR positive and negative tumors with regard to response rate in those patients in the ER positive group. Furthermore, AR positivity did not alter the low response rate in the ER negative tumors.

Table 19. Objective response rate to endocrine therapy as a function of estrogen receptor and androgen receptor status

	ER Positive		ER Negative	
	AR positive	AR negative	AR positive	AR negative
Response rate	11/15 (73%)	10/16 (63%)	0/4 (0%)	1/19 (5%)

Of the 44 patients who had a glucocorticoid receptor assay performed on their tumors, 34 were GR positive and 10 were GR negative. These two groups were similar with regard to age, menopausal status, Karnofsky performance index, disease free interval, and proportion of patients with visceral disease. Twenty of 34 patients whose tumors contained greater than 10 fmols of GR/mg cytoplasmic protein had an objective response to endocrine therapy compared to 2 of 10 patients in the GR negative group. Although this is of borderline statistical significance (p equals 0.07) it is important to note that there is no difference in the

Table 20. Objective response rate to endocrine therapy as a function of estrogen receptor and glucocorticoid receptor status

	ER positive		ER negative	
	GR positive	GR negative	GR positive	GR negative
Response rate	19/23 (82%)	2/5 (40%)	1/11 (9%)	0/5 (0%)

districution of GR values when responders and non-responders are
compared by Wilcoxon rank-sum analysis.

Table 20 examines the ability of the GR to increase the predictive index of the ER.   Nineteen of 23 patients (82%) whose
tumor contained both receptors responded to endocrine therapy.
The comparison group of patients with ER positive and GR negative
tumors is too small at the present time to perform a meaningful
comparison.   Unfortunately, GR positivity did not alter the low
response rate in ER negative tumors.

Multiple Assays and the Effects of Intervening Therapy

All of the above data strongly suggest that receptor status
is important in making therapeutic decisions.   Thus, knowledge of
site-to-site variability and the influence of time and therapy on
receptor concentration is quite important.   A brief summary of our
results in this area follows.

Sixty-one patients had more than one specimen assayed.   Four
groups are defined: GROUP 1 - 27 patients with simultaneous assays from different metastatic sites: GROUP 2 - 5 patients with
2 assays over time without intervening therapy;   GROUP 3 - 10 patients with 2 assays over time with intervening hormonal therapy;
GROUP 4 - 19 patients with 2 asays over time with intervening
chemotherapy.

GROUP 1:   SIMULTANEOUS BIOPSIES AND RECEPTOR DETERMINATIONS

Twenty-seven patients had simultaneous biopsies and receptor
determinations.   All assays were performed on metastatic tissue.
In 23 patients (85%) concordant results were obtained, i.e. the
ER determination between the 2 sites agreed with respect to clas-
sifying the tumor as ER positive or ER negative.   There was dis-
agreement between the 2 sites in only 4 cases.   (Case #1 - mediastinal node ER positive, 97 fmols but supraclavicular node ER
negative, 4 fmols; Case #2 -Breast ER negative, 0 fmols but node
ER positive, 22 fmols; Case #3 - Breast ER negative, 6 fmols but
node ER positive, 30 fmols; Case #4 - Cervical node ER negative,
6 fmols but axillary node ER positive, 62 fmols).   Of the 23 patients in whom concordant ER determinations were obtained, 10 were
ER positive and 13 ER negative.

GROUP 2:   ASYNCHRONOUS BIOPSIES AND RECEPTOR DETERMINATIONS -
            NO THERAPY

Five patients had asynchronous biopsies and assays without
intervening therapy.   One patient had an ER positive tumor which
remained ER positive at the time of the second biopsy.   Four patients had ER negative tumors.   Three remained ER negative over
time; however, one patient had an ER positive tumor at the time
of the second biopsy.   This patient had a breast biopsy which was
ER negative (0 fmols) but a subsequent mediastinal node biopsy 3
months later was borderline ER negative (13 fmols).   In this small
group of 5 patients, no change was noted over time in the mean ER
concentrations.

GROUP 3:   ASYNCHRONOUS BIOPSIES AND RECEPTOR DETERMINATIONS -
            INTERVENING HORMONAL THERAPY

Ten patients had asynchronous biopsies and assays with intervening hormonal therapy.   A marked change in ER status was noted

in this group of patients. The individual receptor assays for
this group are listed in Table 21. The mean ER concentration
pre-therapy was 66 fmols and this decreased to a mean ER concentration of 8 fmols post-therapy (p less than 0.05). In patients
1-8, all of whom had ER negative tumors, the second ER determination after hormonal therapy is markedly lower as compared to the
pre-therapy level. Four of these 9 patients had a change in ER
status going from ER positive to ER negative after hormonal therapy. ER levels did not change after hormonal therapy in the 2 patients who were ER negative pre-therapy.

Table 21. Asynchronous estrogen receptor determinations in patients
with intervening hormonal therapy

Patients	Assay #1 (fmol/mg cytoplasmic protein)	Assay #2 (fmol/mg cytoplasmic protein)
1	46	0
2	75	9
3	13	0
4	87	5
5	200	17
6	217	50
7	132	14
8	40	11
9	4	5
10	0	0

GROUP 4:   ASYNCHRONOUS BIOPSIES AND RECEPTOR DETERMINATIONS -
INTERVENING CHEMOTHERAPY

Nineteen patients had asynchronous biopsies and assays with
intervening chemotherapy. The mean ER concentrations pre- and
post-therapy were similar (2 fmols pre-therapy versus 5 fmols
post-therapy). No patient had a change in ER status from ER positive to ER negative; however, 3 patients who were ER negative
tumor pre-therapy had ER positive metastases post-chemotherapy.
(Case #1 - 6 fmols pre-therapy but 10 fmols post-therapy; Case
#2 - 6 fmols pre-therapy but 11 fmols post-therapy; Case #3 - 4
fmols pre-therapy but 14 fmols post-therapy).

The results of this study show that receptor determinations
performed from multiple metastatic sites simultaneously are highly
concordant. Our 85% rate of agreement compares favorably with
the 80% incidence of concordance (12/15) reported by Kiang and
Kennedy (15), the 62% concordance reported by Webster et al. (16)
and the 85% concordance rate reported by Rosen et al (17).

Although the reliability of a single biopsy has been questioned in the past, these high concordance rates appear to indicate that a single biopsy is highly reliable.

The most striking finding in this study is the marked decrease in ER concentration following hormonal therapy. In our small group of patients, the mean ER concentration decreased from 66 fmols pre-therapy to 8 fmols post-therapy. Of the 8 ER positive patients, 8 decreased their ER levels while no change was seen in the 2 ER negative patients after hormonal therapy. These data strongly suggest that hormonal therapy selectively eliminates ER positive tumor cells.

It is also interesting to note that in the 19 patients having receptor assays performed over time with intervening chemotherapy that although mean receptor concentrations were not significantly different pre- and post-therapy, there was a trend toward more ER "rich" tumors after chemotherapy with 3 patients exhibiting a change in ER status (ER negative to ER positive). A similar trend was also reported by Kiang and Kennedy (15). In their study, the incidence of ER positivity post-chemotherapy was 67% as compared to a 57% incidence of ER positivity in patients not treated by chemotherapy. Chemotherapy exposed tumors had a median ER value of 82 fmols versus 46 fmols in those patients who had received no prior chemotherapy. These trends suggest some selection in favor of ER positive cells post-chemotherapy and these results are consistent with a major cytotoxic effect of chemotherapy against rapidly proliferating ER negative cells.

Receptors and Male Breast Cancer

Finally, it is worth outlining our preliminary data with respect to male breast cancer. Unlike female breast cancer, male breast cancer responds to endocrine therapy about two-thirds of the time (18). Because this disease is so rare (about 1% of the incidence of the disease incidence in females), we were fortunate to obtain the cooperation of Drs. J. Wittliff, W.L. McGuire, E.V. Jensen, and S. Brooks. Their data combined with our own are summarized in Table 22. Clearly, virtually all patients with male breast cancer have some detectable estrogen receptor activity in their tumors (87%). A smaller proportion have detectable progesterone (77%), glucocortocoid (67%) and androgen (33%) receptor

Table 22. Steroid receptors in male breast cancer*

	ER	PR	AR	GR
Positive	54 (84)	16 (73)	2 (22)	4 (67)
Borderline	2 (3)	1 (4)	1 (11)	0
Negative	8 (13)	5 (23)	6 (67)	2 (33)
Total	64	22	9	6

*Number (percent) of specimens positive, borderline, or negative.

activity. Unfortunately, at the present time, although there are trends toward a positive correlation between estrogen receptor concentration and disease free interval and response to endocrine therapy and duration of response, none of the correlations are statistically significant.

All of these studies taken ensemble clearly establish some of the uses (and limitations) of steroid receptor analyses. Space precludes a consideraton of the potential role for such analyses in predicting response to chemotherapy. Pro (19) and con (20) views of this controversial area are published. Also omitted from this discussion is a consideration of the relationship between disease free interval and ER status. Studies of Meyer and colleagues (21) suggest that ER negative tumors are less well differentiated and tend to be more rapidly dividing. From this one might guess that ER negative tumors might tend to recur earlier. We (22) and others (23,24) have made this observation.

Further work in many areas will be required to improve the accuracy of these data and to extend them to other hormone dependent neoplasia.

References

1. Beatson, G.T.: On the treatment of inoperable cases of carcinoma of the mama: suggestions for a new method of treatment, with illustrative cases. Lancet 2: 104-107, 1896.

2. Steroid Cell Interactions. Edited by R.J.B. King, WIP Mainwaring, London, Butterworth, 1974.

3. Jensen, E.V., DeSombre, E.R., and Jungblut, P.W.: Estrogen receptors in hormone-responsive tissues and tumors. Endogenous factors influencing host-tumor balance. Edited by R.W. Wissler, T.L. Dao, S. Wood, Jr., Chicago, Univ. of Chicago Press, pp. 15-30, 1967.

4. Terenius, L.: Selective retention of estrogen isomers in estrogen-dependent breast tumors of rats demonstrated by in vivo methods. Cancer Res 28: 328-337, 1968.

5. Estrogen Receptors in Normal and Neoplastic Tissues. Edited by W.L. McGuire, P.P. Carbone, E.P. Vollmer, New York, Raven Press, 1974.

6. Progesterone Receptors in Normal and Neoplastic Tissues. Edited by W.L. McGuire, J.P. Raynaud, E.E. Baulieu, New York, Raven Press, 1977.

7. Allegra, J.C., Lippman, M.E., Thompson, E.R., Simon, R., Barlock, A., Green, L., Huff, K., Do, H.M.T., and Aiken, S.C.: The distribution frequency and quantitative analysis of estrogen, progesterone, androgen, and glucocorticoid receptors in human breast cancer. Cancer Research 39: 1447-1454, 1979.

8. McGuire, W.L.: Physiologic principles underlying endocrine therapy of breast cancer. In: W.L. McGuire (ed.), Advances in Research and Treatment, p. 238. New York, Plenum Medical Book Co., 1977.

9. Persijn, J.P., Korsten, C.B., and Engelsman, E.: Oestrogen and androgen receptors in breast cancer and response to endocrine therapy. Br. Med. J. 4: 503, 1975.

10. Lippman, M.E., Bolan, G., and Huff, K.: Human breast cancer responsive to androgen in long-term tissue culture. Nature 258: 339-341, 1975.

11. Horwitz, K.B., Costlow, M.E., and McGuire, W.L.: MCF-7: A human breast cancer cell line with estrogen, androgen, progesterone, and glucocorticoid receptors. Steroids 26: 785-795, 1975.

12. Goldenberg, I.S., Waters, N., Ravdin, R.S., Ansfield, F.J., and Segaloff, A.: Androgenic therapy for advanced breast cancer in women. J. Am. Med. Assoc. 223: 1267-1268, 1973.

13. Teulings, F.A.G. and Van Gilse, H.A.: Demonstration of glucocorticoid receptors in human mammary carcinomas. Horm. Res. 8: 107-116, 1977.

14. Pollow, K., Sinnecker, R., Gollwitzer, M.S., Boquoi, E., and Pollow, B.: Binding of (3H) progesterone to normal and neo-plastic tissue samples from tumor bearing breast. J. Mol. Med. 2: 69-82, 1977.

15. Kiang, D.T. and Kennedy, B.J.: Factors affecting estrogen receptors in breast cancer. Cancer 40: 1571-1576, 1977.

16. Webster, D.J.T., Bronn, D.G., Minton, J.P.: Estrogen receptor levels in multiple biopsies from patients with breast cancer. Am. J. Surg. 126: 337-338, 1978.

17. Rosen, P., Mendenez-Botet, C.J., Urban, J.A. et al.: Estrogen receptors protein (ERP) in multiple tumor specimens from individual patients with breast cancer. Cancer 39: 2194-2196, 1977.

18. Everson, R.B., Lippman, M.E., Thompson, E.B., McGuire, W.L., DeSombre, E.R., Wittliff, J.L., Singhakowinta, A., and Neifeld, J.P.: Steroid receptors in male breast cancer. Cancer Research (In press).

19. Lippman, M.E., Allegra, J.C., Thompson, E.B. et al.: The relation between estrogen receptors and response rate to cytotoxic chemotherapy in metastatic breast cancer. N. Engl. J. Med. 298: 1223-1228, 1978.

20. Frennings, D.G., Kennedy, B.J., Vosika, G.J., et al.: Correlation of estrogen receptors and response to chemotherapy in advanced breast cancer. Proc. Am. Soc. Clin. Oncol. 19: 347, 1978.

21. Meyers, J.S., Rao, B.R., Stevens, S.C., et al: Low incidence of estrogen receptor in breast carcinomas with rapid rates of cellular replication. Cancer 40: 2290-2298, 1977.

22. Persijn, J.P., Korsten, C.B., Engelsman, E.: Oestrogen and androgen receptors in breast cancer and response to endocrine therapy. Br. Med. J. 4: 503, 1975.

23. Knight, W.A., Livingston, R.B., Gregory E.J., et al: Estrogen receptor as an independent prognostic factor for early recurrence in breast cancer. Cancer Res. 37: 4669-4671, 1977.

24. Maynard, P.V., Blamey, R.W., Haybittle, J.L., et al.: Oestrogen receptor assay in primary breast cancer and early recurrence of the disease. Cancer Research (In press).

Perspectives in Steroid Receptor Research,
edited by F. Bresciani.
Raven Press, New York © 1980.

Steroid Receptors and Clinical Breast Cancer

William D. McGuire

*Department of Medicine/Oncology, University of Texas Health Science Center,
San Antonio, Texas 78284, U.S.A.*

Considerable progress has been made in the last decade in our approach to patients with breast cancer. Endocrine therapy for advanced disease has now progressed to the point where physicians can confidently select patients who are likely to respond. New information is emerging regarding the use of estrogen receptor (ER) assays to predict which patients will have an early recurrence. It is the purpose of this chapter to present data from my own laboratory on the use of ER and Progesterone receptor PgR) assays in the management of both primary and advanced breast cancer.

Estrogen Receptor in the Primary Breast Tumor

It is well appreciated that only about one half of breast cancer patients are cured by surgical and/or radiation therapy of the primary tumor. The majority of these patients have tumors confined to the breast without extension to the axillary lymph nodes (1). Those patients with regional lymph node involvement will usually present with metastitic disease at some later date. Until the pat few years, axillary node positive patients were simply observed following surgery with the hope, albeit slim, of cure. Upon recurrence, pallative endocrine and cytotoxic therapies provided prolongation of life but eventually all patients died of the disease. More recently, the concept of adjuvant therapy with the goal of cure has emerged, particularly in the case of axillary node positive patients. The reasoning is that extension of tumor to regional lymph nodes is operationally equivalent to finding distant microscopic tumor metastases. Rather than waiting until these foci are clinically evident, systemic anti-tumor therapy begun soon after surgery might be very successful since tumor burden is relatively low. There is considerable experimental animal tumor data to support this concept and now many large clinical trials are underway with some preliminary reports showing early success (2,3,4,). The question is not whether to use adjuvant therapy but rather which drugs, which patients, and for how long! Since there are considerable arrays of systemic agents available and undoubtedly many subsets of patients with varying degrees of risk of recurrence and potential response to these agents, a method to select patients at risk and the proper adjuvant therapy for particular subsets of these patients is needed.

In San Antonio, we had begun to measure ER in primary breast tumors in hopes of eventually correlating these data with the response to endocrine therapy at some later date. In many of these patients we had follow up data including time to recurrence and survival. So we decided to look at the natural history of our patient population to see if the ER status was correlated with any particular outcome. To our surprise, we found that regardless of axillary node status, age, size of the primary tumor, or location of the tumor in the breast, those patients with ER- tumors recurred earlier than ER+ patients (5). Approximately a year later we reanalyzed our data with the addition of more patients and the elimination of patients who had received any systemic endocrine or cytotoxic therapy. Our earlier conclusions were confirmed and extended to show that ER- patients not only recurred earlier but had worse survival than ER+ patients (6). These data are illustrated in Table I.

Table I

Estrogen Receptor and Recurrence

| Characteristic | | Recurrence at 20 months | | |
		ER-%	vs	ER+%
Age:	<50	32		0
	>50	36		16
Nodes:	Negative	19		6
	Positive	59		26
	1-3	36		25
	>4	72		27
Primary Size:	<2 cm	40		5
	>2 cm	37		16
Primary Location:	Outer	31		9
	inner and central	50		19

Adapted from Knight et al. (ref. #5).

Subsequently, similar data has been recently reported from other centers around the world which substantiates the results of our pilot study (7,8,9,10). The implications of these findings are considerable. First, we now can identify a subset of axillary node positive patients who have an extremely poor prognosis if left untreated. Second, the ER assay results indicate that the latter group should receive intensive combination chemotherapy and that the ER+ axillary node positive patients should receive an endocrine therapy as part of the adjuvant therapy. In fact, this approach is now being tested. In collaboration with Drs. Hubay, Pearson, and colleagues in Cleveland, we have been assaying ER in primary breast tumors of patients randomized to receive combination chemotherapy with or without antiestrogen therapy. The preliminary data are very encouraging (4). ER+ patients are recurring less frequently if they receive a combination of chemo-endocrine therapy compared to chemotherapy alone. ER- patients recur at the same rate whether or not antiestrogens are added to the chemotherapy. Independent trials from other centers are needed to confirm these data but the approach is based upon sound physiological principles and the use of ER assays in the primary tumor for prognostic information as well as therapeutic strategy seems assured.

As will be discussed later, the presence or absence of ER in a biopsy of metastatic breast cancer correlates well with the response of that cancer to endocrine therapy. The question remains, however, whether ER assay results at the time of primary surgery are valuable, perhaps years later, if the patient develops metastatic disease. This is of considerable importance since less than 50% of patients presenting with advanced disease have readily accessible lesions for biopsy and assay -- whereas practically all patients undergoind primary breast surgery have tissue available for this purpose. The theoretical objection to this approach is that the ER status of a tumor could change between the time of primary surgery and the clinical presentation of advanced disease. This has been examined by various investigators and in the great majority of cases, the ER status is unchanged when comparing pirmary and metastatic biopsies in the same patient. The most direct test, of course, is to measure ER in the primary tumor and correlate the results with subsequent endocrine therapy for metastatic disease; data from Jensens laboratory clearly supports such a correlation (11). Our own data is illustrated in Table II. We find approximately the same response rate to endocrine therapy of advanced disease in ER+ tumors regardless of whether ER determination was made on the original primary tumor or a subsequent metastatic lesion.

Table II

ER and Response to Endocrine Therapy

	Primary Biopsy	Metastatic Biopsy
ER-	1/6 = 17%	4/47 = 8%
ER+	22/44 = 50%	48/101 = 48%

The Value of Quantitative Estrogen Receptor Assays

In the early days of ER correlations, few laboratories reported quantitative data. It seemed sufficient to merely indicate whether the receptor was present or absent. Our earliest analysis, however, though based on a limited number of patients, indicated that the response rate was the highest in those patients with the highest quantitative tumor ER content (12). As we examine in Table III the actual values in primary vs metastatic biopsies and younger vs older patients, certain features stand out. First, metastatic ciopsies are more often ER- than primary biopsies regardless of age. Second, the older patient is much more likely to have a high receptor content than the younger patient regardless of whether the biopsy is from a primary or metastatic lesion. This might be expected since the older patient is more likely to have a favorable response to endocrine therapy. Our actual clinical correlations are shown in Table IV. In almost 200 endocrine trials we find that the response rate is proportional to the absolute receptor content.

Table III

Quantitative ER Values in Primary
and Metastatic Breast Cancer

Age	<50		>50	
Biopsy	1°	2°	1°	2°
ER Value				
<3	162 (37%)	49 (52%)	279 (23%)	75 (31%)
3-10	90 (20%)	13 (14%)	176 (15%)	39 (16%)
11-100	183 (41%)	28 (29%)	432 (35%)	67 (27%)
100-2000	10 (2%)	5 (5%)	312 (26%)	63 (26%)
Total	445	95	1199	244

Table IV

Quantitative ER and the Response
to Endocrine Therapy

| ER fm/mg | Response | |
	1^{O} Biopsy	2^{O} Biopsy
<3	1/6 = 17%	4/47 = 8%
3-10	3/7 = 42%	11/24 = 45%
11-100	14/31 = 45%	15/41 = 36%
>100	5/6 = 83%	22/36 = 61%

Progesterone Receptor and Response to Endocrine Therapy

Despite the success of ER assays for prediction, a large number of ER+ patients fail to respond to endocrine therapy. Several years ago we reasoned that since cytoplasmic binding of estrogen to receptor was only the first step in a complex biochemical pathway leading to growth and specific protein synthesis in a breast tumor cell, perhaps certain ER+ tumors failed to respond because of defects distal to the binding step. We hypothesized that progesterone receptor (PgR) might be an ideal marker of estrogen action in breast tumor cells as it had been shown to be estrogen dependent in normal reproductive tissue (13). We developed an assay for PgR which was quite specific and sensitive in breast cancer tissue (14) and demonstrated that PgR synthesis was strictly controlled by estrogen in both experimental (15) and human breast cancer cells (16). The distribution of PgR in a large number of human breast cancer biopsies is shown in Table V.

Table V

Distribution of ER and PgR
in 1366 Breast Cancer Patients

	Premenopausal	Postmenopausal
ER-, PgR-	30%	19%
ER-, PgR+	9%	3%
ER+, PgR-	12%	23%
ER+, PgR+	49%	55%

As anticipated PgR is rarely found in those tumors lacking Er. Conversely, the likelihood of finding PgR in a tumor was proportional to the absolute amount of ER in the tumor. Thus it was likely that PgR would correlate with a faborable response to endocrine therapy. Our own data on clinical response is illustrated in Table VI. As anticipated, those tumors without ER and

Table VI

Objective Remission of Metastatic Breast Cancer
As a Function of ER and PgR

	Objective Response
ER-, PgR-	3/20 = 15%
ER-, PgR+	-
ER+, PgR-	14/45 = 31%
ER+, PgR+	16/20 = 80%

PgR are unlikely to respond. Tumors containing only PgR are rare and not enough information is available to reach any conclusions. Those patients with both ER and PgR have a remarkably high response rate. The interesting group is that with ER but without PgR. We would have anticipated that few if any of these patients would have responded. Yet the response rate is appreciable even though far below those patients with both receptors. We have considered several possibilities to explain the behavior of this group. First, the assays for PgR are imperfect and it is possible that a few patients in this group are false negative. However, it is doubtful that this could explain the whole result. Second, we must consider the influence of endogenous progesterone in premenopausal women. Saez and colleagues have reported that PgR cannot be found in breast tumor cytosols of women with high circulating levels of progesterone during the luteal phase of the menstrual cycle (17). Presumably all of the cytoplasmic PgR sites have been translocated to nuclei. A nuclear exhange assay might solve this problem. Finally, since PgR synthesis is estrogen dependent, could some postmenopausal women have insufficient circulating estrogen to stimulate PgR in the tumor even when the appropriate biochemical pathways are present? Degenshein and associates (personal communication) have, in fact, biopsied patients before and after a few days of estrogen therapy and found several women who converted to PgR+. So it appears that many of the ER+, PgR-cases who respond to endocrine therapy can be explained.

Quantitative Estrogen Receptor Assays vs Progesterone Receptor Assays

Although the merits of PgR assays are now well documented, one could take the position that since the likelihood of finding PgR in a tumor is correlated with the amount of ER in the tumor and that the likelihood of faborable response is proportional to the amount of ER in the tumor, perhaps PgR is just a signal that a high level of ER is present. If so, PgR measurements would be redundant. Fortunately, the matter can be resolved by direct analysis of the data. We have studied 65 ER+ patients where we have quantitative ER and PgR data as well as objective response to endocrine therapy. The data are illustrated in Table VII.

Table VII

Quantitative ER vs PgR

		Objective Response Rate		
PgR	+	16/20	=	80%
	-	14/45	=	31%
ER	>100	17/27	=	63%
	3-100	13/38	=	34%

If we use quantitative ER alone to discriminate between low and high response rates in ER+ patients, we find that the best separation obtained is 34% vs 63%. If we use the presence of PgR, the discrimination becomes 31% vs 80%. So we must conclude from our own data that the measurement of ER and PgR is superior to just quantitating ER alone. The implications for therapy are just emerging. In those patients with both ER and PgR, endocrine therapy is the therapy of choice. The group ER+, PgR- is a little more difficult in that about 30% of these patients will still have a good response. Perhpas many of these responders could be reclassified as ER+, PgR+ if nuclear exchange assays are employed or estrogen stimulation were used. At present, we would not recommend withholding endocrine therapy from this group but would suggest that only those therapies with low morbidity be used (e.g., antiestrogens); this group might be ideal candidates for combined chemo-endocrine therapies.

Acknowledgments

This work was partially supported by the National Cancer Institute (CA 11378, CB 23682) and The American Cancer Society. This review chapter was prepared as a requirement for attending both the 1st International Congress on Hormones and Cancer, Rome,

October 1979 and the Satellite Symposium on Perspectives in Steroid Receptor Studies, Sorrento, October 1979.

REFERENCES

1. Fisher, B. (1977). In Breast Cancer: Advances in Research and Treatment (W.L. McGuire, ed.) p. 1. Plenum Press, New York.
2. Fisher, B., and Wolmark, N. (1977). In Breast Cancer: Advances in Research and Treatment (W.L. McGuire, ed.), p. 25. Plenum Press, New York.
3. Bonadonna, G., Rossi, A., Valaqussa, P., Banfi, A., and Veronesi, U. (1977). The CMF Program for Operable Breast Cancer with Positive Axillary Nodes. Cancer, 39:22904.
4. Hubay, C.A., Pearson, O.H., Marshall, J.S., Rhodes, R.S., DeBanne, S.M., Mansour, E.G., Herman, R.E., Jones, J.C., Flynn, W.J., Eckert, C., and McGuire, W.L. (1980). Submitted.
5. Knight, W.A., Livingston, R.B., Gregory, E.J., and McGuire, W.L. (1977). Cancer Research, 37:3667-4671.
6. Knight, W.A., Livingston, R.B., Gregory, E.J., Walder, A.I., and McGuire, W.L. (1978). Proceedings of the American Society of Clinical Oncology, 19:392.
7. Rich, M.A., Furmonski, P., and Brooks, S.C. (1978). Cancer Research, 38:4296.
8. Maynard, P.V., Davies, C.J., Blamey, R.W., Elston, C.W., Johnson, J., and Griffiths, K. (1978). Brit. J. Cancer, 38:745.
9. Allegra, J.C., Lippman, M.E., Simon, R., Thompson, E.G., Barlock, A., Green, L., Huff, K., Do, H.M.T., Aitken, S.C., and Warren, R. (1979). Cancer Treatment Reports, in press.
10. Hahnel, R., Woodings, T., and Vivian, A.B. (1979). Cancer, 44:325.
11. Block, G.E., Ellis, R.S., DeSombre, E., and Jensen, E. (1978). Ann. Surg., 188:372.
12. McGuire, W.L., Carbone, P.P., and Vollmer, E.P., eds.(1975). In: Estrogen Receptors in Human Breast Cancer, Raven Press, New York.
13. Horwitz, K.B., and McGuire, W.L. (1975), Science, 189:726-727.
14. Horwitz, K.B., and McGuire, W.L., (1975), Steroids, 25:497-505.
15. Horwitz, K.T., and McGuire, W.L., (1977), Cancer Research, 37: 1733-1738.
16. Horwitz, K.B., and McGuire, W.L. (1978), J. Biol. Chem., 253: 2223-2228.
17. Saez, S., Martin, P., and Chouvet, C. (1978), Cancer Research, 38:3468.

Perspectives in Steroid Receptor Research,
edited by F. Bresciani.
Raven Press, New York © 1980.

Steroid Hormone Receptors in Human Breast Cancer

A. J. M. Koenders, *L. V. M. Beex, and Th. J. Benraad

*Departments of Experimental Endocrinology and *Medicine, Division of Endocrinology,
University of Nijmegen, Nigmegen, The Netherlands*

In normal target tissues the concentrations of estradiol and progesterone receptors are regulated by steroid hormones (1). There is ample evidence that also in DMBA-induced rat mammary tumors steroid hormones exert acute control over the production of ER and PgR. In DMBA-tumors estradiol receptors are stimulated by estradiol and prolactin, whereas progesterone inhibits ER synthesis (2,3,4). On the other hand PgR synthesis in these tumors is induced by estradiol (5,6). Tumors from premenopausal patients appear to have lower ER levels than tumors from post-menopausal patients, which suggests that receptor levels in human breast tumors may be modulated by circulating steroid hormones (7).

In the present report the distributions of ER and PgR in primary and metstatic human breast cancers are presented. The data were evaluated with special emphasis on the menopausal status and the use of contraceptive steroids. To our knowledge no studies have been reported regarding the influence of contraceptive steroids on ER and PgR levels in human breast cancer.

Recently it has been questioned whether receptor assays performed in the primary tumor at time of mastectomy can be used to guide endocrine therapy at time of recurrence (8). In other words, is there a relation between receptor activity in the primary tumor and in metastatic lesions? This would be of clinical importance because many patients have metastatic lesions that are inaccessible for excision. To investigate this attractive possibility, sequential receptor assays were performed in the primary breast tumor and metastases of the same patient.

MATERIALS AND METHODS

Tumor specimens

Breast tumor specimens were obtained from the Canisius/Wilhelmina

247

Hospital (Nijmegen) and the Radboud Hospital (Nijmegen). As far as macroscopically possible excised breast cancer tissue speci- mens were freed from fat, connective and necrotic tissue by the pathologist. A representative part was used for histological examination, the remaining tissue was immediately deep frozen (dry ice) and stored at -70 C. Within two weeks the tissue was transferred to our laboratory and stored in liquid nitrogen. Almost all metastatic biopsy specimens, after removal of a re- presentative part for histological examination, were immediately placed on dry ice and within a few hours stored in liquid nitro- gen. All biopsies were analysed within 2 to 3 weeks after arrival at the laboratory.

Dextran-coated Charcoal Assay

All receptor assays were performed in microtiter plates, as published (6). Shortly, 50 1 of cytosol was incubated with six different concentrations of ^3H-E_2 (1-8 nM) or ^3H-R5020 (1-10 nM). The nonspecific binding for ^3H-E_2 and ^3H-R5020 was determined in the presence of $10^{-6}M$ Diethylstilbestrol and R5020, respectively. After equilibrium was reached (16-20 hr at 0-4 C), the unbound steroid was removed by the addition of a dextran-coated charcoal suspension. Scatchard-analysis was performed to determine the concentration of receptor binding sites and the equilibrium dissociation constant (K_d).

RESULTS

Estradiol and Progesterone Receptors in Primary and Metastatic Breast Tumors

Biopsies of 297 primary and 91 metastatic breast tumors have been analysed for the presence of estradiol receptor (ER) and progesterone receptors (pgR). The incidence of both receptors in primary and metastatic breast tumors is presented in Table 1. Biopsies of metastases obtained within six weeks after tamoxifen withdrawal were excluded.

Table   1. Incidence of ER and PgR in human breast cancer.

	Total	Primary	Metastatic
ER-positive	71% (277/388)	74% (219/297)[a]	64% (58/91)[a]
PgR-positive	51% (199/388)	55% (165/297)[b]	37% (34/91)[b]

[a] $\chi^2 = 3.41$; DF = 1 ; $0.1 > p > 0.05$

[b] $\chi^2 = 9.23$; DF = 1 ; $p < 0.01$

Of all tumors (n=388) analysed 71% were ER-positive and in 51% of the tumors PgR could be detected. The frequency of PgR-positive tumors was significantly higher (p 0.01) in primary (55%) than in metastatic tumors (37%). Primary breast tumors were also more likely to be ER-positive than metastases, the difference being close to statistical significance (0.1 p 0.05). The distribution of PgR-positive tumors, in relation to the presence or absence of ER, can be seen in Table 2.

Table   2 Distribution of PgR-positive human breast tumors.

		Total	Primary	Metastatic
ER+	PgR+	68% (189/277)	72% (157/219)[a]	55% (32/58)[a]
ER-	PgR+	9% (10/111)	10% (8/78)	6% (2/33)

[a] $\chi^2 = 5.77$; DF = 1 ; p<0.02

It appeared that the presence of PgR was essentially restricted to ER-positive tumors. In the group of ER-positive tumors 68% were also PgR-positive whereas only 9% of the ER-negative tumors were PgR-positive. The frequency of ER+ PgR+ tumors was significantly (p 0.02) higher in primary (72%) as compared to metastatic breast tumors (55%). In these series of patients, 10 (2.6%) showed PgR, whereas no ER could be detected. Most (7/10) of these tumors had very low PgR levels (20 fmoles/mg protein). Six out of these 10 patients appeared to be premenopausal.

Estradiol and Progesterone Receptors in Primary Breast Tumors

1. Influence of Menopausal Status on Steroid Hormone Receptors

The influence of the menopausal status on the receptor distributions and the receptor levels was examined. A woman was considered as postmenopuasal when menses had ceased at least one year prior to biopsy. The receptor distributions of these groups of patients is presented in Table 3. It appeared that postmenopausal patients were more likely ($\chi^2=3.57$; 0.1 p 0.05) to have ER-positive tumors (78%) than premenopausal women (67%). The frequency of PgR-positive tumors however was not different for these two groups of women.

Table   3   ER and PgR distributions in primary breast tumors of
            pre- and postmenopausal patients.

	number of patients analysed	ER+ PgR+	ER+ PgR-	ER- PgR+	ER- PgR-
premenopausal	76	57%	10%[a]	7%	26%
postmenopausal	167	53%	25%[a]	2%	20%

[a] $\chi^2 = 6.83$; DF = 1 ; p<0.01

The difference in ER distribution between pre- and postmenopausal
patients was due to ER+ PgR- tumors being significantly (p 0.01)
more frequent in postmenopausal patients (25%) as compared to
premenopausal patients (10%). The mean receptor levels of the
receptor-positive tumors of these two groups of women are collected
in Table 4.

Table   4   ER and PgR levels in primary breast tumors of pre- and
            postmenopausal women (ER- PgR- tumors excluded).

Patients	Estradiol Receptor		Progesterone Receptor	
	mean ± S.E.	range[a]	mean ± S.E.	range[a]
premenopausal	62 ± 7 (51)[b]	9-220	193 ± 29 (48)[c]	8-1250
postmenopausal	202 ± 19★(131)	20-1400	190 ± 28 (92)	8-1230

[a] all values are expressed as fmoles/mg protein

[b] the number of estradiol receptor-positive tumors is indicated
in parentheses

[c] the number of progesterone receptor-positive tumors is indicated
in parentheses

★p<0.01 (pre-vs. postmenopausal women, Wilcoxon rank test).

The mean receptor level of the estradiol receptor-positive tumors
of premenopausal patients was significantly lower than the
corresponding mean receptor level of postmenopausal patients.   No
such difference was observed for the mean level of PgR.

2. Influence of Age on Steroid Hormone Receptors

   In Figs. 1 and 2 the ER and PgR levels of primary breast tumors
are plotted against the age of the patient.

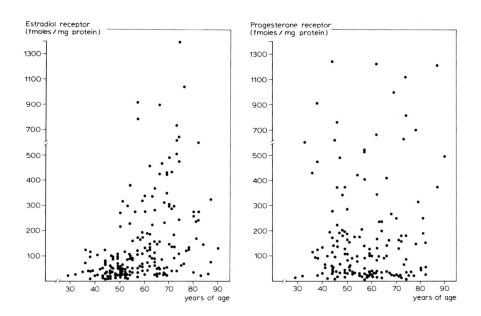

Figs. 1 and 2.   ER and PgR levels in primary breast tumors plotted
               against the age of the patient.

It is noteworthy that frequently ER levels of patients older than
50 years of age (predominantly postmenopausal) were higher than
the upper level obtained in younger patients (predominantly premenopausal).   No such difference was observed for PgR values.
As Table 5 shows the frequency of ER-positive tumors increased
with age.   The difference between the percentage of ER-positive
tumors in the group of women younger than 40 and older than 60
was close to statistical significance (X^2=3.51; DF=1; 0.1 p 0.05).
There appeared to be no consistent influence of the age of the
patient on the incidence of PgR-positive primary breast tumors.

Table   5   ER and PgR distribution in primary breast tumors:
Influence of age.

age (years)	number of patients analysed	ER-positive (%)	PgR-positive (%)
<40	23	61	52
40-50	59	69	66
50-59	77	71	49
>60	115	79	57

3. Influence of Contraceptive Steroids on Steroid Hormone Receptors

Some of the premenopausal patients used contraceptive steroids (Lyndiol[R], Stediril d[R], Neogynon[R], Microgynon[R], and Orthonovum[R]) just prior to tumor biopsy excision. Receptor distributions and levels were compared in two groups of premenopausal women; contraceptive steroid users and non-users. The ER levels of the non-users ranged from 0 to 120 fmoles/mg protein. Interestingly 6 out of 23 users with ER-positive tumors showed values above this level (120-220 fmoles/mg protein). The range of PgR levels was similar for both types of patients (0 to about 1000 fmoles/mg protein). No statistically significant differences in the frequency of ER-positive and PgR-positive tumors between these two groups of patients were observed (Table 6).

Table   6   ER and PgR distribution in primary breast tumors of premenopausal women in relation to use of contraceptive steroids.

	ER-positive	PgR-positive
patients using contraceptive steroids	74% (23/31)[a]	72% (13/18)[b]
patients not using contraceptive steroids	61% (34/56)[a]	61% (34/56)[b]

[a] $\chi^2 = 1.06$; DF = 1 ; p>0.1

[b] $\chi^2 = 0.36$; DF = 1 ; p>0.5

4. Correlation Between Estradiol and Progesterone Receptor Binding Sites in Primary Breast Tumors

Estradiol receptor levels have been plotted against the corresponding progesterone receptor levels separately for pre- (Fig.3)

and postmenopausal patients (Fig. 4). No correlation was observed between the levels of ER-positive and PgR-positive tumors in either category of patients.

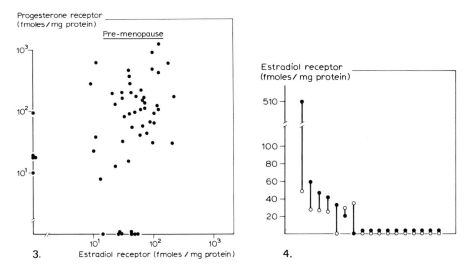

Figs. 3 and 4. Correlation between estradiol and progesterone receptor levels in primary breast tumors from pre-(n=76) and postmenopausal (n=167) patients.

When both receptors were present, premenopausal women generally (74%) had a PgR/ER ration above 1, whereas 61% of the postmeno-pausal women had a ration below 1 ($X^2=13.74$; DF=1; p 0.001). Al-though no correlation between the quantitative ER and PgR values was observed, there was a positive relation between the incidence of PgR-positive tumors and the concentration of estradiol receptor binding sites (Table 7).

Table 7 Comparison of estradiol receptor binding sites and the incidence of PgR-positive primary breast tumors.

ER (fmoles/mg protein)	number of patients analysed	PgR-positive
0	78	10%
<30	41	54%
31−50	29	66%
51−99	51	73%
>100	98	82%

Estradiol Receptors in Sequential Biopsies of Primary and
Metastatic Breast Tumors

   During the course of this investigation there was opportunity
with 17 patients to obrain a tumor specimen as well from the
primary tumor, as at various time intervals, from a metastatic
lesion.   The ER values of these patients are collected in Fig. 5.
It appeared that ER-positive primary tumors generally give rise
to ER-positive metastases (5 out of 6 patients), whereas ER-negative primary tumors generally give rise to ER-negative metastases
(10 out of 11 patients).

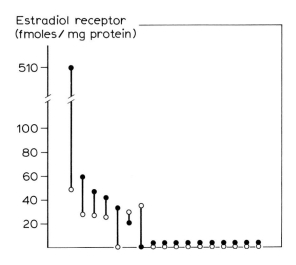

Fig. 5.   Comparison of ER levels in sequential biopsies of the
          primary breast tumor (•) and metastases (○) of the same
          patient (n=17).

Only in 2 out of these 17 patients (12.0%) the receptor classification of the primary tumor and of the metastasis at time of recurrence was not in agreement.   One patient had an ER value of
35 fmoles/mg protein in the primary breast tumor, 29 months later
a lymph node metastasis appeared to be ER-negative, however with
a PgR value of 55.   This patient was still menstruating and the
biopsy specimen was excised during the follicular phase of the
cycle.   The other patient showed an ER- PgR- primary tumor, the
assay of which however was not reliable, because of a protein
content in the cytosol of 1.4 mg/ml.   Six months later a metastasis
revealed an ER value of 35 and a PgR value of 110 fmoles/mg protein.   Five out of 6 patients with ER-positive primary tumors
showed lower ER values in the later appearing metastases.

DISCUSSION

In accordance with several reports from other laboratories it was observed that the presence of PgR was essentially restricted to ER-positive tumors (9-14). Of all ER-positive tumors 68% contained also PgR, whereas in only 9% of the ER-negative tumors PgR could be detected. Actually the incidence of PgR-positive tumors was strongly positively related with increasing ER levels (11-13, Table 7). Primary tumors with high ER levels were more likely to be PgR-positive than tumors with low ER levels. These findings suggest that in human breast tumors, as in normal target tissues and in DMBA-induced rat mammary tumors (5,6) the synthesis of PgR is still under estrogen control.

Interestingly several investigators (13,14) as in the present study, observed that ER-positive primary breast tumors were significantly more frequent PgR-positive than metastatic breast tumors. From this finding one could speculate that the ability to synthesize PgR is gradually lost when the tumor tissue dedifferentiates. In line with this are a few observations that PgR became undetectable in sequential biopsies of the same patients during the metastatic period of their disease (manuscript in preparation).

In has consistently been observed that tumors from premenopausal patients have on the average lower ER values than tumors from postmenopausal patients (7, Table 4). In addition it appeared that some of the premenopausal patients using contraceptive steroids showed sometimes much higher ER values than premenopausal patients not using these types of hormones. Furthermore Saez et al. (11) recently reported that no PgR could be detected in human breast tumors from premenopausal patients showing plasma progesterone levels above 100 ng/ml. These observations illustrate that receptor levels in human breast tumors may be modulated by circulating steroid hormones. Therefore there is a need for receptor measurements of both free and occupied receptor sites in the cytoplasmic as well as the nuclear compartment.

Several investigators have performed sequential ER assays in the primary breast tumor and from a metastatic lesion at time of recurrence (15-17). It appeared that an ER-positive primary breast tumor generally gives rise to an ER-positive metastasis; whereas an ER-negative primary breast tumor gives rise to ER-negative metastasis. In this study 15 out of 17 patients (88%) showed concordant tumor receptor classifications. Therefore it can be expected that ER assays performed in the primary tumor can be used to guide endocrine treatment or other treatments, when a patient subsequently develops metastatic disease. In fact DeSombre and Jensen (18) recently reported that the ER-value of the primary breast tumor predicted response to endocrine therapy much later, at time of recurrence.

REFERENCES

1. Bayard, F., Damilano, S., Robel, P., andBaulieu, E.E. (1978):
Cytoplasmic and nuclear estradiol and progesterone receptors
in human endometrium. J. Clin. Endocrinol. Metab., 46:635-648.
2. Sasaki, G.H. and Leung, B.S. (1975): On the mechanism of
hormone action in 7,12 Dimethylbenz(a)anthracene-induced
mammary tumor. Cancer, 35:645-651.
3. Leung, B.S. (1978): Hormonal dependency of experimental breast
cancer. In: Hormones, Receptors, and Breast Cancer, edited by
W.L. McGuire, pp. 219-257. Raven Press, New York.
4. Kelly, P.A., Asselin, J., Labrie, F., and Raynaud, J.P. (1977):
Regulation of hormone receptor levels and growth of DMBA-induced
mammary tumors by RU16117 and other steroids in the rat. In:
Progesterone Receptors in Normal and Neoplastic Tissues, edited
by W.L. McGuire, J.P. Raynaud, and E.E. Baulieu, pp. 85-101.
Raven Press, New York.
5. Horwitz, K.B. and McGuire, W.L. (1977): Progesterone and pro-
gestone receptors in Experimental breast cancer. Cancer Res.,
37:1733-1737.
6. Koenders, A.J.M., Geurts-Moespot, A., Zolingen, S.J., and
Benraad, Th.J. (1977): Progesterone and estradiol receptors in
DMBA-induced mammary tumors before and after ovariectomy and
after subsequent estradiol administration. In: Progesterone
Receptors in Normal and Neoplastic Tissues, edited by W.L.
McGuire, J.P. Raynaud, and E.E. Baulieu, pp. 71-84. Raven Press,
New York.
7. McGuire, W.L. Carbone, P.P., and Vollmer, E.P. (eds.) (1975):
Estrogen Receptors in Human Breast Cancer. Raven Press, New
York.
8. Block, G.E., Jensen, E.V., and Polley, T.Z. (1975): The prediction of hormonal dependency of mammary cancer. Ann. Surg.,
182:342-351.
9. McGuire, W.L., Raynaud, J.P., and Baulieu, E.E. (eds.) (1977):
Progesterone Receptors in Normal and Neoplastic Tissue. Raven
Press, New York.
10.May-Levin, F., DeLaRue, J.C., Bohuon, C., and Contesso, G.,
(1978): Estrogen and progesterone cytosol receptors in human
malignant and benign breast lesions. In: Hormone Deprivation
in Breast Cancer, edited by M. Mayer, S. Saez, and B.A. Stoll,
pp. 68-75. ICI.
11.Saez, S., Martin, P.M., and Chouvet, C.D. (1978): Estradiol and
progesterone receptor levels in human breast adenocarcinoma in
relation to plasma estrogen and progesterone levels. Cancer
Res., 38:3468-3473.
12.Pichon, M.F. and Milgrom, E. (1977): Characterization and assay
of progesterone receptor in human mammary carcinoma. Cancer
Res., 37:464-471.
13.Horwitz, K.B. and McGuire, W.L. (1977): Estrogen and progesterone: their relationship in hormone-dependent breast cancer.
In: Progesterone Receptors in Normal and Neoplastic Tissues,

edited by W.L. McGuire, J.P. Raynaud, and E.E. Baulieu, pp. 103-124. Raven Press, New York.

14. Leclercq, G., Heuson, J.C., Deboel, M.C., Legros, N., Longeval, E., and Mattheiem, W.H. (1977): Estrogen and progesterone receptors in human breast cancer. In: Progesterone Receptors in Normal and Neoplastic Tissues, edited by W.L. Mcguire, J.P. Raynaud, and E.E. Baulieu, pp. 141-154. Raven Press, New York.

15. Jensen, E.B., Polley, T.Z., Smith, S., Block, G.E., Ferguson, D.J., and DeSombre, E.R. (1975): Prediction of hormone dependency in breast cancer. In: Estrogen Receptors in Human Breast Cancer, editedy by W.L. McGuire, P.P. Carbone, and E.P. Vollmer, pp. 37-56. Raven Press, New York.

16. Rosen, P.P., Menendez-Botet, J.M., Urban, J.A., and Schwartz, M.K. (1977): Estrogen receptor protein (ERP) in multiple tumor specimens from individual patients with breast cancer. Cancer, 39:2194-2200.

17. Nomura, Y., Kobayashi, S., Tokatani, O., Sugano, H., Matsumoto, K., and McGuire, W.L. (1977): Estrogen receptor and endocrine responsiveness in Japanese versus American breast cancer patients. Cancer Res., 37:106-110.

18. DeSombre, E.R. and Jensen, E.V. (1978): Hormone dependency in breast cancer. In: Hormone Deprivation in Breast Cancer, edited by M. Mayer, S. Saez, and B.A. Stoll, pp. 15-28. ICI.

ACKNOWLEDGMENT

The authors wish to thank Anneke Geurts-Moespot for her skillful technical assistance.

Perspectives in Steroid Receptor Research,
edited by F. Bresciani.
Raven Press, New York © 1980.

Application of Steroid Receptor Analyses to Clinical and Biological Investigations of the Postmenopausal Endometrium

R. J. B. King and *M. I. Whitehead

*Hormone Biochemistry Department, Imperial Cancer Research Fund, London WC2A 3PX, England; and *Department of Obstetrics and Gynaecology, King's College Hospital, London SE5 8RX, England*

Receptor assays are now an established tool in the clinician's armamentarium for the treatment of human breast cancer (14, 22). In this guise their use is based on two facts; if any part of the estradiol receptor (RE) machinery is present in a tumor that tumor has a good probability of responding to endocrine therapy and, because of the estrogen inducibility of progesterone receptor (RP), the presence of RP is indicative of the estrogen sensitivity of the tumor. Similar logic has been applied to endometrial carcinomata with results that are essentially similar to those obtained with breast cancer (15,32). Clinical uses of receptor assay outside the area of tumor prognosis are virtually nil. The present paper will describe a new use of receptor assays in determining the optimal form of steroid treatment to alleviate symptoms of the climacteric in women. Such treatments are frequently referred to as hormone replacement therapy (HRT) or menopausal estrogen treatment. HRT is highly efficacious in relieving menopausal symptoms but has found some disfavor because of reports of an attendant increased risk of developing endometrial cancer (2, 4, 20). The validity of the epidemiological evidence on which the last statement was based has been much discussed (2, 4, 20) but, at our present state of knowledge it would be prudent to assume that

Estrogen preparations:- Premarin-estrone (50%), equilin (25%) 17α dihydroequilin (15%), other components (10%) all as sulfates (Ayerst International Ltd., Farnborough, England); Harmogen-estrone sulfate (Abbot Laboratories Ltd., Queensborough, England); Progynova-estradiol valerate (Schering U.K. Ltd., Burgess Hill, England); Mestranol-17α ethinyl estradiol 3 methyl ether (Syntex Pharmaceuticals, Maidenhead, England); Norethisterone (Primolut N, Schering U.K. Ltd., Burgess Hill, England).

administration of estrogens alone is unwise. This has lead to
the development of various estrogen plus progestin therapies on
the basis that progestins are known to counteract some effects
of estrogen. In many cases, a sound scientific background to
the proposed therapy is lacking and a somewhat bewildering array
of compounds and treatment schedules are currently in use.

In an attempt to answer the question of whether estrogens
unopposed by progestins are more likely to generate endometrial
abnormalities than if a progestin is included, Whitehead et al.
(30, 31) set up a prospective study in which endometrial
histology was studied in women receiving either estrogen
(Premarin) alone (cyclical therapy) or Premarin to which the
progestin, norethisterone was added for 7 days each month
(sequential therapy). The conclusion from this and other (27)
studies was that estrogen unopposed by a progestin produced
hyperplasias in up to 30% of women as compared with about 5% in
women taking sequential estrogen plus progestin. In the main,
histology was performed on endometrial samples obtained by
vacuum curettage; portions of these samples were also available
for biochemical analysis. The present paper describes the
background and results of such analyses that have been made
thus far.

The original questions we posed ourselves related to clinical
aspects of the therapy such as measuring the estrogenic potency
of the various forms of medication, determining whether all
types of estrogen were equivalent and assessing the most
efficient form of progestin treatment. It soon became clear
that additional biological data of a fundamental nature could
also be obtained about the mode of action of estrogens and
progestins and about possible mechanisms in the development of
hyperplasias. All of these points will be discussed. Clinical
and methodological details will be found in refs. 19 and 31.

CLINICAL STUDIES

Estrogenic potency on the endometrium

Estrogen preparations used in HRT can be divided into three
categories depending on whether they are based on estrone
(Premarin, Harmogen), estradiol (Progynova, estradiol implant) or
other compounds (Mestranol, estriol). The majority of our
patients were receiving Premarin. As indices of biological
potency we chose to measure the amount of nuclear estrogen
receptor (REN) by an exchange assay with ^{3}H estradiol and also
cytoplasmic RP (19). In these tissue samples, REN values only
give a very approximate idea of estrogenicity as they do not
indicate what estrogen is complexed with the receptor. Therefor,
it was important to measure RP as an index of biological
effectiveness of the REN.

Initially we compared receptor levels in women receiving

cyclical treatment (3 weeks of daily oral Premarin, 1 week of
nothing) with those in endometria from women on a sequential
regime (continuous daily Premarin supplemented with daily norethisterone during the fourth week). Due to the diminishing use
of estrogen-only treatments, the number of analyses in the
cyclical group are small. However, it is clear that the cyclical
group do not have higher REN contents than their sequential
counterparts (Fig. 1) despite the higher incidence of hyperplasias
in the former group. Indeed, the statistically significant
difference in REN content seen in week 3 specimens indicates a
greater receptor content in the group with a lower incidence of
hyperplasia. The week 4 samples are not directly comparable as

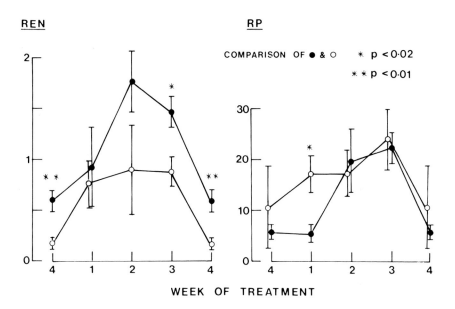

REN   **RP**

COMPARISON OF ● & ○   ＊ p < 0·02

＊＊ p < 0·01

WEEK OF TREATMENT

FIG.1. Nuclear estradiol receptor (REN) and soluble progesterone
receptor (RP) content (p mole/mg DNA) of endometria from postmenopausal women receiving oral Premarin daily during weeks 1, 2
and 3. During week 4, the cyclical group (0) receiving nothing
whilst the sequential group (●) received Premarin plus
norethisterone. Results are given as mean ± SEM. The p values
were derived by Student's t-test.

the sequential group were ingesting estrogen whereas the cyclical
group were not. Interestingly, the fall in REN with Premarin
plus norethisterone during week 4 was due to a lower proportion
of cellular RE being in the nucleus (19). This is discussed

further below. Differences between the two types of endometria
were noted with the RP assays; norethisterone diminished the
measurable cytoplasmic RP (Fig. 1). Interpretation of this
observation is difficult and highlights one of the problems of
using RP as an index of estrogenicity in cases where progestins
are also being given. Any receptor carried into the nucleus
would be lost to the assay procedure. Methods are available for
measuring nuclear RP which would obviate the problem but their
quantitative aspects are still suspect (3, 29). Hence at
present, RP assay is of limited use in determining estrogenic
potency when progestins are also present. This criticism does
not apply when estrogens alone are being given. Hence
comparison of different estrogen preparations is possible (Fig.2).
Two general conclusions can be made. Firstly, comparison of
the estrogen-treated postmenopausal endometria with the premenopausal specimens shows that all the HRT treatments subject
the endometrial cells to an estrogenic stimulus at least as

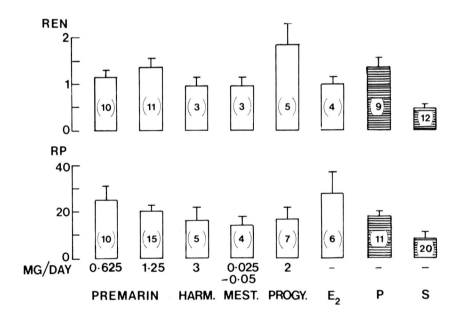

FIG.2. Receptor content (p mole/mg DNA) of post (☐) and
premenopausal (▤) endometria. HARM = Harmogen; MEST =
Mestranol; PROGY = Progynova; E_2 = estradiol; P = proliferative
phase; S = secretory phase. Results are given as means ± SEM
with no. observations in parentheses.

great as that encountered during the proliferative phase of the
menstrual cycle. Secondly, there were no significant differences

between the various estrogen therapies. With the main preparation tested, Premarin, the low dose pill (0.625 mg/day) was as potent as the higher dose (1.25 mg/day).

So, in relation to the first two clinical questions we posed above, receptor assays have provided evidence as to the biological effects of the different HRT preparations on the endometrium and a tentative conclusion would be that the type of HRT preparation does not matter. However, the latter conclusion cannot be substantiated if one takes duration of estrogenic stimulation and the mechanism by which progestins act in human endometrial cells into account. The latter point is fully discussed below but the former point needs comment at this stage. Although comparison of cyclical and sequential therapy (Fig. 1) does not allow, for methodological reasons, one to conclude that differences exist, they might be present. Thus, in week 1, RP levels were higher in cyclical than sequential endometria (Fig. 1) which might indicate a more prolonged estrogenic stimulus on cyclical therapy. One point is clear: the receptor levels at the times we have measured them do not adequately reflect the different efficacies in producing endometrial hyperplasias. Duration of treatment may be a missing factor but it is also possible that receptor levels give only an incomplete picture of endometrial response to prolonged estrogen and progestin administration. If one adopts the very simplified attitude that progestin effects can be divided into those that counteract estrogen (anti-estrogenic) action and those that are either independent of or synergise with estrogen (non anti-estrogenic effects) then REN and RP would mainly be a measure of the former response. Examples of the latter category would be secretion and menstruation and certainly menstrual loss of potentially abnormal cells could be very important (6, 30).

Type of estrogen preparation to use for HRT

The tentative conclusion was reached from the REN and RP data that all of the estrogen preparations studied had similar effects on the endometrium. The majority of patients providing data for that conclusion were receiving either estrone- or estradiol-based therapy. An additional body of data support the view that as far as estrone and estradiol medications are concerned, their endometrial effects are similar. Analysis of estrone and estradiol in nuclei from endometria of women on HRT indicates that both estrone and estradiol-based treatments result in a preponderance of estradiol in the nucleus (Table 1 and ref. 16). The body interconverts orally administered estrone and estradiol and the endometrial cells selectively accumulate estradiol. This conclusion would not apply to estrogens such as estriol or synthetic compounds such as ethinylestradiol that do not give rise to estrone or estradiol. Our experience with the

TABLE 1. Estrogen content of nuclei of endometria from postmenopausal women receiving estrogens

Type of therapy[+]	Nuclear content (p mole/mg DNA)	
	Estradiol	Estrone
'Estrone'	1.45 ± 0.22 (10)	0.45 ± 0.09 (10)
'Estradiol'	5.87 ± 3.36 (4)	0.35 ± 0.11 (4)

+ Estrone - Premarin or Harmogen; Estradiol - Progynova or estradiol implant.
  For practical details, see ref. 16.

synthetic compounds is too limited for detailed comment but one point should be made. Results are discussed below indicating that the progestin-induced enzyme estradiol dehydrogenase is very important in the detoxification of estradiol. It follows that only estrogens capable of acting as substrates for the enzyme should be used in HRT. Thus, treatments based on estrogens, such as estriol or ethinylestradiol which are not substrates for the dehydrogenase would theoretically not benefit from the detoxifying effect of the enzyme. The same point has been made by Gurpide (8).

Progestin administration

The inclusion of progestin in HRT regimens has been done on the same empirical basis as the original estrogen-only treatments. As progestins counteract many of the beneficial estrogen effects for which the patients attend the clinic it is desirable that progestin exposure be minimised to that required for optimal suppression of hyperplasias and neoplasias of the endometrium. Clinical trials to establish optimum type, dose and duration of progestin treatment would be very difficult to set up although some successes have been reported (5, 28). We are attempting to simplify matters by studying the biochemistry of endometrial samples from women receiving different progestin treatments (18). The logic behind this approach is that by establishing treatment schedules that have optimum effects on endometrial biochemistry one can rule out sub- and supra-optimal regimes and thus limit the number of clinical trials.

The choice of biochemical parameters has been determined by availability of tissue and a desire to assess both the anti-estrogenic and non-antiestrogenic effects of the progestins. The latter category includes a range of progestin-sensitive enzymes such as acid and alkaline phosphatase, isocitric

dehydrogenase and glucose-6-phosphate dehydrogenase. These
results are only pertinent to the present communication in that
the results obtained thus far indicate that the activities of
these enzymes are induced by the progestin, norethisterone in a
dose-dependent manner (18). Antiestrogenic effects are
monitored with ^{3}H thymidine labeling index, REN and estradiol
dehydrogenase activity. The physiological interrelationship of
these components will be discussed later. As indices of progestin
effects on the endometrium, the preliminary data look
interesting. The dehydrogenase is very progestin-sensitive and
provides data indicating that 5 mg/day norethisterone is
optimally effective (Fig. 3). The REN values are more variable
than the dehydrogenase but the indications are that REN
estimation is a useful index of the antiestrogenic potency of
norethisterone when given together with estrogens. RP assays

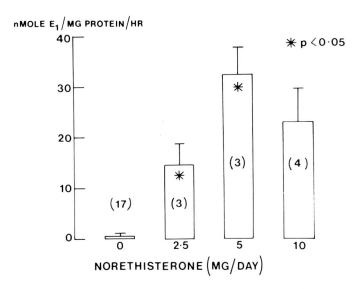

FIG. 3. Estradiol dehydrogenase activity of endometria from
postmenopausal women receiving daily oral Premarin plus the
stated dose of norethisterone. Curettage was performed after 6
days of norethisterone. Enzyme activity was calculated from the
amount of estrone (E_1) formed from estradiol. Results are
expressed as mean ± SEM with no. observations in parentheses.
The p value was derived by Student's t-test.

in this type of study are not worthwhile because of the dubious
quantitative interpretation of results obtained from norethis-
terone-treated endometria (see above). Undoubtedly, the assay of
nuclear progesterone receptors would be worthwhile but have not
yet been achieved by us.

BIOLOGICAL STUDIES

Mode of action of estrogens

Two sets of data have derived from our studies that contribute
to our understanding of estrogen action in the human endometrium,
namely the nature of the active intracellular estrogen and the
characteristics of the nuclear estradiol receptor.

Intracellular estrogen

It is well established in the rodent that when estradiol is
administered, the same estrogen is the active intracellular
compound. Estrone works largely by metabolic conversion to
estradiol (13) although it does have low activity in its own
right (23). The situation in women is less clear. In
premenopausal women, substantial evidence exists that estradiol
is more important than estrone (1, 7, 24). However, in postmenopausal women, estrone is the predominant plasma estrogen
(12, 21) and an hypothesis has been formulated that estrone
may be the active postmenopausal estrogen (21, 25). This
hypothesis could be tested by direct analysis of tissue estrone
and estradiol levels but this is impracticable in postmenopausal
endometrium because of paucity of tissue. Postmenopausal women
receiving either estradiol- or estrone-based HRT have estrone as
the main plasma estrogen (12, 30) and abundant endometrium. We
have accordingly used this tissue for estrogen analysis (16).
The results are clearly in favor of the view that, despite the
excess of estrone over estradiol in the plasma, nuclear estradiol
is quantitatively more important than estrone in women taking
estrogen alone (Table 1, Fig. 4). It seems reasonable to
conclude that in these postmenopausal endometria estradiol is
the active intracellular estrogen but one caveat must be applied
to that conclusion. Most of our samples were taken from women
receiving Premarin which contains equine estrogens in addition to
estrone (26). As we did not quantitate the ring B unsaturated
compounds we may have missed some biologically active estrogen
although this seems unlikely from the known behaviour of the other
Premarin components (26).

Nuclear receptor complex

Accepted writ says that estrogen is necessary for the
transference of receptor into the nucleus and that the estrogen
receptor complex is the active component (17). This well-

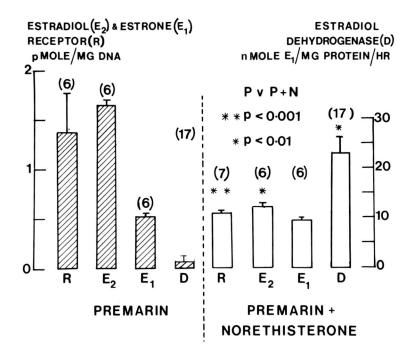

FIG. 4. Nuclear estradiol, estrone and estradiol receptor
content (left hand ordinate) and total estradiol dehydrogenase
activity (right hand ordinate) of endometria from postmenopausal
women receiving oral Premarin (▨) or Premarin plus
norethisterone (☐). Results are expressed as mean ± SEM
with the no. observations in parentheses. The p values were
derived from Student's t-test.

documented view has recently been questioned because of data
obtained in the temperature dependence of REN labeling in
human breast cancer cells (11). In rodent uterine nuclei,
estradiol complexed with its receptor will exchange with added
^{3}H estradiol at elevated temperatures but not at 0-4°. This is
not true for the human breast tumor, MCF7 cell line; good
nuclear labeling is obtained at low temperatures. Our experience
with both pre and postmenopausal endometria is that they behave
more like MCF7 cells than rodent uteri (16). The efficient
labeling at 4° occurs with highly purified nuclei and, with the
limited data at present available, with both estradiol and
estrone-based therapies and untreated premenopausal samples
(Fig. 5 and ref. 16). At present we cannot distinguish between
vacant nuclear receptor and receptor occupied by a low affinity
ligand. The estradiol and estrone content of these samples
(Fig. 4) would seem to be at variance with both of these

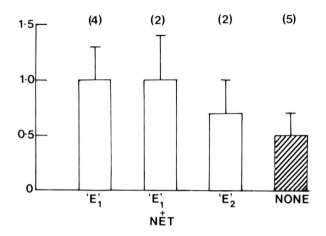

FIG. 5. Ratio of values for nuclear estradiol receptor
obtained by 2 h incubation at 4°C and 30°C. The ordinate is the
ratio values at 4°C/30°C. ☐ - postmenopausal endometria;
▨ - premenopausal endometria; 'E$_1$'- 'estrone' type therapy;
'E$_2$' - 'estradiol' type therapy; NET - norethisterone. For
further definitions see Table 1. Results are expressed as mean
± SEM with the no. observations in parentheses.

postulates. Given the uncertain explanation of the low
temperature labeling of the nuclei, 'available' rather than
'vacant' receptor sites would be the preferred terminology.

Mode of action of progestins

Progestins undoubtedly have multiple effects on the
endometrium, one facet of which is their ability to counteract
estrogenicity by promoting estradiol metabolism. In premenopausal endometria, progestins markedly increase the activity
of estradiol dehydrogenase, an enzyme that predominantly converts
estradiol to estrone thus effectively lowering the estrogenicity
of estradiol (7, 9, 24). Our results indicate that a similar
mechanism is operative in the postmenopausal endometrium (16, 18,
19). There is an inverse relationship between REN and
estradiol dehydrogenase in endometria from women receiving
different doses of norethisterone (Fig. 6) and the presence of
the dehydrogenase is associated with a decline in estradiol but
not estrone content of the nuclei (Fig. 4).

Role of estrogens in the genesis of hyperplasia/neoplasia

There is an increasing body of evidence relating estrogen

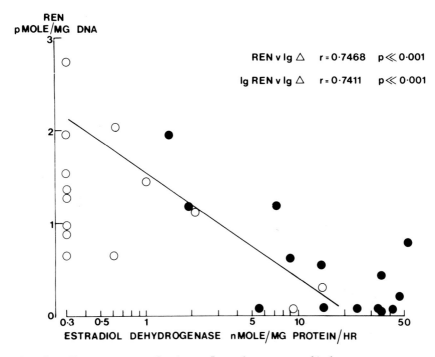

FIG. 6. Inverse correlation of nuclear estradiol receptor content (REN) with estradiol dehydrogenase activity (Δ) in endometria from postmenopausal women receiving either estrogen alone (0) or estrogen plus a progestin (●). Linear correlation coefficients are shown for the two most significant methods of correlation. For REN v Δ, r = 0.5935, p = < 0.001 and for lg REN v Δ, r = 0.5974, p = < 0.001.

action unopposed by progestins with endometrial hyperplasia and neoplasia (2, 5, 10, 27, 31). It is reasonable to associate the mitogenic effect of estrogen with development of cystic hyperplasia but why should cystic hyperplasia with its low attendant risk of generating carcinoma give rise to the more dangerous atypical hyperplasia? No answer is available but one possibility is that a change in end organ sensitivity to estrogen occurs. Receptor analyses can be of use in testing such an hypothesis; increased estrogen sensitivity should manifest itself by an increase in RP relative to REN content. Certainly, the RP:REN ratio is higher in atypical hyperplasia than in normal or cystic hyperplastic endometria (19) but it is not clear if this is due to a change in proportions of cell types making up the endometrial sample or to a genuine change in end organ sensitivity.

GENERAL CONCLUSIONS

RP and REN assays are useful in elucidating both clinical and basic biological features of estrogen and progestin action in the human endometrium. Improved quantitative methodology for the assay of nuclear RP and cytoplasmic RP complexed with very high affinity synthetic progestins will enhance the clinical usefulness of the assays. However, it is clear that receptor estimations on their own give an incomplete picture of endometrial response to the sex hormones and additional parameters should also be quantitated.

REFERENCES

1. Baird, D.T. (1972): In: Endocrinology, Excerpta Medica International Congress Series, No.273, edited by O. Scow, pp.851–856. Excerpta Medica, Amsterdam.
2. Campbell, S., and Whitehead, M.I. (1979): In: Female and Male Climacteric, edited by P.A. van Keep, D.M. Serr and R.B. Greenblatt, pp.111–120. MTP Press, Lancaster.
3. Clark, J.H., Hsueh, A.J.W., and Peck, E.J. (1977): Ann.N.Y. Acad.Sci., 286:161–179.
4. Feinstein, A.R., and Horwitz, R.I. (1978): Cancer Res., 38:4001–4005.
5. Gambrell, R.D. (1978): Maturitas, 1:107–112.
6. Gambrell, R.D., Castenada, T.A., and Ricci, C.A. (1978): Maturitas, 1:99–106.
7. Gurpide, E. (1978): J. Toxicol.Environ.Health, 4:249–268.
8. Gurpide, E. (1978): Pediatrics, 62:1114–1120.
9. Gurpide, E., and Tseng, L. (1974): Gynecol.Oncol., 2:221–227.
10. Gusberg, S.B. (1976): Am.J.Obstet.Gynecol., 126:535–542.
11. Horwitz, K.B., and McGuire, W.L. (1978): In: Breast Cancer, Advances in Research and Treatment, edited by W.L. McGuire, Vol.2, pp.155–204. Plenum Publishing, New York.
12. Jacobs, H.S., Hutton, J.D., Murray, M.A.F., and James, V.H.T. (1977): Curr.Med.Res.Opin., 4 (Suppl.3):58–66.
13. Jensen, E.V., and Jacobson, H.I. (1962): Recent Prog.Horm. Res., 18:387–414.
14. King, R.J.B., editor (1979): Steroid Receptor Assays in Human Breast Tumours: Methodological and Clinical Aspects. Alpha Omega Publishing, Cardiff.
15. King, R.J.B. (1977): In: Tumour Markers, edited by K. Griffiths, A.M. Neville, and C.G. Pierrepoint, pp.162–167. Alpha Omega Publishing, Cardiff.
16. King, R.J.B., Dyer, G., Collins, W.P., and Whitehead, M.I. (1979): J. Steroid Biochem. Submitted for publication.
17. King, R.J.B., and Mainwaring, W.I.P. (1974): Steroid-Cell Interactions. Butterworths, London.
18. King, R.J.B., Townsend, P.T., and Whitehead, M.I. (1980): In: Menopause and Postmenopause, edited by N. Pasetto and N. Paoletti,(in press). MTP Press, Lancaster.

19. King, R.J.B., Whitehead, M.I., Campbell, S., and Minardi, J. (1979): Cancer Res., 39:1094-1101.
20. Mack, T.M. (1978): In: Endometrial Cancer, edited by M.C. Brush, R.J.B. King, and R.W. Taylor, pp.17-28. Baillière Tindall, London.
21. MacDonald, P.C., and Siiteri, P.K. (1974): Gynecol. Oncol., 2:259-263.
22. McGuire, W.L., Zava, D.T., Horwitz, K.B., and Chamness, G.C. (1977): In: Tumour Markers, edited by K. Griffiths, A.M. Neville, and C.G. Pierrepoint, pp.153-161. Alpha Omega Publishing, Cardiff.
23. Ruh, T.S., Katzenellenbogen, B.S., Katzenellenbogen, J.A., and Gorski, J. (1973): Endocrinology, 93:124-134.
24. Schmidt-Gollwitzer, M., Genz, T., Schmidt-Gollwitzer, K., Pollow, B., and Pollow, K. (1978): In: Endometrial Cancer, edited by M.G. Brush, R.J.B. King, and R.W. Taylor, pp.227-241. Baillière Tindall, London.
25. Siiteri, P.K., Schwarz, B.E., and MacDonald, P.C. (1974): Gynecol. Oncol., 2:228-238.
26. Stern, M.D., and Givner, M.L. (1978): In: Endometrial Cancer, edited by M.G. Brush, R.J.B. King, and R.W. Taylor, pp.309-322. Baillière Tindall, London.
27. Sturdee, D.W., Wade-Evans, T., Paterson, M.E.L., Thom, M., and Studd, J.W.W. (1978): Br. Med. J., 1:1575-1577.
28. Thom, M.H., White, P.J., Williams, R.M., Sturdee, D.W., Paterson, M.E.L., Wade-Evans, T., and Studd, J.W.W. (1979): Lancet, ii:455-457.
29. Vu Hai, M.T., Logeat, F., Warembourg, M., and Milgrom, E. (1977): Ann. N.Y. Acad. Sci., 286:199-209.
30. Whitehead, M.I. (1978): Maturitas, 1:87-98.
31. Whitehead, M.I., King, R.J.B., McQueen, J., and Campbell, S. (1979): J. Roy. Soc. Med., 72:322-327.
32. Young, P.C.M., Ehrlich, C.E., Cleary, R.E. (1978): In: Endometrial Cancer, edited by M.G. Brush, R.J.B. King, and R.W. Taylor, pp.258-264. Baillière Tindall, London.

Perspectives in Steroid Receptor Research,
edited by F. Bresciani.
Raven Press, New York © 1980.

Effect of NaSCN on Receptor–Estradiol Interaction and Application to Assay Total Receptor ("Filled" and "Unfilled" Sites) in Tissues and Tissue Fractions, Including Nuclei, by Exchange at Low Temperature With 17β-Estradiol-^{3}H

Francesco Bresciani, Vincenzo Sica, Alessandro Weizs,
Franco Maria Buonaguro, Rudolfo Bova, Giovanni Alfredo Puca,
Anna Maria Molinari, and Laszlo Endrenyi

*Institute of General Pathology, First Faculty of Medicine and Surgery, University of Naples,
80138 Naples, Italy*

In perspective, radioimmunological assay of estrogen receptor will probably become the method of choice in the future. The basic achievements to set up such an assay, i.e. purification of estrogen receptor in tangible amounts and preparation of antibodies to receptor, have already been accomplished (Jensen et al., 1979; Sica and Bresciani, 1979). However, before such method becomes operative and widely available, several years may have to pass. Furthermore, radioimmunoassays able to distinguish between estrogen-free receptor and estrogen-receptor complex may be even more remote. To be able to assess separately receptor free and estrogen-receptor complex is, however, of considerably importance, considering the functional difference between these two states of receptor.

Present methods for measuring estrogen receptor are all based on binding of radioactive hormone by receptor. Because estrogen receptor binding activity is easily inactivated at temperatures higher than those close to 0°C (Peck et al., 1973), the assay is generally carried out at 0-4°C. However, turnover of estradiol complex is very low at 0-4°C and, therefore, during the time of assay there is no significant exchange of added radioactive estradiol with endogenous hormone possibly present and bound to receptor. Thus, preformed complex is overlooked by the

---

This work is dedicated to Elwood V. Jensen, on his sixtieth birthday, in appreciation of his outstanding contribution to progress in the fields of Endocrinology and Oncology.

binding assay method at 0-4°C, a very significant shortcoming especially when dealing with nuclear receptor which is virtually all in the form of complex with estradiol.

The obvious importance of being able to assess total receptor content in tissue and tissue fractions has prompted investigation of how to increase turnover rate of estradiol-receptor complex in order to achieve exchange with added radioactive hormone within reasonable time. Starting from early efforts (Puca and Bresciani, 1968), all methods up to now have been based on carefully controlled increases of temperature (Anderson et al, 1972; Katzenellenbogen et al, 1973; Chamness et al, 1975; Zava et al, 1976; Sutherland and Baulieu, 1976). One must strike a delicate balance between achieving an increase of receptor complex turnover rate sufficient for pratical purposes and keeping to a minimum temperature-induced inactivation of binding sites. Methods which preliminarily decrease heat sensitivity of estrogen--receptor complex by selective extraction and precipitation with protamine (Zava et al, 1976) have, however, the disadvantage that receptor is lost as a consequence of incomplete recovery.

NaSCN, a chaotropic salt which was previously found by us to inhibit receptor aggregation (Sica et al, 1976), has now been found to have other interesting properties. This salt considerably increases the turnover rate of estradiol-receptor complex at 4°C and solubilizes receptor from nuclear pellets much more rapidly and efficiently than KCl. These findings have been exploited to set up a method which measures receptor in tissues and tissue fractions, including the nuclear fraction, regardless of whether the receptor is free or in a complex with hormone. Some preliminary applications of this method will be shown.

MATERIALS AND GENERAL METHODS

All reagents were of analytical grade. NaSCN (ACS) was purchased from C. Erba; 17β-estradiol-6,7-^{3}H (60 Ci/mmole specific activity; 97% pure) from New England Nuclear; dithiothreitol from Calbiochem; Tris (Trizma Base, reagent grade) and EDTA, disodium salt, from Sigma.

Estradiol-17β, testosterone, progesterone, hydrocortisone were from Calbiochem; Tamoxifen (trans-1-(p-dimethylaminoethoxy-

phenyl)1,2-diphenyl-but-1-ene; ICI 46474) was a gift of ICI, Ltd;
Charcoal (Norit A) was from Matheson Coleman and Bell, Norwood,
Ohio; Dextran T 70 from Pharmacia.

Preparation of calf uterus cytosol. Immature calf uteri
weighing not more than 30 gm were collected at the local slaugh-
terhouse as soon as the animals were killed and kept in plastic
bags buried in crushed ice while rushed to the laboratory. The
uteri were stripped of connective tissue and frozen in liquid
nitrogen. Before use they were pulverized in a mortar and homogenized in 4 volumes of TED buffer (0.01 M Tris.HCl, 1 mM EDTA,
1 mM dithiothreitol, pH 7.4) by means of an Ultraturrax homogenizer (Janke and Kunkel, Model TP 18/2) in 4 runs of 30 s each at
60 s intervals. The homogenate was centrifuged at 150.000 g and
the decanted supernatant collected. Cleaning of uteri, homogenization and centrifugation were carried out at 0-4°C.

Preparation of rats. Mature female Sprague Dawley rats (age
45-60 days) were purchased from Charles River Italia, S.p.A..
Animals were ovariectomized under light ether anesthesia 7 days
prior to use and 17β-estradiol was injected i.p. as a solution
in 10% Ethanol-0.9% NaCl. Where indicated, 17β-estradiol-6,7-^{3}H
progesterone, testosterone, hydrocortisone, Tamoxifen or solvent
only were used in place of 17β-estradiol. Rats were killed by
cervical dislocation 2 hours after injection. The uteri were rapidly removed and cleaned of adhering fat and mesentery in the
cold (4°C) room.

Preparation of rat uterus cytoplasmic and nuclear fractions.
All operations at 0-4°C. Uteri were weighed, cut into fine pie-
ces with scissors and homogenized in 4 volumes (w/v) of TED buffer (10^{-2} M Tris-HCl; 10^{-3} M EDTA; 10^{-3} M dithiothreitol, pH 7,4)
by means of an Ultraturrax homogenizer (Janke and Kunkel, Model
TP 18/2) in 4 runs of 15 s each at 60 s intervals. The homogenate
was centrifuged at 1,000 g for 20 min. The pellet was resuspended
twice in TED buffer and centrifuged (1000 g, 20 min). The final
pellet (crude nuclear fraction) was used for nuclear extraction
as described below. The supernatant was centrifuged for 45 min
at 150,000 g (Beckman Spinco L2-65 centrifuge, rotor Ti 50).

Nuclear extraction. All operations at 0-4°C. Fifteen ovariectomized rats were injected with 17β-estradiol-6,7-^{3}H (30 Ci/mmo-
le; 1 μg/100 gm body wt) in 0.5 ml of 10% ethanol in 0.9% NaCl.

After two hours, the rats were killed by cervical dislocation.
The uteri were homogenized and the nuclei sedimented as described above.

The crude nuclear fraction was divided in three aliquots
and resuspended in 10 ml of either ice-cold ethyl ether, or ice-
-cold TED buffer containing the given molarities of either KCl
or NaSCN. The ether suspension was vigorously shaken for 5 min
at 4°C and the ether was decanted in a glass scintillation vial.
The extraction was repeated twice and the pooled ether fractions
were dried. The aqueous suspensions were mixed vigorously, allowed to stand for 30' at 4° and centrifuged at 150,000 g for 30
min. Two ml aliquots of the supernatants were used for radioactivity assay.

General procedures of DCC assays. Separation of free from
macromolecule-bound 17β-estradiol-6,7-^{3}H was accomplished by adsorption of free hormone to an equal volume of a slurry of DCC
(dextran-coated charcoal: 1% Norit A; 0,05% dextran in TED buffer) for 15 min at 4°C, followed by centrifugation at 1500 g for
10 min. Aliquots of 0,5-1 ml of supernatant (2000 g, 15 min)
were added to 6 ml of Insta-Gel and radioactivity measured. The
correction for nonspecific binding was determined in a parallel
incubation in which an excess of unlabeled estradiol had been
added. The difference in the amount of bound ligand in the presence and absence of cold estradiol was taken as a measure of
the specific high affinity binding. Adsorption of free hormone
by DCC was always performed in the presence of NaSCN, by adding
NaSCN to the samples originally without salt. In initial experiments, before DCC adsorption the samples containing NaSCN were,
if necessary, diluted to achieve a 0.1 M NaSCN concentration. Later, this dilution step was eliminated because found to be unnecessary for NaSCN molarities up to 0.5 M.

Radioactivity assay. Aqueous samples (0.1-1 ml) were added
to 5 ml of Insta-Gel liquid scintillation cocktail (Packard) in
glass scintillation vials and the radioactivity was measured in
a Beckman LS-3150 T-counter with 40-50% efficiency. Radioactivity of ether extracted samples was measured by addition of 10 ml
of toluene-phosphor solution containing 3.92 g% of 2,5-diphenyl-
oxazole and 0.18 g% of p-bis (o-methyl-styryl) benzene to the
vials after evaporation of ether.

Protein assay. Protein determinations were performed by the
Bio-Rad protein assay method based on the work of Bradford (1976).
Thiol groups, Tris and EDTA do not interfere with this assay.

RESULTS

1. Effect of NaSCN on receptor-estradiol interaction. Experimental data. Fig. 1 shows that addition of NaSCN 0.5 M to uterus cytosol previously saturated with 17β-estradiol-6,7-^{3}H at 4°C
does not detectably affect the concentration of estradiol receptor complex for at least 23 hrs, i.e. for the whole incubation
period.

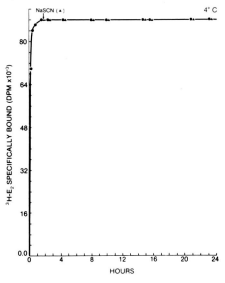

Fig. 1. Effect of NaSCN 0.5 M on
steady-state concentration of
estradiol-receptor complex. Calf
uterus cytosol was incubated with
17β-estradiol-6,7-^{3}H (5 ng/ml) at
4°C. At the given times, 0,2 ml
aliquots were withdrawn and pi-
petted into 0.4 ml of ice-cold
TED buffer pH 7.4. Bound from
free estradiol were separated by
the DCC method as described under Material and Methods. After
90 min (arrow) cytosol was divided into two parts, to one of
which NaSCN was added up to a final concentration of 0.5 M. Experimental points refer to spe-
cifically bound hormone per 0.1 ml of cytosol in the absence (●)
and in the presence (▲) of NaSCN.

However, as show.₁ in fig. 2, NaSCN considerably increases
the rate of dissociation of the estradiol-receptor complex at
4°C, compared to control cytosol. Dissociation rate was visuali-
zed by addition of a 1000-fold excess of non radioactive 17β-
-estradiol to cytosol previously saturated with 17β-estradiol-6,7-
-^{3}H at 4°C, and the decrease of radioactive complex was plotted as
a first order reaction. It can be seen that in untreated cytosol
the dissociation of the estradiol-receptor complex at 4°C is very
slow and follows the well established two-step, first order kinetic pattern (Best-Belpomme et al., 1970; Mester et al., 1970;

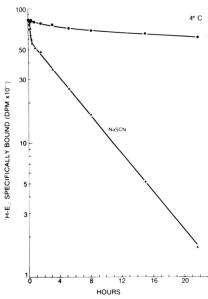

Fig. 2. Effect of NaSCN 0.5 M on dissociation rate of estradiol-receptor complex. Calf uterus cytosol was incubated with 17β-estradiol-6,7-^{3}H (5 ng/ml) at 4°C. After two hours, a 1000-fold excess of 17β-estradiol was added (time 0) and the cytosol divided into two parts, to one of which NaSCN 0.5 M (final concentration) was added. Incubation was continued for 16 hrs. Experimental points refer to specifically bound hormone per 0.1 ml cytosol, in the absence (●) and in the presence (▲) of NaSCN.

Sanborn et al., 1971; Erdos et al., 1971; Truong and Baulieu, 1971; Sala-Trepat and Reti, 1974; Vallet-Strouve et al., 1976; McCormack and Glasser, 1976). In the NaSCN containing cytosol the biphasic pattern persists; however, both rate components are considerably faster, with less than 2% residual radioactive estradiol-receptor complex being left after 22 hrs of incubation at 4°C.

A study of the effect of NaSCN on association rate of 17β-estradiol-6,7-^{3}H with receptor in calf uterus cytosol is shown in fig. 3. Formation of complex in uterine cytosol at 4°C, with or without additional NaSCN 0.5 M, was followed up to 180 min. It can be seen that NaSCN increases the formation rate of the complex and that the maximal concentration reached (asymptote) is slightly lower than that of untreated cytosol. The slight loss of binding activity can be attributed to inactivation of estradiol -free sites exposed to NaSCN during the initial part of the experiment. A study of the effect of NaSCN on binding activity of estrogen free cytosol is shown in the insert in fig. 3. NaSCN 0.5 M was added to calf uterus cytosol which, contrary to the experiment in fig. 1, was not previously saturated with 17β-estradiol. One can see that, contrary to the case of filled sites (fig. 1), receptor unfilled sites are affected by NaSCN, with irreversible loss of estrogen binding activity. Therefore, from a practical point of view, in order to avoid losses of binding activity, NaSCN should always be added to receptor preparations previously saturated with hormone.

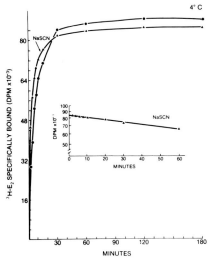

Fig. 3. Effect of NaSCN on association rate of estradiol-receptor complex. 17β-estradiol-6,7--^{3}H (5 ng/ml) without or with 0.5M NaSCN (final concentration) were added to calf uterus cytosol at time 0. Formation of complex was followed by measuring specifically bound hormone as described in legend to fig. 1. Experimental points refer to specifically bound hormone per 0.1 ml of cytosol in the absence (●) and in the presence (▲) of NaSCN.

Insert: Effect of NaSCN on estrogen-free receptor. NaSCN 0.5 M (final concentration) was added to estrogen-free calf uterus cytosol. Experimental points refer to binding activity of cytosol assayed with the DCC method (see Material and Methods) after variable length of incubation with NaSCN

2. Effect of NaSCN on receptor-estradiol interaction. Analysis of experimental data. In the control experiment (fig. 1) performed without thiocyanate, association of hormone with receptor takes place according to

$$E + R \xrightarrow{k_1} ER \quad ,$$

where E is estradiol, R is receptor and k_1 is the association rate constant. The rate of association, i.e. the rate of complex (ER) formation, is then

$$d\left[ER\right]/dt = k_1\left[E\right]\left[R\right]$$

which is subjected to the limitation of the total receptor concentration:

$$R_t = \left[R\right] + \left[ER\right] \quad .$$

In the presence of thiocyanate (fig. 1), the association proceeds with a modified rate constant, k_1':

$$E + R \xrightarrow{k_1'} ER \qquad .$$

In addition, the receptors available for binding is depleted (inactivated) according to

$$R \xrightarrow{k_2'} R' \qquad .$$

In this case, the rate of association is

$$d[ER]/dt = k_1'[E][R] \qquad ,$$

and the disappearance rate of free receptor is

$$d[R]/dt = -k'[R] \qquad ,$$

which is subject to the limitation of

$$R_t = [R] + [R'] + [ER]$$

and where

$$k' = k_1'[E] + k_2' \qquad .$$

In both cases, the solution of the differential equations is, on the assumption of approximately constant hormone concentration,

$$[ER] = [ER]_\infty - ([ER]_\infty - [ER]_0)e^{-kt} \qquad ,$$

where, in the presence or absence of thiocyanate, $k=k'$ or $k=k_1[E]$, respectively, and the asymptotic complex concentration is

$$[ER]_\infty = k_1[E]R_t/k \qquad .$$

If, in a binding experiment, there is no endogenously bound hormone, then the initial complex concentration is zero,

$$[ER]_0 = 0$$

and

$$[ER] = [ER]_\infty (1-e^{-kt}) \quad .$$

Rearrangement of the expression yields

$$-\ln(1 - [ER]/[ER]_\infty) = kt \quad .$$

Therefore, the slope of a line in a diagram plotting the left-hand side of this relationship against time yields k. In the absence of thiocyanate, k_1 is obtained directly. In the presence of thiocyanate, k_1' and k_2' can be calculated from k and from

$$[ER]_\infty / [ER]_\infty' = 1 + k_2'/(k_1' [ER]) \quad .$$

Here the left-hand side is the ratio of asymptotes observed in the absence and presence of thiocyanate, respectively. The observed value is 1.038.

The binding takes place in two phases. For both lines, the least-squares slopes (k_1) could be calculated on the assumption of their common intersection. As a result, with $[E] = 1.8 \times 10^{-8}$ M, the association and depletion (inactivation) rate constants could be evaluated. These values are reported in table 1. The tabulation includes also the dissociation rate constant (k_{-1}) observed in separate experiments and the consequently calculated dissociation equilibrium constants, $k_d = k_{-1}/k_1$.

The calculated depletion rate constants, k_2', can be compared with the value of 3.9×10^{-3} min^{-1} measured directly in separate observations (Fig. 3, insert). Since in any case the depletion inactivation constant was much less than $k_1' [E]$, its actually calculated value had very little effect on the estimated association rate constant, k_1'.

Finally, a few remarks should be made about the shape of the association curve (fig. 3) and, in particular, about possible misinterpretations of its two segments. The points in the linearized plot could be affected by the incorrect assignment of the asymptotic $[ER]_\infty$ values. These were obtained by averaging the very close 120- and 180-minute observations. It is conceivable that these readings may slightly underestimate the asymptote. In this case, however, the true values would not eliminate the second segment.

Rather they would accentuate it.

TABLE 1. Effect of NaSCN on receptor-estradiol interaction

PARAMETER	CONTROL	NaSCN
1st Phase		
$10^{-6}\ k_1$ ($M^{-1}min^{-1}$)	7.4	12.7
$10^3\ k_{-1}$ (min^{-1})	1.1	11.4
$10^3\ k_2'$ (min^{-1})	---	8.7
$10^{10}\ k_d$ (M)	1.4	9.0
2nd Phase		
$10^{-6}\ k_1$ ($M^{-1}min^{-1}$)	4.3	5.2
$10^3\ k_{-1}$ (min^{-1})	0.098	2.7
$10^3\ k_2'$ (min^{-1})	---	3.6
$10^{10}\ k_d$ (M)	0.23	5.1

It is also possible that the assumption of approximately constant hormone concentration may not be entirely valid. This possibility is raised by noting the initial estradiol concentration of
$1.8x10^{-8}$ M and the final, asymptotic concentration of the complex
of $6.6x10^{-9}$ M. Consequently, if for the case of no receptor depletion, i.e. in the absence of thiocyanate, an additional constraint
for the total hormone concentration (E_t) is imposed

$$E_t = [E] + [ER]$$

then, again, with $[ER]_o = 0$,

$$[ER] = \frac{H_t - AE_t}{1 - A}$$

where

$$A = \frac{H_t e^{k_1 (H_t - R_t) t}}{R_t}$$

Application of these expressions to the observed data by non linear regression revealed systematic deviations. Therefore, the inconstancy of the hormone concentration does not account for the observed time course of estradiol binding.

3. Search of optimal conditions for an exchange assay of e-stradiol receptor at low temperature exploiting the effect of NaSCN on receptor-estradiol interaction. Based on the above results, an exchange method to asses both filled and unfilled sites of estrogen receptor at 0-4°C is feasible. Optimization of assay parameters is thus in order.

Fig. 4 shows an experiment carried out for the purpose of establishing the optimal concentration of NaSCN, i.e. the lowest concentration of the chaotropic salt which gives an increase of estradiol-receptor complex turnover rate sufficiently high for practical purposes. One can see that when uterine cytosol is presaturated with cold estradiol and then incubated at 4°C in the presence of 17β-estradiol-6,7-^{3}H (15 nM) and varying concentrations of NaSCN, there is virtually 100% exchange of radioactive for cold estradiol after 16 hrs with 0.5 M NaSCN.

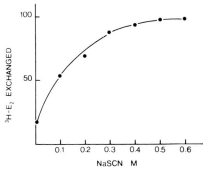

Fig. 4. Exchange of 17β-estradiol -6,7-^{3}H for 17β-estradiol at 4°C in calf uterus cytosol as a function of NaSCN concentration. Cytosol was saturated with 17β-estradiol for 2 hrs at 4°C, the excess hormone was then adsorbed on DCC and the cytosol incubated for 16 hrs at 4°C in presence of 17β-estradiol-6,7-^{3}H (15 nM) and different concentrations of NaSCN. Experimental points refer to radioactive bound hormone at end of incubation. Binding is expressed as percent of cytosol binding

activity measured by the DCC method (see Material and Methods) on untreated cytosol from the same preparation.

Another important point in an exchange assay is the choice of the concentration of radioactive estradiol (Katzenellenbogen et al., 1973; Sutherland and Baulieu, 1976). The concentration of labeled hormone must be high enough to make the decrease of specific activity, due to release of bound endogenous hormone during incubation, negligible; and, at the same time, it must be not so high as to increase aspecific binding to a level which interfers with sensitivity of the assay. The experiment in fig. 5 shows that 10 nM is the lowest concentration of ^{3}H-estradiol which, under our experimental conditions, saturates binding sites. However, specific activity of added 17β-estradiol-6,7-^{3}H would decrease about 7,5% at the end of incubation, due to release of endogenous estradiol from pre-formed complexes. The best choice, therefore, is 20 nM ^{3}H-estradiol, a concentration about 25 times higher than that of endogenous cold estradiol (0,75 nM) which makes it possible to keep dilution of specific radioactivity below 4% and produces a still acceptable level of non-specific binding.

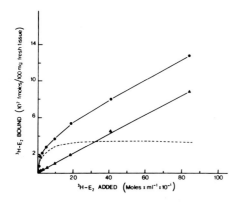

Fig. 5. Exchange of 17β-estradiol-6,7-^{3}H for 17β-estradiol at 4°C in calf uterus cytosol containing NaSCN 0.5 M as a function of 17β-estradiol-6,7-^{3}H concentration. Cytosol, pre-saturated with 17β-estradiol as described in legend to fig. 4, was incubated for 16 hrs at 4°C in presence of NaSCN 0.5 M and different concentrations of 17β-estradiol-6,7-^{3}H. At the given times, amount of bound radioactive 17β-estradiol were assessed as described in legend to fig. 1. Experimental points refer to radioactive hormone bound in presence of a 100-fold excess of 17β-estradiol over 17β-estradiol-^{3}H (aspecific binding,▲) or in absence of excess cold estradiol (total binding, ●). Specific binding (broken line) is derived by subtracting aspecific binding from total binding.

An actual exchange assay at 4°C, 0,5 M NaSCN, 20 nM estradiol-^{3}H , using uterine cytosol of known receptor binding activity, pre-saturated with cold estradiol, (fig. 6) shows that after 16 hours ("overnight") there is already virtually complete exchange (over 95%) of radioactive for cold hormone, with no loss of binding activity: the less than 5% underestimate of binding activity is indeed accounted for by dilution of label due to release of bound cold hormone (see above). Of course one can introduce a correction factor for dilution of label. However, such a correction appears to be unnecessary for most purposes.

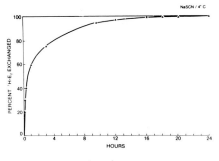

Fig. 6. Time-course of exchange of 17β-estradiol-6,7-^{3}H for 17β--estradiol in calf uterus cytosol at 4°C in presence of NaSCN 0.5 M. Cytosol, presaturated with 17β-estradiol as described in legend to fig. 4, was incubated for 24 hrs at 4°C in presence of NaSCN 0.5 M and 17β-estradiol--6,7-^{3}H 15 nM. Experimental points refer to specifically bound hormone, assessed as described in legend to fig. 1. Binding is expressed as percent of cytosol binding activity previously measured by the DCC method (see Material and Methods) on untreated cytosol from the same preparation.

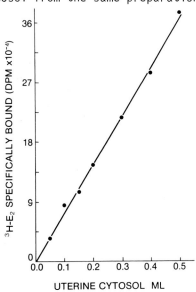

Fig. 7. Correlation between amount of calf uterus cytosol and amount of estradiol binding activity found by the NaSCN exchange method. The exchange assay was carried out as described in legend to fig. 6 for 16 hrs at 4°C, 0.5 M NaSCN, but varying the amount of cytosol.

The exchange assay also shows, within the range tested, a linear relationship between binding activity and amount of cytosol (fig. 7). Furthermore, the assay is highly precise and accurate, as shown by the low standard error and the non-significant difference between the true content of estradiol receptor assessed by direct incubation with 17β-estradiol-6,7-^{3}H and the content assessed by the NaSCN exchange method after previous saturation of the same cytosol with cold hormone (Table 2). Also, the exchange is specific: as shown in table 3, there is exchange only with estrogenic molecules, while testosterone, cortisone, deoxycorticosterone and progesterone are ineffective.

TABLE 2.   Accuracy and precision of the NaSCN exchange method

SPECIFIC BINDING OF E_2-^{3}H BY UTERINE CYTOSOL INCUBATED WITH E_2-^{3}H FOR 2 HRS AT 4°C.	SPECIFIC BINDING OF E_2-^{3}H BY UTERINE CYTOSOL PRE-SATURATED WITH E_2 THEN INCUBATED WITH E_2-^{3}H IN PRESENCE OF NaSCN 0.5M FOR 16 HRS AT 4°C.

ASSAY NO.	CPM/50 µl CYTOSOL		ASSAY NO.	CPM/50 µl CYTOSOL	
1	18588		1	17923	
2	18157		2	18415	
3	15363		3	16333	
4	16821	m = 17456	4	17615	m = 17093
5	16860	S_X = 1053	5	19393	S_X = 1283
6	17488	S_X' = 999	6	16815	S_X' = 1217
7	17124	$S_{\bar{X}}$ = 333	7	15941	$S_{\bar{X}}$ = 405
8	17243	$S_{\bar{X}}'$ 316	8	16318	$S_{\bar{X}}'$ = 384
9	19131		9	15003	
10	17791		10	17810	

Δ = 363; t = -.039; DF = 18.

m = mean; S_X = standard deviation by n-1 method; S_X' = standard deviation by n method; $S_{\bar{X}}$ = standard error of the mean by n-1 method; $S_{\bar{X}}'$ = standard error of the mean by n method; Δ = difference between the means; t = t statistic; DF = degrees of freedom.

TABLE 3. Specificity of NaSCN induced exchange of E_2-^{3}H for E_2 in uterine cytosol

	% OF E_2-^{3}H COMPLEX (a) IN PRESENCE OF COMPETITOR
None	100
17β-ESTRADIOL	2
ESTRONE	46
ESTRIOL	72
TESTOSTERONE	98
CORTISONE	116
DEOXYCORTICOSTERONE	96
PROGESTERONE	91

(a) Mean of triplicate determinations.

4. Extraction of receptor from nuclei by NaSCN vs. KCl. Based on previous experiments showing that NaSCN inhibits the estradiol receptor-nuclear acceptor interaction, the ability of NaSCN to solubilize nuclear receptor was investigated. One can see from fig. 8 that NaSCN is more efficient than KCl on a molar basis in extracting receptor from nuclei. But, more important, NaSCN,unlike KCl, extracts nuclear receptor quantitatively. In fact,as shown in table 4, NaSCN releases 802 fmoles of bound 17β-estradiol-6,7--^{3}H from nuclei of 100 mg of uterus, compared to 812 fmoles extracted by ethyl ether; that is, NaSCN solubilizes 98% of total nuclear radioactivity. KCl, on the other hand, solubilizes 680 fmoles, or only 83% of total.

These experiments were carried out with crude nuclear pellets from uteri of ovariectomized rats injected i.p. with 1 μg of 17β-estradiol-6,7-^{3}H (30 Ci/mmole)/100 gm of body wt two hours before sacrifice. The presence of uterine nuclear binding sites resistant to KCl extraction has already been described by several research workers (Zava et al., 1976; Clark and Peck, 1976; Baudendistel and Ruh, 1976; Ruh and Baudendistel, 1977; Barrack et al., 1977).

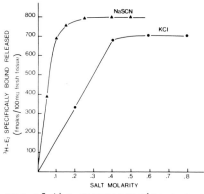

Fig. 8. Solubilization by NaSCN vs. KCl of receptor from nuclear fraction of uteri from rats injected i.p. with 17β-estradiol 1 μg/100 gm body wt) 2 hrs before sacrifice. Nuclear pellets were resuspended in TED buffer pH 7.4 containing either KCl or NaSCN at the given molarities. The final volumes of nuclear suspensions were equal to the volumes of the corresponding amounts of homogenate . After incubation with shaking for 30 min at 4°C, suspensions were centrifuged at high speed for 30 min and receptor in supernatant assessed according to the standard NaSCN method (see Results). NaSCN 0.25 M solubilizes over 98% of nuclear receptor vs. 83% by KCl 0.4 M (see table 4).

TABLE 4.   Salt extraction of nuclear estradiol receptor

	E_2 BOUND	PERCENT
	(FMOLES/100 mg OF TISSUES)	
ETHER EXTRACTION	812	100
KCl EXTRACTION	680	83
NaSCN EXTRACTION	802	98

Ovariectomized rats were injected in vivo with 17β-E_2-^{3}H (1 μg//100 gm body wt). After two hours animals were sacrificed and crude nuclear fraction, prepared as described in Materials and Methods, was extracted with either ethyl ether, KCl (0.4 M), or NaSCN (0.5 M).

5. Extraction and exchange of nuclear receptor in a single step. Based on the above results, the extraction and exchange steps for assay of nuclear receptor were unified. Nuclei were directly incubated with 0.5 M NaSCN at 4°C for 16 hrs (overnight) in the presence of increasing amounts of 17β-estradiol--6,7-^{3}H (fig. 9). The experiment was carried out using the uterine nuclear fraction from ovariectomized rats injected with cold 17β-estradiol (1 μg/100 of body wt) 2 hrs before. Parallel in vitro tests were carried out with and without addition of a 500-fold excess of unlabelled estradiol, in order to measure total and specific binding and to derive aspecific binding by subtraction. As expected, the number of nuclear binding sites apparently increased as a function of the amount of 17β-estradiol-6,7-^{3}H added, and it reached a plateau beginning at about 10 nM ^{3}H--estradiol. Identical results were obtained in a parallel experiment (not shown) in which nuclei were first quantitatively extracted with 0.5 M NaSCN for 30 min at 4°C and then extract assayed for estradiol receptor by the NaSCN assay method.

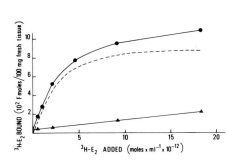

Fig. 9. Exchange of 17β-estradiol-6,7-^{3}H at 4°C in rat uterus nuclear fraction in presence of NaSCN 0.5 M as a function of 17β-estradiol-6,7-^{3}H concentration. The nuclear fraction from homogenates of uteri from rats injected i.p. with 1 μg/100 g body wt of 17β-estradiol were incubated with NaSCN 0.5 M and 17β-estradiol-6,7-^{3}H according to the standard NaSCN exchange method (see Results) except that concentration of radioactive hormone was varied. Experimental points refer to total binding (●), aspecific binding (▲) and the broken line to specific binding, i.e. total minus aspecific.

6. Description of recommended standard NaSCN method for assaying total estrogen receptor ("filled" and "unfilled" sites) in tissue or tissue fractions at 0-4°C. All procedures are carried out at 0-4°C (temperature of melting ice or temperature of refrigerator). Tissue homogenate is prepared with TED buffer pH

7.4 and filtered through a nylon filter in order to eliminate gross residues; cytosol and nuclear fractions are also prepared according to standard methods (see Material and Methods). The nuclear fraction is resuspended in TED buffer pH 7.4, in a final volume equal to the original volume of homogenate. The method described below applies equally well to (1) homogenate, (2) cytosol, and (3) nuclear fraction.

To 0.1-0.2 ml of homogenate, cytosol or nuclear suspension (duplicate samples), ice-cold TED buffer pH 7.4 containing 17β-estradiol-6,7-^{3}H of high specific activity, with or without a 500-fold excess of non radioactive hormone, was added to bring the volume of sample to 0.3 ml. The amount of 17β-estradiol-6,7--^{3}H to be added to samples should be about 25 times the estimated amount of endogenous hormone in the sample. Under usual operating conditions, 15-20 nM 17β-estradiol-6,7-^{3}H (60 Ci/mmole) is the amount of choice. After 1 hr, 0,3 ml of ice-cold TED--buffer pH 7.4 containing NaSCN 1 M was further added to each sample, thus achieving a final volume of 0.6 ml and a final NaSCN concentration of 0.5 M. After incubation for 16 hrs (overnight) in the refrigerator, the samples are shaken briefly and 0.6 ml of ice cold dextran-coated charcoal suspension is added to each sample; after an additional 15 min, free estradiol is separated from bound by centrifugation. Specific binding activity is computed by subtracting the binding activity of samples with radioactive hormone only, from binding activity of samples with labelled and excess unlabeled hormone (aspecific binding). The method is simple, precise, accurate and very reliable. When parallel measurements of binding activity of homogenate and of nuclear and cytosol fractions were made, a precise correspondence was found between binding activity of whole homogenate and binding activity of cytosol+nuclei.

7. Examples of application of the standard NaSCN exchange method.

A. Assay of nuclear and cytosol receptor in ovariectomized rats after injection of unlabelled E_2 (1 μg/100 gm of body wt) or other steroid hormones (5 μg/gm of body wt) or Tamoxifen (200 μg/100 gm of body wt).

Two hrs after injection of above compounds, the ovariecto-mized rats were killed and uterine cytosol and nuclear fraction assayed by the standard NaSCN method described above. Results are shown in fig. 10 and confirm that only estrogens as well as Tamoxifen (Jordan and Koemer, 1975; Horwitz and McGuire, 1978c) induce translocation of receptor from cytoplasm to nuclei.

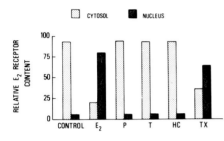

Fig. 10. Distribution of estro-gen receptor in cytosol and nu-clei of uteri from ovariectomi-zed rats injected 2 hrs before sacrifice with 17β-estradiol (E_2) or Progesterone (P) or Te-stosterone (T) or Hydrocortiso-ne (HC) or Tamoxifen (Tx). To-tal receptor content of tissue fractions was assayed by the standard NaSCN exchange method (see Results).

B. Total content of estradiol receptor in uterus nuclear and cytosol fractions 2 hrs after i.p. injection of 17β-estra-diol into ovariectomized rats.

This experiment is shown in fig. 11. The rats were injected i.p. with different doses of non-radioactive hormone two hours before sacrifice. If receptor content of cytosol and nuclei is expressed as a function of total (fig. 11 A), one can see that, regardless of the estradiol dose injected, about 80% of receptor is found in nuclei and 20% in the cytosol. However, when absolu-te values are considered (fig. 11 B), one can see that the total tissue content of receptor two hrs after estradiol treatment de-creases progressively as a function of the dose of estradiol injected. This is the first time that estradiol was found to in-duce decrease of total receptor content in vivo. A similar fin-ding has been described by Horwitz and McGuire (1978 a,b,c) in experiments with cell cultures. This phenomenon is presently under further scrutiny.

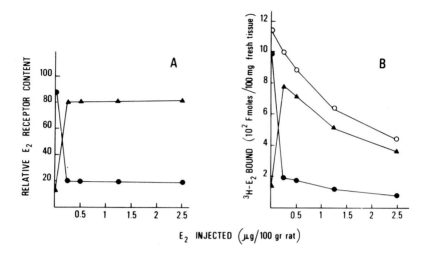

Fig. 11. <u>Total receptor content of uteri and of uterus nuclear</u>
<u>and cytosol fractions 2 hrs after injection of 1 µg/100 gm of</u>
<u>body wt of 17β-estradiol into ovariectomized rats</u>. Receptor con-
tent of tissue and tissue fractions was assessed by the standard NaSCN exchange method (see Results). A. Receptor content
of cytosol (●) and of nuclear fraction (▲) are expressed as percent of total receptor in uterus. B. Receptor content of whole
uterus (○), nuclear fraction (▲) and cytosol (●).

DISCUSSION

NaSCN, a chaotropic salt previously applied in our laboratory to prevent age-dependent aggregation of receptor (Sica et al.,
1976) and for eluting receptor from estradiol containing agarose
supports used in affinity chromatography (Bresciani et al., 1978,
Sica and Bresciani, 1979) was found to increase the turnover rate
of estradiol receptor complex at 0-4°C. Both, the dissociation
rate and the association rate of the complex increase, with no
detectable change in steady-state concentration of estradiol-receptor complex. The increase of turnover rate is sufficient

to achieve a virtually complete exchange of bound estradiol within 16 hrs at 4°C. This finding has been exploited to set up a method for assessing receptor in tissue and tissue fractions regardless of whether the receptor is or is not interacting with ligand. The method is simple, precise and accurate and, in the case of nuclear receptor, there is no need for preliminary extraction of receptor from nuclei. In fact, quantitative extraction from nuclei and exchange is achieved in a single step consisting of incubation of the nuclear fraction with radioactive 17β-estradiol and NaSCN 0.5 M at 4°C overnight (16 hrs).

Previous methods for measuring estrogen receptor complexed to hormone are all based on carefully controlled temperature increases. The first demonstration of the feasibility of an exchange between receptor bound estradiol with added radioactive 17β--estradiol was reported for the rat uterus nuclear receptor (Puca and Bresciani, 1968). In further work, Anderson et al (1972) described an estradiol exchange assay by direct incubation of nuclear fraction at 37°C. However, noting the several shortcomings of the Anderson et al.,(1972) method, i.e. high nonspecific labeled 17β-estradiol binding, instability of receptor at 37°C and low precision (high standard error), Zava et al (1976) proposed a method by which nuclear receptor is extracted with KCl 0.6 M, precipitated with protamine sulphate and the precipitate subjected to ligand exchange with radioactive estradiol for 2.5 hrs at 37°C. This test for nuclear receptor is an application of a previously developed method by the same group (Chamness et al., 1975) to assay preformed endogenous estrogen receptor complex in cytosol. After very detailed investigation, Katzenellenbogen et al (1973) suggested that exchange assay of cytoplasmic estradiol-filled binding sites be conducted by incubation of cytosol for 18-24 hrs at 25-30°C. They noticed a significant loss of binding sites at 37°C, even in presence of large excess of hormone. Indeed, the fundamental limitation of all these methods is the well known sensitivity of receptor to temperatures higher than those close to 0°C. The higher the temperature the faster the rate of inactivation, which is irreversible (Peck et al., 1973). Furthermore, in the case of crude preparation, there is a definite possibility of considerable proteolytic destruction of receptor.

The results of Zava et al.,(1976) suggest that when complexed to protamine sulphate, the receptor is less sensitive to higher temperatures. However, if there is little or no loss of receptor by temperature in this method, there is still considerable loss of receptor due to incomplete recovery after salt extraction and protamine precipitation.

The unquestionable advantages of our method are: 1) that is performed at 0-4°C, thus avoiding any possible temperature inactivation and proteolytic destruction of receptor; 2) that is equally applicable, without modification, to whole homogenate as well as nuclei or cytosol; 3) that there is complete extraction of nuclear receptor, vs. incomplete with KCl, and that this extraction occurs during the incubation with radioactive 17β-estradiol; 4) that is very simple and, at the same time, reliable, precise and accurate.

The ability of NaSCN 0.5 M to extract nuclear receptor quantitatively is an interesting finding in itself. Up to now, KCl has been the standard salt used by many research groups to extract receptor from nuclear pellets (Puca and Bresciani, 1968; Giannopoulos and Gorski, 1971; Zava et al, 1976). However, a single extraction with KCl always failed to remove all nuclear receptor. Indeed, Clark and Peck (1976) suggested the existence of two types of nuclear receptor in rat uterine nuclei. One type, accounting for about 10% of the total, is not removed by a single KCl extraction, is retained for a longer period in the nucleus and is thought to be related to long term stimulation of uterine growth. The second type accounts for the rest of nuclear receptor, is salt extractable, is retained by nuclei for a shorter time and is not related to uterine growth. Barrack et al (1977) postulated that the tightly bound component may represent high affinity sites associated with the nuclear matrix. However, Juliano and Stancel (1976) and Muller et al. (1977) question the concept of two distinct classes of nuclear receptor and describe results contrary to those of Clark and Peck (1976). The ability of NaSCN to release from nuclei even the KCl extraction resistant receptor not only furnishes a useful tool for a complete quantitation of nuclear receptor but also allows fast and easy preparation of KCl resistant nuclear receptor.

Finally, the finding described in this paper that the content of total receptor in uterine tisssue decreases two hours after injection of estrogen into ovariectomized rats should be briefly commented upon. While a similar finding has been described by Horwitz and McGuire (1978 a,b,c) in a human breast cancer cell culture (MCF-7), such a phenomenon had not previously been found in vivo. Our findings thus open the way to in vivo study of the so-called "nuclear processing" of receptor (Horwitz and McGuire, 1978 a,b,c).

CONCLUSION

In conclusion, we report that NaSCN considerably increases the turnover of estradiol-receptor complex at 0-4°C, without detectably affecting the steady-state concentration of the complex. Furthermore, NaSCN solubilizes receptor from the nuclear pellet much more efficiently than KCl; extraction by NaSCN is in fact complete, i.e. no more radioactivity is extracted from nuclei by ether. Based on these findings, a simple assay method has been set up which measures receptor in tissue and tissue fractions, including nuclei, at 0-4°C, regardless of whether the receptor is interacting with endogenous hormone or not. The procedure consists of a single incubation step at 0-4°C, overnight (16 hrs), of total homogenate, nuclear fraction or cytosol in the presence of excess radioactive estradiol and NaSCN 0.5 M. The assay is very easy to carry out, accurate and precise, and avoids loss of binding sites from the heating procedures of previous exchange methods.

Among other results, demonstrative application of the method shows that two hours after injection of estradiol into ovariectomized rats total receptor content of uterus decreases proportionally to the amount of hormone injected.

ACKNOWLEDGMENT

These investigations were supported by Progetto Finalizzato "Controllo della Crescita Neoplastica" del Consiglio Nazionale delle Ricerche, Roma.

REFERENCES

1. Anderson, J., Clark, J.H. and Peck, Jr., E.J. (1972): Biochem. J., 126:561.
2. Barrack, E.R., Hawkins, E.F., Allen, L.S., Hicks, L.L. and Coffey, D.S. (1977): Biochem. Biophys. Res. Commun., 79:829.
3. Baudendistel, L.J. and Ruh, T.S. (1976): Steroids, 28:223.
4. Best-Belpomme, M., Fries, J. and Erdos, T. (1970): Europ. J. Biochem., 17:452.
5. Bradford, M.M. (1976): Anal. Biochem., 72:248.
6. Bresciani, F., Sica, V. and Weisz, A. (1978): Biochem. Action Horm., 6:461.
7. Chamness, G.C., Huff, K. and McGuire, W.L. (1975): Steroids, 25:627.
8. Clark, J.H. and Peck, E.J. (1976): Nature, 260:635.
9. Erdos, T., Bessada, R., Best-Belpomme, M., Fries, J., Gospodarowiez, D. and Menahem, M. (1971): In Advances in the Biosciences (Raspèe G., ed). Vol. 7 p. 119. Pergamon Press, Oxford.
10. Giannopoulos, G. and Gorski, J. (1971): J. Biol. Chem. 246:2524.
11. Horwitz, K.B. and McGuire, W.L. (1978a): J. Biol. Chem. 253:2223.
12. Horwitz, K.B. and McGuire, W.L. (1978b): J. Biol. Chem. 253:6319.
13. Horwitz, K.B. and McGuire, W.L. (1978c): J. Biol. Chem. 253:8185.
14. Jensen, E.V., Greene, G.L., Closs, L.E. and De Sombre, E.R. In: Steroid Hormone Receptor Systems (Leavitt, W.W. and Clark, J.H., eds.; Plenum, N.Y. pp. 1:16, 1979).
15. Jordan, V.C. and Koerner, S. (1975): Europ. J. Cancer, 11:205.
16. Juliano, J.V. and Stancel, G.M. (1976): Biochemistry, 15:916.
17. Katzenellenbogen, J.A. and Charlson, K.E. (1973): Biochemistry, 12:4092.
18. McCormack, S.A. and Glasser, S.R. (1976): Endocrinology, 99:701.
19. Mester, G., Robertson, D.M., Feherty, P.J. and Kellie, A.E. (1970): Biochem. J. 120:831.
20. Muller, R.E., Traish, A.M. and Wotiz, H.A. (1977): J. Biol.

Chem., 252:8206.

21. Peck, Jr, E.R., De Libero, J., Richards, R. and Clark, J.H. (1973): Biochemistry, 12:4603

22. Puca, G.A. and Bresciani, F. (1968): Nature, 218:967.

23. Ruh, T.S. and Baudendistel, L.J. (1977): Endocrinology, 100:420.

24. Sala-Trepat, J.M. and Reti, E. (1974): Biochim. Biophys. Acta, 338:92.

25. Sanborn, B.M., Ramanth Rao, B., Korenman, S.G. (1971): Biochemistry, 10:4955.

26. Sica, V., Nola, E., Puca, G.A. and Bresciani, F. (1976): Biochemistry, 15:1915.

27. Sica, V. and Bresciani, F. (1979): Biochemistry, 18:2369.

28. Sutherland, R.L. and Baulieu, E.E. (1976): Eur. J. Biochem. 701:513.

29. Truong, H. and Baulieu, E.E. (1972): Biochim. Biophys. Acta, 237:167.

30. Vallet-Strouve, C., Rat, C. and Sala Trepat, J.M. (1976): Eur. J. Biochem., 66:327.

31. Zava, D.T., Harrington, N.Y. and McGuire, W.L. (1976): Biochemistry, 15:4292.

Perspectives in Steroid Receptor Research,
edited by F. Bresciani.
Raven Press, New York © 1980.

Histochemical Assay of Steroid Hormone Receptors

Louis P. Pertschuk, *Ellis H. Tobin, Eric Gaetjens,
**David J. Brigati, †Anne C. Carter, Dong S. Kim,
‡George A. Degenshein, and ‡Norman D. Bloom

*Departments of Pathology and †Medicine, Division of Endocrinology, and *School of
Medicine, State University of New York Downstate Medical Center, Brooklyn,
New York 11203; **Department of Pathology, Memorial Sloan-Kettering Cancer Center,
New York, New York 10021; and ‡Department of Surgery, Maimonides Medical Center,
Brooklyn, New York 11219, U.S.A.*

In the past decade, scientific investigations in the
area of molecular endocrinology have revealed the
presence of steroid hormone receptor proteins in both
normal and abnormal human and animal tissues. Steroid
hormone receptors have been described in breast cancer
(3,11,14), prostatic carcinoma and hyperplasia (2,12),
lung (1), kidney (16), and central nervous system (24)
among others. With the exception of autoradiography,
all current techniques for the detection of steroid
hormone receptors require homogenization of tissue for
assay of cytosol or nuclear receptor proteins. As a
consequence, there is total specimen disruption which
precludes anatomical localization of the receptor site.
Recent developments of histologic methods for detection
of steroid receptor in intact tissue sections provides
a means for exact anatomical localization of these
proteins.

In this laboratory, histochemical assays have been
developed for the detection of estrogen (ER), progesterone (PgR) and androgen (AR) receptors. These methods
utilize ligand-conjugates composed of steroid hormones
linked to a carrier bovine serum albumin (BSA) molecule
which is then labeled with fluorescein isothiocyanate
(FITC)(4,17-19,22,23).

Synthesis of Ligand-Conjugates

17β -estradiol, 17 β -testosterone and 11 α -hydroxy-
progesterone were each covalently linked to BSA by a

modification of Erlanger's technique (10) so as to achieve a lower steroid/albumin stoichiometry in the resulting conjugate. This was accomplished by reacting 60 μmoles hemisuccinate, 60 μmoles tri-n-butylamine and 60 μmoles isobutylchlorocarbonate in 1.0 ml of anhydrous dioxane at 10°C for 45 minutes. The reaction mixture was added in one step, with rapid stirring, to 270 mg BSA dissolved in 32 ml of 50% aqueous dioxane at 10°C and pH 9.0. Stirring was continued for one hour while the pH was maintained at 9.0 by the addition of 1N NaOH. The reaction mixture was dialyzed against cold phosphate buffered saline (PBS) for 30 hours at pH 7.4, then against cold distilled water for an additional 30 hours prior to lyophilization to dryness. Incorporation of steroid was determined from each extinction coefficient using UV spectrophotometry.

The steroid-albumin conjugates were reacted with FITC in a ratio of 1.0 mg FITC/10.0 mg conjugate in 0.1M sodium carbonate buffer for 24 hours at 0°C and pH 9.5. The reaction mixture was then dialyzed against cold distilled water for 72 hours prior to lyophilization to dryness. A BSA-FITC conjugate was prepared containing the same number of moles FITC/mole BSA but not bound to steroid. Incorporation of FITC/mole BSA was determined based upon its extinction coefficient of 495 nm.

The conjugates were soluble in water and in PBS, pH 7.4. Upon chromatography on a column of Sephadex G-25, the conjugates eluted as sharp peaks in the void volume. UV spectra showed strong absorption between 240 and 250 nm corresponding to absorption maxima of steroid. The difference spectra, obtained by subtracting absorption of BSA from those of the conjugates at various wavelengths, corresponded to those of the steroids. It was found that ligand-conjugates composed of 4 to 10 moles of steroid hormone and 4 to 6 moles FITC/mole BSA gave the most satisfactory results in histochemical receptor assays.

Specificity of Ligand-Conjugates

The specificity of each ligand-conjugate was determined by extensive competition binding studies employing various steroids, anti-steroids and non-steroidal synthetic agents. These studies were performed on frozen sections prepared from pellets of the MCF-7 mammary carcinoma cell line, known to be positive for ER, PgR and AR (9). Results are shown in Figure 1a-c. In addition, each conjugate was tested on similarly

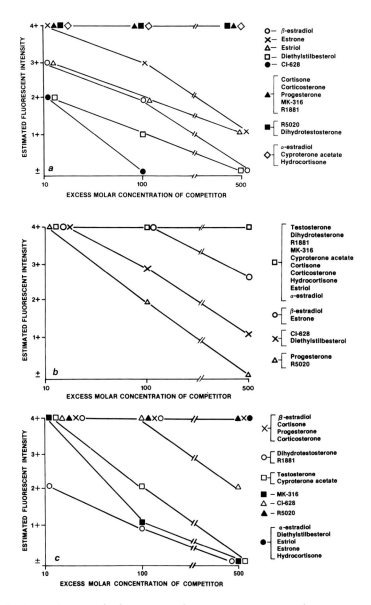

FIGURE 1. Competition studies performed with the ligand-conjugates plus excess molar concentrations of various steroids, anti-steroids and non-steroidal synthetic agents. a) With the exception of α-estradiol the estrogens successfully compete with the estradiol ligand-conjugate for ER. b) Progesterone and R5020 exhibit the most successful competition with the progesterone ligand-conjugate for PgR although some competition is also shown by some of the estrogens. c) The androgens and antiandrogens compete most successfully with the testosterone ligand-conjugate for AR. Some competition is also displayed by CI-628.

prepared sections of the ZR-75-31A cell line known to
be negative for ER, PgR and AR (9). No cytoplasmic
fluorescence was produced in the latter cells with any
ligand-conjugate, whereas bright cytoplasmic staining
was seen in the MCF-7 cell line with all conjugates.

Histochemical Processing

Tissue in excess of the amount required for adequate
histologic diagnosis was divided into two portions and
frozen in liquid nitrogen within 15 minutes of removal.
One portion of each breast cancer was subjected to
standard biochemical ER and PgR assay by dextran-
coated charcoal (DCC) or sucrose gradient assay (SGA)
(3,13,15). Prostate specimens were assayed for ER and
AR by DCC (15,25) with or without protamine sulfate or
salt extraction. Corresponding tissue blocks were
stored in liquid nitrogen for histochemical studies.

In brief, histochemical analyses were performed on
frozen tissue sections 4μ thick. These were incubated
in 50 pmoles of each ligand-conjugate while serial
sections were additionally exposed to a 200 to 500 fold
molar excess of competitor. For this purpose CI-628
or diethylstilbesterol were used for ER, R5020 was
employed for PgR, and MK 316, cyproterone acetate,
R1881 or flutamide were used for AR. For PgR, unlabeled cortisol and androgen were added to inhibit nonspecific binding of progesterone to AR and glucocorticoid receptor. A parallel tissue section was exposed
to the same concentration of BSA-FITC not steroid
linked, to monitor nonspecific binding of BSA. After
2 hours in a humidifying chamber at 24°C, the sections
were rinsed in PBS, fixed in acetone-ethanol for 10
minutes and triple washed in PBS for 30 minutes (19,22).

Prepared sections were mounted in buffered glycerol,
pH 7.0, and examined by incident light UV microscopy
employing an FITC interference-excitation dichroic
mirror filter and a K530 barrier filter.

Interpretation of Histochemical Assay Results

Specimens were designated as receptor positive when
sections exposed to ligand-conjugate plus the appropriate competitor showed significantly less fluorescence
than sections exposed to ligand-conjugate alone.
Sections exposed only to BSA-FITC were expected to show
little to no staining.

Breast and prostate specimens were classified as
receptor rich when the majority of tumor cells showed

clear cytoplasmic (Figure 2) or nuclear fluorescence
(Figure 3), or both. They were designated as receptor
poor if less than 10% of constituent tumor cells
displayed staining or if the overall intensity of
fluorescence was low. The majority of tumors exhibited tumor cell receptor heterogeneity evidenced by a
wide range of fluorescent intensities graded from ± to
++++. The latter specimens were designated as receptor
positive, heterogenous.

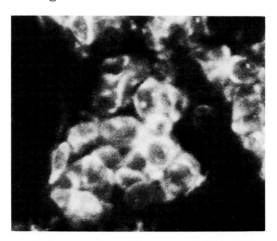

FIGURE 2. Infiltrating duct cell mammary carcinoma
after exposure to estrogen ligand-conjugate. The tumor
cells show primarily cytoplasmic fluorescence. X500.

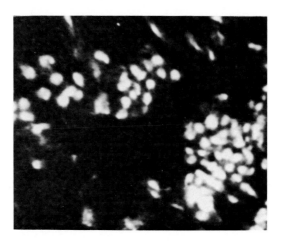

FIGURE 3. Intraduct and infiltrating duct cell breast
cancer showing predominantly nuclear ER. X200.

Comparison of Histochemical and Biochemical Assay Results

Histochemical and biochemical assay results correlated in 92% of 314 breast cancer specimens assayed for ER, and in 86% of 86 specimens assayed for PgR (20). Assay results of prostatic tissue correlated in 89% of 66 specimens for AR and in 80% for ER (23). A chi-square test performed on these data show that histochemical assay results correlate well with those of conventional biochemical assays (p <0.01). Biochemical results are pending for an additional 96 breast and 154 prostate specimens.

Correlation of Histochemical Assay Results and Clinical Response to Endocrine Therapies

Results of histochemical and biochemical receptor studies were correlated with clinical response to ablative and additive endocrine therapies in 40 women with Stage IV breast cancer. These results are shown in Table I and indicate that the histochemical assay for ER and PgR has the same potential for correlating clinical response to such treatment as do standard biochemical assays. A favorable response to therapy was seen in 65% of 23 patients with ER+PgR+ tumors, whereas progression occurred in 94% of 16 ER-PgR- cases (20).

Renal Cell Carcinoma

Utilizing the estradiol ligand-conjugate, 36 renal cell carcinomas were analyzed for ER. Nuclear ER was seen in 8 while 2 exhibited foci of cytoplasmic binding. Two other tumors had a mosaic pattern of both nuclear and cytoplasmic fluorescence. Such tumors have been shown by biochemical assay to occasionally possess steroid hormone receptor proteins (5,6) and there is some evidence that they occasionally may be hormone responsive (7).

Localization of Receptor Proteins in Other Tissues

In studies of over 100 human and animal kidneys, ER, PgR and AR were localized exclusively to the glomerular capillary loops (Figure 4) in rats, mice, ferrets and guinea pigs. However, in man and rabbits, receptor was present in tubular epithelium in addition to the glomeruli.

In rat and human lung, receptor predominated in the lining cells of the bronchial and bronchiolar mucosa.

TABLE I

HISTOCHEMICAL AND BIOCHEMICAL ASSAY RESULTS FOR ER/PGR: COMPARISON WITH CLINICAL
RESPONSE TO ADDITIVE OR ABLATIVE ENDOCRINE THERAPIES

Results	#	Histochemical Assay			#	Biochemical Assay		
		Clinical Response		%		Clinical Response		%
		Yes	No	correlate		Yes	No	correlate
ER+PgR+	23	15	8	65	14	9	5	64
ER+PgR-	1	0	1	100	10	4	6	60
ER-PgR-	16	1	15	94	8	0	8	100

Includes one responder with pleural effusion. No biochemical assay performed.
Two responders and 5 non-responders had insufficient solubilized cytosol protein
for PgR by DCC/SGA.

In the central nervous system of rats, nuclear receptor
was predominantly localized within the limbic system.
Receptor was also observed in the endometrium, myo-
metrium and oviduct epithelium.

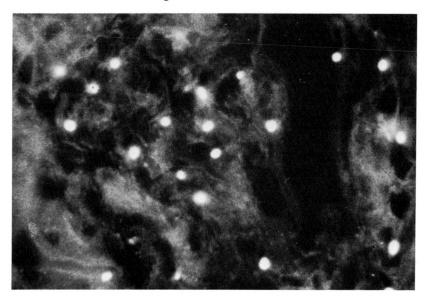

FIGURE 4.   Adult male rat kidney after incubation with
estradiol ligand-conjugate.   There is bright, nuclear
fluorescence localized to the glomerular capillary
loops with a distribution indicating that it is limited
to epithelial cells.   X500.

Conclusion

Histologic receptor protein analysis in intact tissue has been accomplished using ligand hemisuccinate
bound to BSA and labeled with FITC.   Fluorescent microscopy of labeled tissue sections reveals that both
cytoplasmic and nuclear fluorescent patterns as well as
receptor heterogeneity can be identified.   This rapid
and inexpensive method requires small amounts of tissue and correlates quite well with standard biochemical
procedures.   The histochemical assay also correlates
well with breast cancer response to endocrine therapy.
The simplicity of the technique lends itself to widespread application.   Furthermore, since the process
permits the exact localization of minute amounts of
steroid receptor protein it should be of considerable
basic investigative value.

Acknowledgments

Supported in part by USPHS grants Nos. CA23623 and CA25760 and Contract No. N01-CN-45139 from NCI, and the Jack R. Aron Foundation.

We thank J. P. Raynaud of Roussel UCLAF for the gift of R5020 and R1881. Schering AG donated cyproterone acetate and Schering Corporation, flutamide. Merck, Sharp & Dohme donated MK 316 and Warner-Lambert/Parke Davis, CI-628. Drs. J. Allegra and N. Young, NCI, supplied the ZR-75-31A cell line. Ms. E. Rainford, L. Autuoro and E. Jones provided technical expertise.

The majority of breast cancer specimens were assayed for ER in the laboratory of Dr. W. L. McGuire, University of Texas Health Sciences Center at San Antonio. Dr. D. T. Zava performed the biochemical prostate assays in Dr. McGuire's laboratory. ER and PgR biochemical assays on other breast cancers were done in the Surgical Research Laboratory, Maimonides Medical Center, Brooklyn.

References

1. Agarwal M. K., and Philippe M. (1977): Biochim.et Biophys. Acta 500:42-48.

2. Bashirelahi, N., O'Toole, J. H., and Young, J. D. (1976): Biochem. Med. 15:254-261.

3. Bloom, N., Tobin E., and Degenshein, G. A. (1977): In: Progesterone Receptors in Normal and Neoplastic Tissues, edited by W. L. McGuire, J-P. Raynaud, and E-E. Baulieu, pp. 125-139. Raven Press, New York.

4. Brigati, D. J., Bloom, N. D., Tobin, E. H., Kim, D. S., Gaetjens, E., Degenshein, G. A., and Pertschuk, L. P. (1979): Breast 5:27-33.

5. Concolino, G., Marocchi, A., Conti, C., Tenaglia, R., DiSilverio, F., and Bracci, U. (1978): Cancer Res. 38:4340-4344.

6. Concolino, G., Marocchi, A., DiSilverio F., and Conti, C. (1976): J. Steroid Biochem. 7:923-927.

7. Concolino, G., Marocchi, A., Tenaglia, R., and Bracci, U. (1976): Conference on Biochemistry in Clinical Medicine, Innsbruck, January 28.

8. DeSombre, E. R., Carbone, P. P., Jensen, E. V., McGuire, W. L., Wells, S. A., Wittliff, J. L., and Lipsett, M. B. (1979): N. E. J. M. 301:1011-1012.

9. Engel, L. W., and Young, N. A. (1978): Cancer Res. 38:4327-4339.

10. Erlanger, B. F., Borek, F., Beiser, S. M., and Lieberman, S. (1959): J. Biol. Chem. 228:713-727.

11. Folca, P. J., Glascock, R. P., and Irvine, W. T. (1961): Lancet i:796-798.

12. Hawkins, E. F., Nijs, M., and Brassine, C. (1977): Clin. Chim. Acta 75:303-312.

13. Horwitz, K. B., and McGuire, W. L. (1977): In: Progesterone Receptors in Normal and Neoplastic Tissues, edited by W. L. McGuire, J-P. Raynaud. and E-E. Baulieu, pp. 103-124. Raven Press, New York.

14. McGuire, W. L. (1979): In: Advances in Internal Medicine, edited by G. H. Stollerman, pp. 127-140.

15. McGuire, W. L., De La Garza, M., and Chamness, G. C. (1977): Cancer Res. 37:637-639.

16. Pasqualini, T. R., Sumida, C., Gelly, C., Nguyen, B. L., and Tardy, J. (1979): Cancer Res. 38:4246-4250.

17. Pertschuk, L. P., Gaetjens, E., Brigati, D. J., and Kim, D. S. (1979): Ann Clin. Lab. Sci.9:225-229.

18. Pertschuk, L. P., Gaetjens, E., Brigati, D. J., Kim, D. S., and Carter, A. C. (1979): Ann. Clin. Lab. Sci. 9:219-224.

19. Pertschuk, L. P., Gaetjens, E., Carter, A. C., Brigati, D. J., Kim, D. S., and Fealey, T. A (1979) Am. J. Clin. Pathol. 71:504-508.

20. Pertschuk, L. P., Tobin, E. H., Gaetjens, E., Carter, A. C., Degenshein, G. A., Bloom, N. D., and Brigati, D. J. (in press), Cancer.

21. Pertschuk, L. P., Tobin, E. H., Gaetjens E., Degenshein, G. A., Autuoro, L. M., Brigati, D. J., Bloom, N. D., Carter, A. C., and Rainford, E. A. (1979): Res. Commun. Chem. Pathol. Pharmacol. 23: 635-638.

22. Pertschuk, L. P., Zava, D. T., Gaetjens, E., Macchia, R. J., Brigati, D. J., and Kim, D. S. (1978): Res. Commun. Chem. Pathol. Pharmacol. 22: 427-430.

23. Pertschuk, L. P., Zava, D. T., Tobin, E. H., Brigati, D. J., Gaetjens, E., Macchia, R. J., Wise, G. J., Wax, S. H., and Kim, D. S. (1979): In: Prostate Cancer and Hormone Receptors, edited by G. P. Murphy and A. A. Sandberg. Alan R. Liss, New York, pp. 113-132.

24. Stumpf, W. E., and Sar, M. (1978): Amer. Zool. 18: 435-445.

25. Zava, D. T., Landrum, T. B., Horwitz, K. B., and McGuire, W. L.(1978): Clin. Res. 26:31a.

Subject Index

A

Actinomycin D, 104–106, 169, 173, 175

Activation step, DNA binding of glucocorticoid receptor, 113–129

Adenosine triphosphate, 103 and glucocorticoid binding, 124, 125

Affinity labeling, androgen receptor purification, 89–96

Age, role in breast disease, 218–236, 240–242, 251

Alkaline phosphatase of endometrium, 264 inactivation of steroid binding, 124–127

Androgen receptors in breast disease, 221–236 histochemistry, 299–307 and hyaluronidase, 54, 57 interaction with chromatin, 99–110 purification, 89–96

Androgens, structure, 4, 5, 14, 18

Androstanediol, 7

Antibodies to estradiol, 67 to estrophilin, 23–35 to uterine peroxidase, 179

Antiestrogens, 173–174, 220, 241 263, 265

Aprotinin, 53

B

Binding sites androgen–receptor complex interaction with chromatin, 99–110

cytochemistry of steroid–target cell interaction, 61–71

estradiol in uterine nuclei, 143–163, 273–295

estrogen and progesterone in breast tumor, 252–253 in fetus and newborn, 183–192 general properties, 1–3 indirect mapping, 3–18

Breast cancer, human cytochemistry of steroid binding sites in membrane of, 61–71 estradiol–receptor complex, 105 histochemistry of hormone receptors, 302–307 immunology, 27–30, 34 steroid receptor analysis and endocrine therapy, 217–236, 239–245, 247–255

17β-Bromoacetoxytestosterone, affinity label for androgen receptor purification, 89–96

C

Chemotherapy in breast cancer, 217, 228, 234–235, 240–245

Chloroquine, 104, 109

Chromatin, 23 estradiol effect, 148, 163, 168, 180 interaction with androgen–receptor complex, 99–110

Compound B19, 14, 18

Compound J, 18

Conformation of steroids, 3–16 role in interaction with chromatin, 99–101

1,2-Cyclohexanedione, 118

Cycloheximide, 169, 173